KINESIOLOGY

KINESIOLOGY

JOHN M. COOPER, Ed.D.

Professor of Physical Education,
Indiana University, Bloomington, Indiana

MARLENE ADRIAN, P.E.D.

Professor of Physical Education,
Washington State University, Pullman, Washington

RUTH B. GLASSOW, M.A.

Professor Emeritus of Physical Education,
University of Wisconsin, Madison, Wisconsin

FIFTH EDITION

With **528** illustrations

The C. V. Mosby Company

ST. LOUIS • TORONTO • LONDON   1982

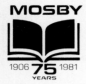

MOSBY

1906 **75** 1981
YEARS

A TRADITION OF PUBLISHING EXCELLENCE

Editor: Charles K. Hirsch
Manuscript editor: Sue Jane Smith
Design: Susan Trail
Production: Margaret B. Bridenbaugh

The C.V. Mosby Company
11830 Westline Industrial Drive, St. Louis, Missouri 63141

Library of Congress Cataloging in Publication Data

Cooper, John Miller, 1912-
    Kinesiology.

    Bibliography: p.
    Includes index.
    1. Kinesiology.   I.   Adrian, Marlene, 1933-
II. Glassow, Ruth Bertha.
QP303.C565   1982   612'.76   81-11116
ISBN 0-8016-1040-0   AACR2

AC/VH/VH   9   8   7   6   5   4   3   2   1   02/C/267

To
the curious, inquiring students
who are not satisfied with existing knowledge
but strive to gain new understanding and insights,
who will be the future analysts and explorers into
the mysteries of human and animal movement

Preface

The teacher, rehabilitator, researcher, and student of human movement will find this book to be a balanced blend of theory and application, thus providing a basic and holistic approach to the study of kinesiology (biomechanics).

Some readers will remember the 1950 kinesiology book by one of us (Cooper) and Lawrence Morehouse. That book is considered by many to have been the first to depart from the traditional applied-anatomy approach of the then-current kinesiology books by emphasizing analyses of human movements. In 1963 Ruth B. Glassow replaced Lawrence Morehouse and joined in developing more scientific material to support or refute previous concepts that in the earlier edition had been based more on observation and experience than on research. This author partnership continued through four editions. The field of kinesiology is deeply indebted to Ruth Glassow for her pioneer work.

Now in this fifth edition there is another change in authorship. This change represents a continuation of the tradition of providing the newest concepts and newest research, both domestic and foreign. This fifth edition is truly a complete revision synthesizing mechanics and biology, incorporating the guidelines and standards proposed by the Kinesiology Academy, introducing and utilizing the International System of Units of measurement (metric distances, for example), and emphasizing the analysis and improvement of human movement based on both a holistic and an individualized approach. The student of animal movement also will find this book helpful.

The contents of this edition have been designed to challenge the thinking of the reader and yet provide the reader with a logical and meaningful progression from the presentation of a model for studying movement to the future utilization of knowledge for assessment, improvement, and prediction of performance.

One important feature of this fifth edition is the inclusion of mini laboratory exercises inserted at frequent intervals within and at the end of each chapter. These exercises provide learning experiences that require the use of problem-solving techniques, the application of knowledge, and the reinforcement of concepts.

Part I, Approaches to Efficient and Effective Movement, develops a rationale for studying and understanding human movement. Classifications of movement are mentioned relative to position and environment. The similarities and differences in movement patterns are discussed. Efficiency and safety factors are included. A theoretical model is presented that consists of describing the movement, setting the performance goal, identifying the elements to consider in accomplishing the goal, determining the quantitative principles involved in the movement, and, finally, assessing the performance in view of these principles. Tools at the disposal of kinesiologists are listed and evaluated, and mention is also made of some of those persons who have contributed to the development and utilization of these analysis tools.

Part II, Moving in a Gravitational World, lays the foundation for movement on earth. The most important concepts are concerned with the effects of gravity and friction on movement. Mechanical, anatomic, and neurologic considerations, as well as muscle-bone lever systems, are described in detail, with numerous examples of their significance to the movement outcome. In addition, a description of forces acting on the body tissues is presented to provide the valuable linkage between safe and dangerous effects of forces and movement.

Part III, Analyzing and Improving Performance, begins with a discussion of qualitative and quantitative assessment procedures. Then many human movements, primarily in the sports area, are analyzed. Less traditional sports, both recreational and competitive, are presented. Inclusion of chapters on activities of daily living and on exercises from a biomechanical perspective provides the much-needed analysis of activities vital to human and animal existence. These chapters provide specific information for teachers of adults and children, persons working in fitness and health clubs, and researchers investigating muscular and neurologic dysfunction.

Part IV, Moving Beyond to Future Utilization and Prediction, completes the main portion of the book. This section encapsulates the theme of this book—that the student of human or animal movement must learn, above all, to utilize an analysis model to scientifically and creatively analyze skills of the future and patterns of movement that are unfamiliar or that will be performed under varying environmental conditions. However, it is not enough to merely analyze; one must understand the meaning of the analysis and be able to act on its implications.

We believe sincerely that this edition incorporates virtually all of the current material available to kinesiologists that is pertinent to the modern student. We believe that the wise teacher and thoughtful student will wish to look to the future in planning the learning experiences of the present. This edition presents such an approach. Facts are presented as a vehicle to learning. Facts can be classified into three types: those which appear to be absolute, those which are relative, and those which are discovered to be false. The perceptive student must always be critical of "facts" and must always strive to discover ways to synthesize and utilize accurate information.

Gratefully, we wish to acknowledge many hours of typing of the manuscript by Charlianna Cooper. We also extend our appreciation to Sue Yeager and Michael Allan Purcell, who helped in the development of many of the illustrations, and to Nancy Guillaume, who not only served as a subject in some of the photographs but also aided in collecting literature information. Finally, we wish to offer our thanks to those who reviewed the manuscript— Kathleen Miller, Ph.D., of the University of Montana, and Larry D. Hensley, Ed.D., of the University of Northern Iowa—as well as the many friends and students who submitted suggestions for improvements, acted as subjects for the illustrations, and generally provided support for this endeavor.

John M. Cooper
Marlene Adrian

Contents

KINESIOLOGY

PART ONE

Approaches to efficient and effective movement

CHAPTER 1

Introduction

Movement is basic to life. There can be no life without movement, whether that movement is extrinsic or intrinsic to the organism. To survive, one must move: move to eat, to breathe, to reproduce, to defecate, to develop bone and muscle, and to continue all the life processes. Movement allows human beings, birds, fish, quadrupeds, and other life forms to achieve a degree of independent living. Through the acquisition of skilled movement patterns, human beings are able to work and to play more effectively and more efficiently. The thrill of being able to tie one's shoes, saw wood, hit a baseball, kick a soccer ball, swing an axe, ride a horse, shovel snow, peel and slice potatoes, hoe a garden, sing a song, play a piano, swim or walk a mile, play a game of racquetball, or jump from an airplane and form a free-fall skydiving pattern is part of the joy of life. These overt movement patterns, however, do not arise spontaneously at birth. Overt movement patterns must be learned, although some movements are more reflex based and therefore are easier to learn than others. Nevertheless, there is always some trial and error involved in every attempt at locomotion, manipulation, or a combination of these and other types of movements.

One of the underlying goals of any human being, then, might well be to learn to perform skilled movement patterns with the least amount of frustration, failure, and danger. Another important goal may be that of helping others, humans or animals, to develop effective, efficient, and safe movement skills. Additionally, one might be merely curious about movement: how it occurs and how it can be changed. All these goals are best accomplished by receiving instruction from persons who have conducted a scientific study of movement. This scientific study of movement is termed kinesiology, which literally means the science of motion.

In its purest form kinesiology consists of the study of the physics of motion of living beings and is synonymous with the term *biomechanics*. Studying biomechanics includes studying the temporal and spatial characteristics of motion, which are referred to as the *kinematics* of motion. The spatial characteristics of motion include (1) the direction of the motion with respect to the three-dimensional world in which all things move and (2) the path of the motion. Temporal characteristics include the time span needed to execute the motion or selected phases of the motion. These characteristics can be described in qualitative or quantitative terms. Thus some of the words and phrases used to denote the kinematics of motion are as follows: fast, slow, right, left, forward, diagonally, in a straight line, in a circle, 30 m/sec, 200 rad/sec, 4 kmph, 6 m, 180 degrees/sec, and 5 m at a 60-degree angle with the horizontal. Biomechanics also include the study of the *kinetics* of motion, which refers to the forces causing, modifying, or otherwise facilitating or inhibiting motion. Force, work, kinetic and potential energy, momentum, and power are some of the terms used to describe the force aspects of motion.

An expanded definition that can be used by the student of kinesiology (biomechanics) is as follows:

Kinesiology is that branch of science concerned with the understanding of the interrelationships of structure and function of living beings with respect to the kinematics and kinetics of motion. Thus concepts from anatomy, physics, and mathematics are used to determine and measure the quantities of motion—time, space, and force—and to fully understand movement of living things.

Historically, kinesiology did not comprise the investigation of deformation and stresses to the human and animal body or their parts. This limitation, however, may have been a result of three factors: (1) inadequate instrumentation, (2) a primary interest in the analysis of movement patterns, and (3) a movement-effects approach toward the analysis of muscle force. Steindler, however, did include discussion of pressures within the hip joint and structural deformities of bones in his treatment of kinesiology. Therefore in this book no differentiation will be made between kinesiology and biomechanics. For persons who wish to pursue this topic farther, Atwater provides an informative discussion of various meanings of kinesiology and of biomechanics.

WHAT IS MOVEMENT?

Based on the spatial characteristics of motion described previously, movement patterns can be categorized as planar or general. A planar movement occurs in one plane; that is, if the movement occurs in a vertical plane, there will be no horizontal deviation. If the movement occurs in a horizontal plane, there will be no vertical deviation. One

might liken planar movement to movement on a sheet of paper (one plane). One might then tilt the paper to produce a multitude of planes of motion, including diagonal planes of motion. Rarely does human or animal motion occur in a single plane. Although locomotion tends to be in a vertical plane known as the sagittal, or anteroposterior (AP), plane, the anatomy of the body is such that some horizontal motion occurs as the body alternates between right-leg support and left-leg support. Only during imposed conditions and during limited single-limb movements used in exercising is pure planar motion likely to occur. Motion tends to occur in two or more planes and is termed general motion, or it might also be referred to as three-dimensional motion.

If movement is primarily in one plane and movement in a second plane is negligible, the movement may be analyzed as a planar movement for ease of analysis. For example, many movements of humans and quadrupeds are sagittal-plane movements primarily, since anatomically the flexor and extensor muscle groups are the principal locomotor muscles. Birds use their wings in the frontal plane, a vertical plane with movements right and left of body center. Fish move their caudal appendage in a horizontal plane. Thus these three planes (sagittal, frontal, and horizontal) are considered to be the basic planes of motion in our three-dimensional world. Logan and McKinney have defined several diagonal planes of motion because many human arm motions occur in diagonal planes. Two of these diagonal planes are (1) right high to left low and (2) right low to left high. Additional planes of motion have been identified in human-factors engineering and in aerospace research. The complexity of spatial description of motion increases as the need for more precision in locating the path of movement arises. Knowledge of the path of movement enables the movement

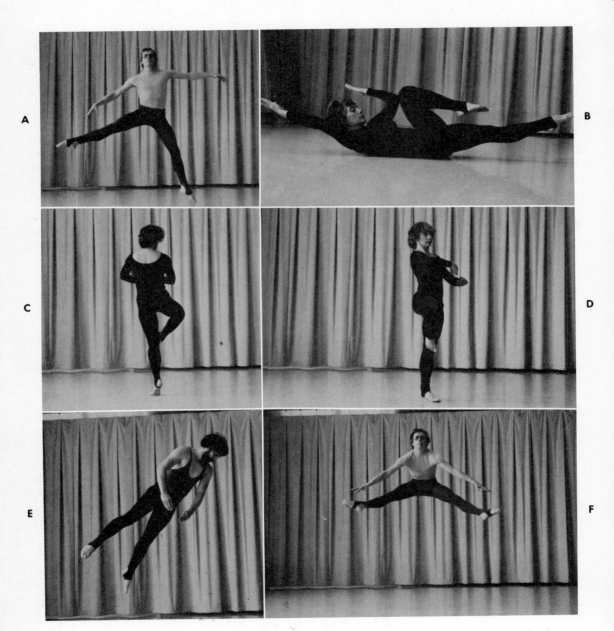

Fig. 1-1. Planes of motion. **A,** Arms and legs have moved in frontal plane. **B,** Arms, legs, and head have moved in sagittal plane. **C** and **D,** Turning movement has been performed in transverse plane. **E** and **F,** Movements have been performed in diagonal planes (two or more of the basic planes).

analyst to determine the probable muscles involved in producing the movement (Fig. 1-1).

The three types of motion that occur within a plane or through several planes may be described as follows.

Translatory motion is motion of a body from one place to another, with each part of the body moving an equal distance. The movement may be linear, that is, occur in a straight line, as in the movement by which a child is carried. Since we live in a gravitational world, many of the observed translations of objects are curvilinear, or parabolic, such as the flight of a ball. The translation path may have any direction; the only criterion is that each particle of the body must move the same distance.

Contrast translation with the second type of motion, *rotatory motion*. This type of motion differs from translation in that the body or body segment rotates about an axis, causing each part of the body to move a distance proportional to its position from the axis. For example, a person performing a giant swing on the high bar (Fig. 1-2) will experience only slight movement of the wrists, whereas the hips will move a distance equal to $2\pi r$, with r equal to the length of the body from hands to hips. Logically the feet travel the greatest distance of all the body parts, a total of $2\pi r$, with r now being the length of the body from hands to feet ($\pi = 3.1416$).

Many limb-segment exercises utilize pure rotation; however, human and animal movements tend

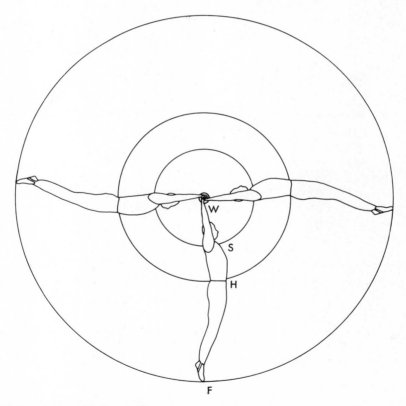

Fig. 1-2. Giant swing on high bar: an example of rotatory motion. Bar is fixed axis of rotation. Wrist (*W*) travels circumferential distance of $2\pi r_W$ where r_W represents radius of rotation of wrist. Hip (*H*) travels $2\pi r_H$, and foot (*F*) travels $2\pi r_F$.

to be complex, and a third type of motion, a *combination of translation and rotation,* is the more common type of motion produced voluntarily. The human anatomy consists of a number of body parts attached by means of joints, which act as axes of rotation. Locomotion occurs, and the body translates as a result of rotations of two or more body segments. Therefore one or more of the axes of rotation translate, and only one axis is stationary, or fixed. The complexity of locomotion is illustrated again when one notes that the same axis does not remain fixed during locomotion. At one point in time the fixed axis is the intersection of the heel of one foot with the ground; next, the axis occurs at the intersection of the metatarsal-phalangeal joint and the ground. Later the fixed axis transfers to the opposite limb. Thus the human body has been referred to as a kinematic link system. Movement of one segment of the body creates movement and a repositioning of another body segment. One can readily see what happens to the position of the forearm and hand when the following movements are executed:

1. Starting in the anatomic position, with the arm vertical at the side of the body, flex the arm at the elbow to an angle of 90 degrees.
2. Abduct the arm at the shoulder and note the position of the forearm and hand.
3. Medially rotate the arm at the shoulder and note the position of the forearm and hand.
4. Extend and flex the forearm from the position described in movement 3.
5. Simultaneously extend the forearm while adducting the arm.

The difficulty of the last movement illustrates the interrelationships of the movements of the limb segments. Adduction at the shoulder also adducts the forearm, which, in this situation, is an opposite movement to that of extension at the elbow.

With respect to the depicted giant swing in Fig. 1-2, the body may not maintain its rigid extended length throughout the swing. A common action is flexion at the hip to assure that a complete revolution can be achieved. Thus the movement now will consist of two axes of rotation, one fixed and one

stationary. A rotation takes place about another rotation without any translation.

Axes of rotation are represented by the joints of the body, by axles of wheels and other inanimate objects, and by imaginary lines within the body or between the living body and another body, living or inanimate. For example, a person pivots (rotates) about an invisible axis at the intersection of the hands with the ground when doing a cartwheel.

Each anatomic axis and each axis external to the living body (external axis) may be described with respect to space. The axis may be represented as a line passing through the plane of motion and at a right angle to that plane. Therefore any rotatory motion in a horizontal plane will occur about a vertical axis. When rotatory motion occurs within one of the two vertical planes of motion, the axis of rotation will be one of the two horizontal axes. The sagittal plane of motion occurs about the horizontal-frontal axis, and the frontal plane of motion occurs about the horizontal-sagittal axis. Rotatory motion occurring in diagonal planes will have diagonal axes.

This description of motion provides the underlying basis for the analysis of motion. From this basis a determination of the sources or forces producing motion can be made. This description also provides an approach to the mathematic evaluation of motion in terms of linear displacement or angular displacement. It must be kept in mind, however, that some aspects of both types of motion almost always occur during a movement pattern.

CLASSIFICATIONS OF MOVEMENT

In addition to the planar-general and rotatory-translatory descriptions of motion, there are several classifications of movement patterns that may be used by the movement analyst. One grouping, according to usage in society, consists of work, activities of daily living (ADL), and leisure. The kinesiologist, biomechanics specialist, or human engineer interested in greater work productivity might well be concerned only with movement patterns relegated to the work situation. The physical therapist might be concerned with ADL and the restoration of independent living for the physically disabled. The physical educator and coach might be concerned only with leisure activities of sports and dance. This broad classification system is not always effective, however, since many movement patterns do not exist solely in only one of each of these categories. For example, walking is an activity of daily living and is also used in the work situation, in folk and disco dancing, and in several sports, including golf.

One might also group movement patterns according to the amount of learning involved—for example, (1) new movements to be learned or to be relearned if rehabilitation is the goal, (2) movements learned in a wrong or unusable manner that need to be unlearned and then learned correctly, (3) movements to be refined that are partially learned, and (4) movements that are automatic, requiring no learning but needing reinforcement. This method of classification does not lend itself to a scientific study of movement, since what is a new skill for one person may not be a new skill for another person. Therefore more definitive classifications of movement that are more useful for the purpose of biomechanical analysis have been developed.

Higgins has grouped movements patterns into three categories: locomotion, manipulation, and a combination of the two. Although these categories are useful, many kinesiologists have preferred to further subdivide movement patterns into more specific, yet rather broad, categories, such as locomotion on land, locomotion in the water, locomotion in the air, projecting oneself into the air, returning to earth, swinging and suspending one's body, projecting external objects, receiving external objects, and manipulating objects. Manipulation has been divided into gross motor skills, such as using long-handled instruments, and fine motor skills, such as piano playing, using a fork and spoon, and typewriting.

Whatever the method selected for categorizing movements, the ultimate purpose is to be able to define general principles of kinesiology (biomechanics) for ease in analyzing many movement

patterns. The cross-country runner, recreational jogger, racehorse, and domestic dog all utilize similar principles in their execution of locomotor patterns.

Categorizing movements enables one to see similarities but may obscure differences. For example, throwing movements that require high accelerations, greater use of muscles, and near-maximal efforts are described analytically in a different manner from throwing movements requiring accuracy but not great speed. Broad categories in the classification of movement patterns do, however, provide the basis for reducing the complexities of possible movements into a workable whole. Specialists may then benefit from knowledge gained in other fields of study. For example, the clinical kinesiologist has provided information related to walking patterns that has proved helpful to the sports kinesiologist investigating the forces produced by and imparted to the jogger and sprinter.

Movement may also be described as being effective or ineffective, efficient or inefficient, and safe or unsafe. If a movement is effective, it is successful, but it is not necessarily the most efficient movement. Efficiency may be determined physiologically, that is, by evaluating the metabolic cost of the movement with respect to the amount of work performed. The relationship of work of the movement or energy input and work or energy output determines the efficiency. When the mechanical work performed by the human body on some object is only slightly less than the mechanical work performed to produce the respective movement of the human body, the movement is considered to be efficient. The formula for the percentage of efficiency from the kinesiologist's point of view is as follows:

$$\text{Efficiency (\%)} = \frac{\text{Work out}}{\text{Work in}} \times 100$$

Rarely does the human body accomplish more than 25% efficiency with respect to a movement task. There are times when efficiency is not as important as effectiveness. For example, in sprinting the expenditure of energy is of little concern. Being effective over a short time is the goal. Utilization of a high rate of energy is expected, and the most efficient pattern may not be the fastest. Long-distance running, on the other hand, requires more efficient movements if the person desires to complete the race.

There are many ways to peform a task effectively. Very young persons and animals usually perform movements using excessive muscle forces and extraneous motions. "Wasted" effort goes unnoticed. To be effective day after day or during movements lasting hours in duration, efficient movements need to be developed. The more efficient a person is in executing a basketball jump shot during the first minutes of a game, the more that person is likely to be able to execute the movement effectively during the last minutes of a strenuous game. On the other hand, a basketball player may be so tense early in the game that unnecessary muscles will be used to perform the task of shooting. As the game progresses and relaxation occurs, the movement becomes more efficient and more effective. The differences between efficiency and effectiveness must be remembered when analyzing movement. They are not the same. Effectiveness is easy to measure; efficiency is not.

Finally, movement may be safe or unsafe. Great concern has arisen concerning the types of movements and the velocities at which these movements are being performed by young athletes. The challenge, the prize, and the glamour of being the best have caused many performers to practice long hours, to exert great forces by the body and on the body, and consequently to reach the pinnacle of human tolerances. What are some of the feats of tolerances that human beings have accomplished? Some remarkable feats are as follows:

1. Persons have been able many times to swim the rough and stormy English channel. It has taken 20 or more hours of continuous swimming to perform this feat. Recently James Counsilman (former U.S. Olympic swimming coach), at age 58, was able to perform **this arduous task.**

2. **Some persons have survived without food for more than 60 days.**

3. Some persons, after becoming quadruple amputees, have still been able to become productive members of society.

4. A few people have fallen to the earth from great heights and lived to tell about it.

5. The entire North American continent has been crossed on foot. Other walking feats, as well as dancing and running, have been performed for record-setting numbers of hours and days.

6. Many humans have been able to survive in equatorial heat and arctic cold.

7. Humans have the ability to pace themselves over a long-distance run. Indians, often in relay fashion, were able to run down a deer.

8. A blind person can play a game of golf. With the aid of an assistant for posture placement, a blind man has obtained a score of 85 on a typical 18-hole course.

9. Humans have attained speeds of 45 kmph (27 mph). When it is realized that the human being has only two legs with which to propel a body designed as a cylinder offering maximum wind resistance, this is truly remarkable.

The fastest and strongest movements tend to be seen in the sports arena. Baseballs are thrown overarm at 167 kmph, and softballs are pitched underarm at a slightly faster speed. The volleyball overarm serves attain speeds of 117 kmph, which must be dissipated by the receiver. Tennis balls are projected at 257 kmph, badminton smashes travel at 400 kmph, and the slap shot in ice hockey has been recorded at 197 kmph. Although locomotor speeds are not as fast, humans ride skateboards at 100 kmph and enter flight at 110 kmph from a ski jump. Contrast these speeds with such ADL movements as walking at 5 to 8 kmph and mopping a floor at 6 to 9 kmph.

Persons do become injured during movements and wonder how to determine the safe limits of movement. This question is of concern to investigators in the animal world as well. The safe limits of animal, and sometimes human, movement in the rodeo events of calf and steer roping and wrestling, bronco and brahma bull riding, and barrel racing are yet unassessed. What are the limits to which horses and dogs may be taken in preparation for and during races? The same question could be, and should be, asked for human racing.

The basic questions, then, can be stated as follows: What is the biomechanically ideal method(s) of performing a particular movement pattern? Is there one biomechanically ideal method of performance? This book may help to answer these questions.

MINI LABORATORY EXERCISES

1. Observe the following movements and name the plane of motion, the axes of rotation, and which part, if any, translates.
   a. Bicyclist and bicycle
      (1) Anatomic axes in bicyclist
      (2) Axes in bicycle
      (3) Common plane of motion
   b. Spinning top
      (1) Axis
      (2) Plane of motion
   c. Person lifting box from table and placing box on shelf approximately at the level of the head
      (1) Anatomic axes
      (2) Planes of motion (list each segment motion separately)

   d. Person performing a pushup, with feet and hands on the floor
      (1) Anatomic axes (observe performance)
      (2) External axes
      (3) Planes of motion for each body part (observe motion carefully)
2. Draw a translatory movement and indicate the plane of motion.
3. Draw a rotatory movement and indicate axis and plane of motion. Label the axis with respect to anatomy and space.

REFERENCES

Atwater, A.E.: Kinesiology/biomechanics: perspectives and trends, Res. Q. Exercise Sport **51**:193-218, 1980.

Higgins, J.R.: Human movement: an integrated approach, St. Louis, 1977, The C.V. Mosby Co.

Logan, G.A., and McKinney, W.C.: Anatomic kinesiology, ed. 2, Dubuque, Iowa, 1977, Wm. C. Brown Co., Publishers.

Steindler, A.: Kinesiology of the human body under normal and pathological conditions, Springfield, Ill., 1964, Charles C Thomas, Publisher.

ADDITIONAL READINGS

Bleustein, J., editor: Mechanics and sport, New York, 1973, American Society of Mechanical Engineering.

Roebuck, J.A., Jr.: Kinesiology in engineering, Washington, D.C., 1968, Council on Kinesiology, American Association for Health, Physical Education, and Recreation.

CHAPTER 2

A theoretical model

Movement is a change in position or place, caused by one or more forces and occurring in space with respect to time. This definition is the essence of movement. Coaches, teachers, and other observers of movement have spent many hours attempting to differentiate between skilled and unskilled movements in sport, play, work, and activities of daily living (ADL). This practice relies on the level of skill and the number of subjects available for observation. It represents a trial-and-error approach to movement analysis, since human beings and animals rarely perform a movement with a repetitious precision and timing to exactly reproduce the previous movement.

Movement analysts have therefore constructed theoretical models, that is, a scientific plan, for the determination of a biomechanically ideal performance of a movement. Simplistically, all models define the movement, analyze the movement, and set forth steps to evaluate and improve the actual execution of the movement. The particular model presented here offers a holistic approach and is based on one presented by Higgins. The value of this model is that it can be used with any movement and with any living being. It focuses on the uniqueness of the individual and the movement situation. This model is depicted in Fig. 2-1 and consists of the following steps:

1. Describing the movement
2. Setting the performance goal
3. Identifying the anatomic, mechanical, and environmental considerations
4. Setting forth the biomechanical principles for learning the movement
5. Assessing the performance with respect to these principles

DESCRIBING THE MOVEMENT

Step 1, describing the movement, consists of a qualitative and general depiction of the skill. This description is based on the temporal and spatial characteristics of movement as shown in Fig. 2-2, as well as on a deduction of the forces producing the movement. The displacement of the body and of body parts in space is described with respect to direction and distance. A displacement may also be rotatory, translatory, or a combination of both. Thus the displacement may be expressed in meters or other units of length, or in radians or other units of angular displacement. The speed and velocity of the body or body part may be qualitatively expressed as follows:

1. Since speed is the displacement divided by the time for this displacement to occur, the speed may be termed fast, moderate, or slow, or faster or slower than a preceding movement. Common units of speed are meters per second and radians per second.
2. Velocity includes the addition of a direction to the description of speed. Examples of the expression of velocity would be meters per second forward, meters per second at a 30-degree angle to the ground, and radians per second clockwise.

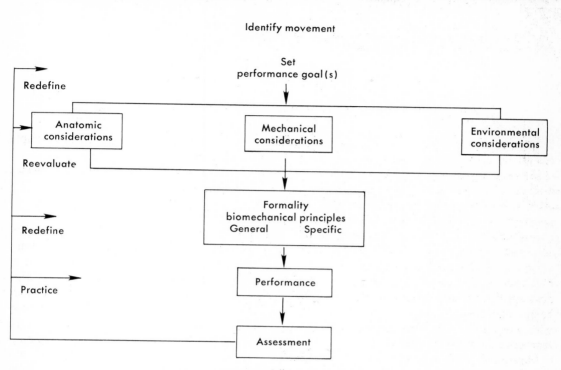

Identify movement

Set
performance goal(s)

Redefine

Anatomic
considerations

Mechanical
considerations

Environmental
considerations

Reevaluate

Formality
biomechanical principles
General   Specific

Redefine

Performance

Practice

Assessment

Fig. 2-1. Theoretical model for movement analyst.

The rate of change of the velocity, termed acceleration, is not as easily observed as are the velocity and displacement. If the velocity changes rapidly, this indicates a high acceleration, either positive or negative. High acceleration indicates large magnitudes of force.

This descriptive approach is applied to bowling to present the reader with an example of the completion of step 1. Bowling would be described as a leisure-sport activity involving locomotion on land plus gross manipulation of a ball that will in turn be projected into space. The movements are pri-

marily in the sagittal plane. Rotations at the hip, knee, and ankle about frontal-horizontal axes cause the body to translate forward four steps. The arm in which the ball is held swings in the sagittal plane, a half circle backward and a half circle forward. The total movement pattern takes approximately 2 seconds to perform. Movements appear to require little muscle force. The fastest movement is the arm swing, which appears to be pendular in nature, that is, influenced primarily by the force of gravity. The hand, fingers, and arm show a diagonally upward and lateral movement at the

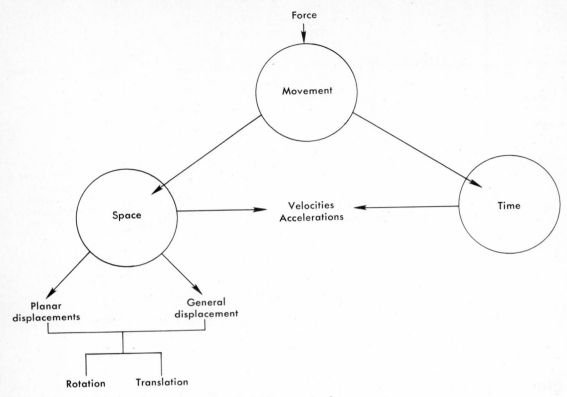

Fig. 2-2. Basic framework of movement.

time of release of the ball. This movement is not precisely described by means of observational techniques. The locomotion shows an increase in speed until the final step, which is a sliding step. The person completes the action of bowling in a rather stable position behind a foul line. The ball rolls along the floor as a result of being released at the low point of the swing during the sliding step.

SETTING THE PERFORMANCE GOAL

The second step, setting the performance goal, is not always simple. The same movement performed by three individuals may have three goals. These goals temper the analysis of the anatomic, mechanical, and environmental considerations. If

in bowling the skill is partially learned, the goal might be to decrease the speed of the arm swing. If the skill is new, the goal might be to swing the arm faster than the first attempts. If the purpose is to "pick up a split," the ball might be given more lateral spin than otherwise. As the goal changes, the expected performance changes. As another example, a competitive breaststroke swimmer will not glide during the stroke cycle, whereas the swimmer desiring maximal stroke efficiency of energy output from each stroke will perform an optimal glide. The competitive swimmer wishes to accelerate from one stroke to the next. In a like manner, the walking pattern of a cat changes when it stalks its prey.

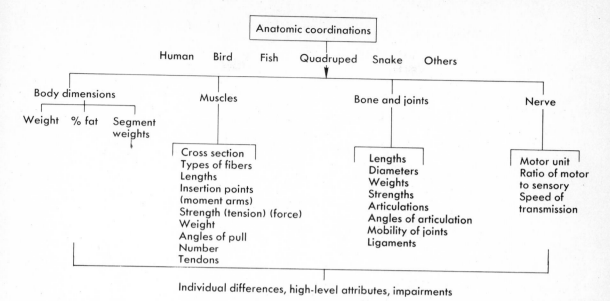

Fig. 2-3. Anatomic considerations in formulation of biomechanical principles by movement analyst.

IDENTIFYING THE ANATOMIC, MECHANICAL, AND ENVIRONMENTAL CONSIDERATIONS

Only after the movement has been identified and the goal established can one execute step 3: identifying the anatomic, mechanical, and environmental considerations for the express purpose of formulating the biomechanical principles. Fig. 2-3 expands the factor under *anatomic considerations*. The first subdivisions, body dimensions, is also termed morphometry (measurement of body) or anthropometry (measurement of human bodies). The general size and shape of the total body is investigated. The body and its parts are measured for girth, breath, depth, and length. Unique characteristics should be noted and comparisons made with respect to age, sex, species, and other subgroups, such as members of a fencing team.

The movement apparatus—muscle, bone, and nerve—comprises the remainder of the anatomic considerations. Here, too, the size, shape, and weight must be considered. In addition, strength

and speed of the movement apparatus need to be estimated or measured to determine whether or not there are unique characteristics that must be considered in the setting of principles for performance. For example, a hemiplegic swimmer and a paraplegic swimmer will perform a swimming stroke differently from each other and especially from an ablebodied and neurologically sound person. Individual differences—whether high-level attributes or impairments—will influence what is biomechanically ideal for the given individual. The biomechanically ideal walking patterns of various species will differ with respect to lengths of bones, types of articulations, angles of articulations, and shapes of bones. Although it is true that within a species one would expect to see described one ideal manner of perfoming one particular movement, slight differences will exist within species because of differences in anatomic factors. In particular, the human individual might be an infant, a physically disabled person, a person over

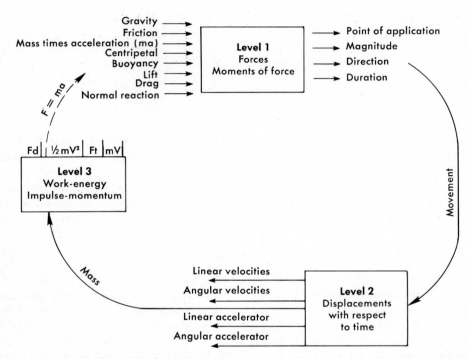

Fig. 2-4. Mechanical considerations in formulation of biomechanical principles by movement analyst.

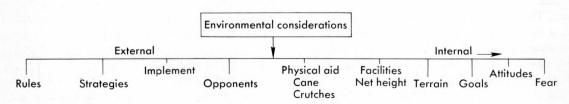

Fig. 2-5. Environmental considerations in formulation of biomechanical principles by movement analyst.

80 years of age, a skilled ballet dancer, a professional tennis player, or some other person of unique or unusual characteristics or performance abilities.

The second set of considerations, *mechanical,* can be expanded in the same way as the anatomic (Fig. 2-4). Some of these considerations are unalterable unless movement takes place in outer space, on the moon, on Jupiter, or on an earth satellite station. Basically the force of gravity rules or controls movements of animals and humans, and even of plants. In addition to gravity, there are other forces as well as moments of forces. A moment of force is a force acting at a point other than through the center of gravity of the body, causing a rotation of that body.

Therefore the first approach to the mechanical considerations is the magnitude, direction, duration, and point of application of force. If rotation is to occur, what is the moment of force required to produce and regulate the rotation? How many forces are present? Which forces facilitate, or can be made to facilitate, the movement? Which forces will inhibit the movement, and how can their inhibitory roles be reduced? An understanding of all forces and moments of forces is necessary in order to analyze their results.

The results of forces and moments of forces acting on a body will be the measurable and predictable velocities and accelerations of the body as it is moved in space. Analysis of these factors provides insight into the kinematics of the movement, but the final approach to the mechanical considerations is holistic. Here the work-energy and impulse-momentum of the body are considered. Thus forces and their kinematic effects are combined to provide insight into the effectiveness of movement. The exchange and generation of energy also allow one to identify levels of safety and human tolerances, and the analysis of work accomplished adds new insight into the efficiency of the movement.

The third set of considerations, *environmental,* often sets forth restrictions or restraints on the proposed movement. What are the implements to be used? What is the climate? What is the terrain? What role do other persons have in a performance by another person? Are there certain rules, strategies, or goals that influence the selection of the type or modification of a movement pattern? Fig. 2-5 depicts these internal and external environmental considerations.

In the work situation the placement of the facilities and equipment to be used offers the greatest restraint to the movement pattern. The expected work output also influences the mode of movement, particularly the speed of the movement. In sports situations the impositions commonly consist of the rules of play. Movements would not be executed, and especially not terminated, in the manner they are if it were not for foul lines, height of nets, and intimidating legal actions by opponents. For ADL, humans and animals are constrained primarily by their physical environment, mainly the terrain. Hyde has shown differences in locomotor patterns of kangaroo rats with respect to soil characteristics of their habitats. Human beings walk differently on iced walkways than on sandy beaches. This last example may not be dependent on the external environment only. Not to be omitted from environmental considerations is the internal environment of the performer. What is his or her motivation, state of mind, level of tension, or level of relaxation? Although difficult to assess, internal environment must be included in this set of considerations.

None of these three sets of considerations, anatomic, mechanical, and environmental, can be isolated in the analysis of movement patterns. Each can be studied separately, but then each must be synthesized with the other two because they are interdependent in a true study of kinesiology (biomechanics). This synthesis of all three sets of considerations is the basis for step 4.

BIOMECHANICAL PRINCIPLES OF MOVEMENT

Step 4 of the theoretical model addresses the formulation of biomechanical principles for the execution or teaching of the performance. A principle denotes a statement of fact about a phenomenon, a person, an object, or an event. Principles are formulated so that the complex movement of living bodies can be effectively reduced to simpler elements and thereby evaluated or described. Principles usually will state a relationship about two factors or will show a cause-and-effect relationship. For example, an understanding of equilibrium is derived from the following basic principle: A body will be in equilibrium (stationary) if the center of mass remains above the base of support of the body.

Selection of the best combination of principles is sometimes necessary, or a compromise or an adaptation of general principles results because of the goal, individual impairments, or uniqueness of the anatomic, mechanical, and environmental considerations. For example, in golf one might sacrifice maximal distance for a gain in accuracy, especially if two moderate-distance shots will equal one long drive and one short chip in distance. In this manner the principles are related to the performance goal. As another example, a person may use a crutch only when walking long distances. The implement and the physical disability determine which principles are formulated for achieving an effective, efficient, and safe performance.

PERFORMANCE AND ASSESSMENT

The final step in the model involves both the performance and the assessment of the performance. Sometimes the assessment becomes a reassessment and redefining of the earlier steps. Therefore one sees that the scientific study of movement, although complex, can be simplified by means of a conceptual framework (model) to gain an understanding of the causes, influences, restrictions, and other components of movement. Only by means of an understanding of movement can prospective teachers coaches, therapists, and other educators of the physical dimension of life assess, improve, and ultimately predict movement. Assessment of movement involves the process of identifying (1) the components that cause the

movement to be effective or efficient and (2) the components that interfere with or hinder the goal—the achievement of the performance. To improve performance one must determine what movement changes need to be made, based on a correct assessment of the performance and the performance goal. The prediction of movement allows one to determine the outcome of an attempt to move. One can then determine whether or not a new style of movement should be utilized, how desirable it would be, and what the components of the new style should include. One might also predict the changes in a movement pattern that would result from a change in environment, implement, or body weight.

This theoretical model underlies the entire contents of this book and is the basis for each of the specific analyses presented in subsequent chapters. Within these chapters, however, an analysis may be primarily one of mechanical considerations, expanding or elaborating on a specific mechanical principle. In other instances a particular analysis tool may have provided limited information about the movement itself or about a particular person's performance of that movement. Specific, narrowly defined analyses may be presented to emphasize a particular typical error, a uniqueness of the particular movement, or a modification of one part of the movement because of an impairment by a performer. The reader must remember, however, that reference to and utilization of Figs. 2-1 to 2-5 (depicting the steps in this theoretical model) will provide the holistic approach to the analysis of the most effective, efficient, and safe manner of performance by a specific individual. In essence, we assess to optimize performance.

MINI LABORATORY EXERCISES

Use the theoretical model to outline your analysis of a movement pattern of your choice. Suggestions are as follows:
1. Select a planar movement.
2. Work in a group.
3. Discuss your outline with others.

REFERENCES

Higgins, J.R.: Human movement: an integrated approach, St. Louis, 1977, The C.V. Mosby Co.

Hyde, M.L.: Analysis and comparison of locomotion in three species of kangaroo rat, genus *Dipodomys,* Lubbock, 1977, Texas Tech University.

ADDITIONAL READINGS

Fitts, P.M., and Posner, M.L.: Human performance, Westport, Conn., 1979, Greenwood Press.

Gowitzke, B.A., and Milner, M.: Understanding the scientific bases of human movement, Baltimore, 1980, The Williams & Wilkins Co.

Hanavan, E.P.: A mathematical model of the human body, Pub. No. AMRL-TR-64-102, Fairborn, Ohio, Oct., 1964, Wright-Patterson Air Force Base.

Marteniuk, R.G.: Information processing in motor skills, New York, 1976, Holt, Rinehart & Winston.

CHAPTER 3

Tools for assessment, improvement, and prediction of movement

Implementation of the previously described theoretical model requires the ability to observe and measure movement. There are several tools available for such observations and measurements. They will be explained briefly and are listed as follows:

1. Human eye and other senses
2. Photography and cinematography
3. Videography
4. Electrogoniometry
5. Electromyography
6. Dynamography
7. Other tools: accelerometry, acoustic tools, and laser and other optical tools
8. Theoretical tools: mathematic modeling and simulation

HUMAN EYE AND OTHER SENSES

Published works and principles based on the analysis of movement of living things have been known in Western civilization since the era of the ancient Greeks. The Greeks were among the first to practice so-called scientific thinking, as opposed to that based on emotional and spiritual ideas. Hippocrates (460-377 B.C.) advocated the concept that people should base their observations on and draw conclusions from only what they perceived through their senses (particularly those of touch, sight, hearing, and smell) without recourse to the

supernatural. One of Hippocrates' contemporaries, the Greek scholar Herodicus, was interested in gymnastics (exercise through active volition) as a means of curing disease. In fact, he prescribed it for fever patients' and was criticized by Hippocrates for doing so.

Aristotle (384-322 B.C.) has been called *the father of kinesiology*. Aristotle made his many observations in almost every field of science. Students of kinesiology are especially impressed with his treatise *Parts of Animals, Movement of Animals, and Progression of Animals*. Today's physical education teachers, athletic instructors, physical therapists, and industrial engineers, along with all persons who are concerned with the observation and study of human beings in motion, use some of the basic principles of Aristotle. In fact, the good modern teacher of movement makes use of the techniques of close observation as a means of evaluation. Certainly Aristotle's concepts of muscular flexion and the part that it plays in movements such as walking are a good foundation for modern studies on gait and other movements involving the transformation of rotatory motion to translatory motion.

Archimedes (287-212 B.C.), a renowned mathematician, established the basic principles that undergird the present knowledge of floating bodies—in water, as well as in outer space.

The scientific awakening known as the *Renaissance* was perhaps initiated and epitomized by the work of Leonardo da Vinci (1452-1519), who is given credit for developing the modern science of anatomy. He studied human structure, especially noting the relation of the center of gravity to balance and motion during different movements. He made these observations while he was developing a treatise on painting. To be sure that his drawings of the body were authentic, da Vinci secured and dissected hundreds of cadavers. He was adept in many fields and blended the artistic with the scientific in a way never since duplicated. According to several historians da Vinci was the greatest engineer, biologist, and artist of his time. Robinson stated that da Vinci was one of the first to break away from the acceptance of Galen, an early Roman physician, as the only authority. He was severely criticized by his contemporaries because he did not blindly follow noted authorities. Leonardo da Vinci said, "I do not know how to quote from learned authorities, but it is a much greater and more estimable matter to rely on experience. They scorn me who am a discoverer; yet how much more do they deserve censure who have never found out anything, but only recite and blazen forth other people's works."*

Da Vinci's ability to draw the muscles of a human body engaged in performing a dynamic act was of great value to medical students and to the science of kinesiology. Da Vinci's intelligence and versatility are exemplified in the following quotations from his treatise *On the Flight of Birds,* as translated by Hart.

When the edge of the point of the wing is opposed to the edge of the wind for an instant, I put this wing under or on this edge of the wind and the same thing happens to the point or sides of the tail, and similarly to the shaft of the shoulders of the wing.

The descent of a bird will always be that (part W) extremity which will be nearest to its center of gravity.

The heaviest part of a bird descending will be always in front of its centre of resistance.

If the wing and the tail are too much on the wind, lower half of the opposite wing, and therewith receive the force of the wind and equilibrium will be restored.*

Modern pilots use the same method of lowering a wing in righting a plane in flight.

Da Vinci's observations on human action in a specific movement show his insight. He said, "He who descends takes short steps because the weight rests upon the hinder foot. And he who mounts takes long steps because his weight remains on the forward foot."†

Even today, observation of motion of living beings, dissection of cadavers, reading of published works, and perusal of clinical records of injury are methods of investigating movement empirically. The data obtained are often limited and qualitative in nature and quite often are erroneous as well. Because of these errors the discarded "facts" of one era are replaced by another set of "facts" in another era of history. The basis for the mechanical analysis of movement was established by Galileo (1564-1642) and Newton (1642-1727). Singer said, "With Newton the universe acquired an independent rationality, and the whole cosmology of Aristotle, of Galen, and of the Middle Ages lay in

---

*Robinson, V.: The story of medicine, New York, 1943, Doubleday & Co., Inc.

*Hart, I.: The mechanical investigations of Leonardo da Vinci, London, 1925, Chapman & Hall, Ltd.
†O'Malley, C.D., and Saunders, J.B. de C.M.: Leonardo da Vinci on the human body, New York, 1952, Henry Schuman, Inc., Publishers.

the dust.''* Conversely, although Newton's laws of motion are in use today and are as valid as they were during his day, they are not applicable for precise measurement of special cases, nor are they applicable in the area of quantum mechanics.

Observation usually provides only qualitative information about movement and therefore enables the observer to note and correct only the most obvious inadequacies of the movement. Observation may be supplemented by means of inexpensive devices to provide some quantification of the motion components. Wetting, dusting, or inking the soles of the feet provides a record of placement and distance between feet during the movement. Relative pressure distribution on the feet can be measured by performing on sand, on layers of corrugated cardboard, or on a surface having an ink pad underneath. Stopwatches and single and multiple electrically powered chronoscopes can be used to time movements and specific segments within each movement pattern.

The extent of devices that may be constructed and used is limited only by one's imagination and knowledge of published literature. For example, Karpovich used a fishing reel to measure the variations in speed within a swimming-stroke cycle. The fishing line was attached to a floating tripod, which was attached to the swimmer. As the swimmer progressed forward, the fishing line uncoiled from the reel. Each time the reel made one revolution, a mark was placed on a paper moving at a predetermined speed. The mark was made possible by a rod attached to the reel, causing the rod to rotate with the uncoiling of the line. A microswitch was contacted by the rod with each turn of the reel. Kluth used this idea for recording the deceleration of the swimmer's body after entry into the water from a racing start.

PHOTOGRAPHY AND CINEMATOGRAPHY

Since the human eye cannot see all particulars of motion, since the eye records motion at 10 to 12

*Singer, C.: A short history of medicine, London, 1928, Oxford University Press, p. 19.

frames/sec, and since the eye may not retain the total motion, persons turned to various devices to provide permanent images of movement.

A French physiologist, Étienne Jules Marey (1830-1904), was so interested in human movement that he developed photographic means for use in biologic research. In his works *Du Mouvement dans les Fonctions de la Vie* and *De Mouvement,* he explained and illustrated how this could be accomplished. Some of the translated works include the history of chronophotography and lectures on the phenomenon of flight in the animal world. Marey, as well as Robinson, was convinced that movement was the important human function and affected all other activities.

Eadweard Muybridge (1830-1904), through his photographic skill, brought a new tool to kinesiologic investigation. He was motivated by the work of Janssen, an astronomer who had been successful in taking sequential pictures of stars. Among the numerous Muybridge publications was an 11-volume work, *Animal Locomotion* (1887). A recent publication called *The Human Figure in Motion* contains much of his original work. Using 24 fixed cameras and 2 portable batteries of 12 cameras each, Muybridge was able to take pictures of animals (Fig. 3-1) and people in action, and by using the zoopraxiscope he could move the pictures fast enough that actual movement was simulated. As an illustration of how an idea may be developed, Muybridge modified this device by mounting transparencies made from a series of his photographs on a circular glass plate. When the plate was rotated, individual transparencies could be projected by a projection lantern in the usual manner. A major refinement of the device was the addition of a second plate, made of metal and mounted parallel to the glass plate on a concentric axis but turning in the opposite direction. The metal plate was slit at appropriate intervals. When the two plates revolved, the metal plate served as a shutter. The persistence of vision between each slit gave the viewer the illusion of motion as each individual picture in the series was projected. As many as 200 transparencies could be mounted on a

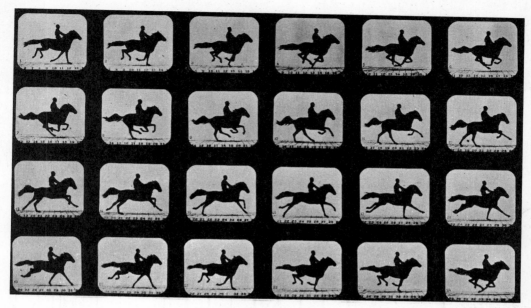

Fig. 3-1. Motion of running horse. Subject is Phryne L, whose length of stride was reported to be 6 m 2 cm (19 ft 9 in). (Courtesy Stanford Museum.)

single plate, and the wheels, or plates, could be revolved endlessly, ''a period limited only by the patience of the spectators.''*

The accomplishments of Marey and Muybridge paved the way for two German scientists, Christian Wilhelm Braune (1831-1892) and Otto Fischer (1861-1917), to study the human gait by means of photographic devices. They also developed an experimental method to determine the center of gravity of the human body. In 1889, these two outstanding German anatomists published a comprehensive paper on an experimental method that they had developed to determine the center of gravity of the human body. Adolf Eugen Fick (1829-1901), who followed, drew on their work; he eventually became one of the outstanding authorities in the field of joint mechanics. Today's concepts on posture appear to have had their origin in the experiments of Braune and Fischer. Earlier methods of

locating the center of gravity of the human body had proved to be ineffective, and Braune and Fischer introduced modifications of some procedures. First, they conceived of a way of freezing a dead body so that it remained unchanged while they made mathematic calculations. Second, they compared the frozen posture of a cadaver with the posture of a living person and found the two postures to be markedly similar. They located the center of gravity not only of the body as a whole but also of each component part. They were the first to estimate the percentage of the weights of body segments. After they located the center of gravity of the total body of the frozen cadavers, they cut two of them into body segments and located the center of gravity of each. Much of their work involved the use of photographic apparatus to obtain the evidence they needed for locating the midpoints of a joint and the axes of rotation, as stated by Hirt and co-workers.

Photography has become sophisticated since those nineteenth-century experiments. Most inves-

*Muybridge, E.: The human figure in motion, New York, 1955, Dover Publications, Inc.

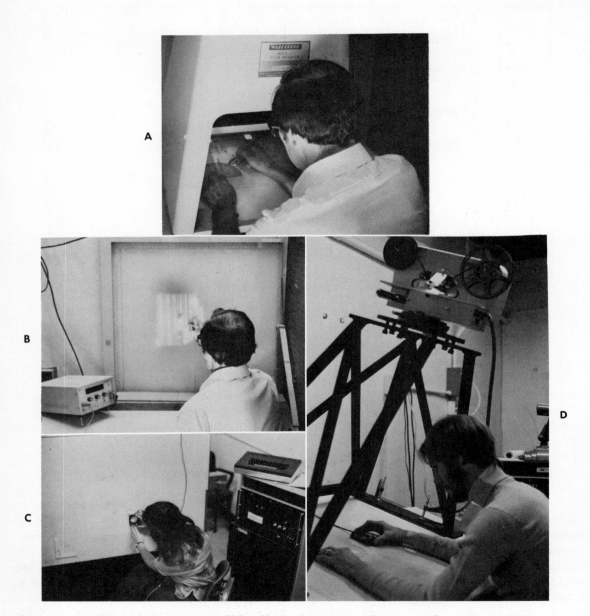

Fig. 3-2. Film analysis systems. **A,** Using film reader to trace and measure 16 mm film. **B,** Using acoustic digitizing system to obtain spatial coordinates. **C,** Computerized digitizing systems. **D,** Vanguard-Bendix film analysis system. The x- and y-coordinate values are transmitted directly to laboratory computer for calculation and analysis. (**A** and **D** courtesy Pennsylvania State University Biomechanics Laboratory; **B,** special equipment, Biomechanics Laboratory, Indiana University; **C,** courtesy Biomechanics Laboratory, Washington State University, Pullman.)

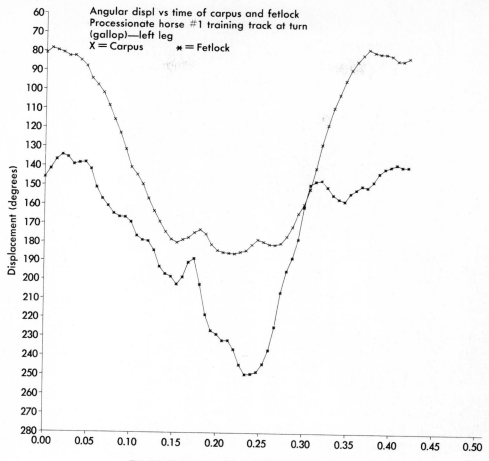

Fig. 3-3. Computer plots of digitized film data.

tigations of human and animal movements are conducted by means of movie cameras, super 8mm or 16mm, capable of filming at rates up to 500 images per second, which is approximately 50 times the number of images the human eye can detect. Other cameras operating at 10,000-plus filming rates are utilized in collision and other impact studies of body deformation (Chapter 6) and destruction. Analysis of the movie films may be conducted by means of manual tracing and measuring of displacements by single-frame projection

of the film and by calculating other motion variables from the displacement data. Since the late 1960s, however, researchers have developed and utilized computerized film analysis systems (Fig. 3-2). These systems provide numerical and graphic printouts of displacements, velocities, accelerations, moments of force, and centers of gravity, as well as statistical and comparative analyses (Fig. 3-3).

Another common type of photography is stroboscopy, or intermittent light photography. Fig.

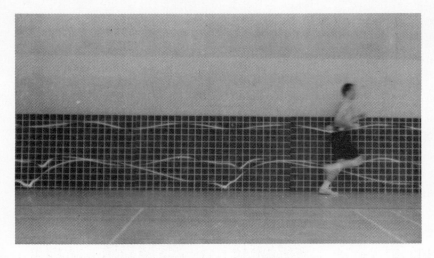

Fig. 3-4. Stroboscopic photography. Film is exposed in semidarkness, while flashing lights record path of lights during action. One instant of illumination of entire field shows position of subject. (Courtesy Biomechanics Laboratory, Indiana University.)

3-4 depicts an example of the results of such a technique. Stroboscopic photography uses multiple exposures on a single negative, which may be exposed to a brightly lighted or a dark background and subject. In the first case the exposures are determined by the opening of the camera shutter at a set rate. In the second, small electric light bulbs are attached to points on the body. These may be lighted continuously, providing a line of light on the photograph, or they may flash at a set rate, providing a series of dots on the photograph.

Another form of photography used in biomechanical research is cineradiography, in which X rays, or fluoroscopic rays, are synchronized with a camera, allowing bones to be filmed in action.

VIDEOGRAPHY

Although developed later than photography, the videotape systems do not have the high framing rates possible with movie cameras. The common rate of total scans on the video monitor (television set) is equivalent to 30 images/sec, slightly greater than the home movie camera. Recently some researchers have reported image speeds higher than 120/sec. When it becomes feasible to manufacture

and produce cameras having this speed, videography will have greater research significance and importance to the general practitioner. The advantages of videography are (1) the ability to synchronize two images on one screen, which is possible by means of a split-image, special-effects generator, (2) the direct and immediate transmission of the image to a computer, thus eliminating the human operator required in photographic analysis, and (3) the direct playback capability, which provides immediate feedback to both the analyst and the performer.

ELECTROGONIOMETRY

Observation of joint action can be facilitated with the use of the electrogoniometer (also called "elgon"), which was devised by Karpovich in the late 1950s. The elgon is essentially a goniometer with a potentiometer substituted for the protractor. The degrees of movement in the joint to which the device has been attached can be read directly from recording paper, thus eliminating laborious measurement. The device has been used with other methods of recording of movement, such as electromyography and cinematography. (An excellent

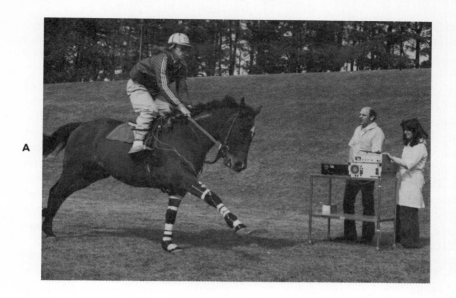

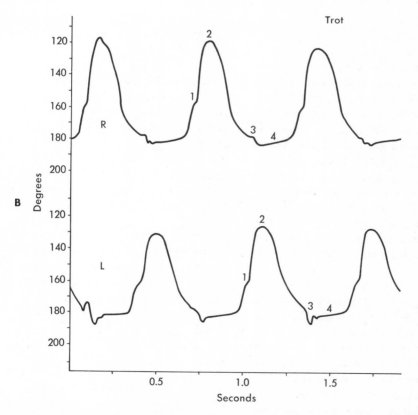

Fig. 3-5. Electrogoniometry. **A,** Electrogoniometers attached to horse. **B,** Goniogram.

description of the elgon and its application is presented by Adrian in the 1968 *Kinesiology Review*.

Three-dimensional electrogoniometers have been used in gait analysis in rehabilitation centers and laboratories and on the sports field. The advantages of electrogoniometry include the ability to record the action at the joint when it is not visible to the observer, such as during swimming and twisting movements. Another advantage is the instantaneous portrayal of angular displacement with respect to time. The electrogoniometry system can be linked to a computer to obtain angular velocities and accelerations. The use of a telemetry system has been used to monitor joint motion of such subjects as racehorses, swimmers, and football players. Fig. 3-5 shows such an electrogoniometry system and the resulting goniogram (recording of angular displacement). The goniogram does not convey any spatial orientation of the limb but solely the angle at the joints.

ELECTROMYOGRAPHY

Muscle analysis based on anatomic position of muscles cannot be accepted as definitive of the action that occurs in the living, moving body. The fallacies of analyzing muscle action on the basis of anatomic position were demonstrated by Duchenne in the middle of the nineteenth century. On the basis of electrical stimulation of muscles, combined with observation of partially paralyzed subjects, he described the movements resulting from contraction of specific muscles as they functioned in living subjects. Unfortunately his findings were not widely used in the United States, since they were published in French and were not readily available until translated in 1949 by Kaplan. By that time investigators in the United States had begun to observe muscle action in living subjects by recording the electrical changes that can be observed as muscles contract. The technique of recording, known as *electromyography,* has been greatly refined and, as complex motor acts are studied, will provide valuable information for the kinesiologist. The major current contributor to this development is J.V. Basmajian; his book *Muscles Alive* is a classic.

Electromyography* is the process of recording electrical changes that occur in a muscle during or immediately before contraction. Necessary equipment includes a device for picking up the electrical activity, a means for conducting the electrical impulses, and a device for translating them to visual form. The pickup devices are metal disks placed on the skin over the muscle or fine wires inserted into the muscle to be observed. Insulated wires conduct impulses from the pickup to the translating devices. Among the latter are ink writers, electromagnetic tape recorders, and oscilloscopes, from which photographs are made during the activity. The final form is a record, an electromyogram (EMG), similar to that shown in Fig. 3-6, *A*.

This brief, simplified statement concerning electromyography does not convey one essential concept—that the competent, trustworthy investigator must have special technical skills. Such skills include the ability to select the best equipment for each study, to use the equipment, and to interpret the EMGs intelligently.

Since the action potentials resulting from muscle contraction do not necessarily occur precisely when muscle contraction is produced, caution is needed in interpretation of the EMG. For example, the EMG signal always occurs before movement and is earlier in phasic than in tonic movements. Phasic movements will show fast-twitch muscle fibers to be active, whereas slow-twitch muscle fibers are active during tonic movements. Thus the magnitude of the EMG sign will be proportional to the velocity of the movement, since the magnitude of fast-twitch fiber action potentials is shown to be greater than that of slow-twitch fiber action potentials. In addition, the EMG magnitude also is directly related to the resistance to be overcome, or

---

*For detailed descriptions of electromyography see Basmajian, J.V.: Electromyographic analysis, Proceedings of Biomechanics Symposium at Indiana University, Chicago, 1971, The Athletic Institute; O'Connell, A.L., and Gardner, E.B.: The use of electromyography in kinesiological research, Res. Q. Am. Assoc. Health Phys. Educ. **34:**166, 1963; and Waterland, J.C., and Shambes, G.M.: Electromyography: one link in the experimental chain of kinesiological research, J. Am. Phys. Ther. Assoc. **49:**1351, 1969.

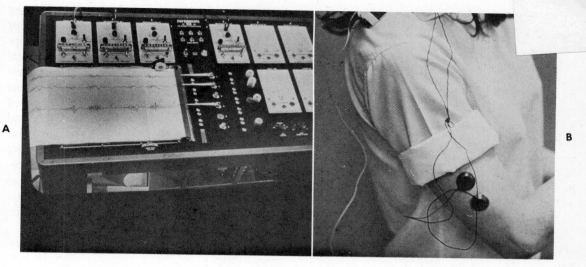

Fig. 3-6. Electromyography. **A,** Electromyogram. **B,** Surface electrodes attached to performer.

the amount of contraction utilized for static loading situations. Therefore the amount of tension in the muscle is not exactly defined by the EMG.

Furthermore, to interpret an EMG it is necessary to know which body segments have moved; in which joints actions have occurred, at what rates, and in what sequence; which muscles pass over these joints; and to which bones these muscles are attached. It is also necessary to know whether other forces were acting on body segments, especially gravitational force. Since EMGs do not provide such information, other records of the action are made at the same time, for example, with photography (biplane is recommended) and electro-goniometry.

DYNAMOGRAPHY

Although dynamography has been used in industry and by engineers for several decades, there has been virtually no use of this technique for the analysis of human forces produced during sports situations prior to the 1960s. Dynamography had been utilized in the measurement of strength, primarily static strength. Since the last decade, strain gauges have been placed on such devices as canoe

and kayak paddles, bicycle pedals, and uneven parallel bars to determine the effectiveness of force production by performers using these devices. Force platforms have been built of many sizes, shapes, and designs to record force-time histories during running, jumping, swimming, walking, and other locomotor patterns of humans, as well as those of cats, dogs, horses, and other animals. Movements of athletes engaged in pole vaulting, shot putting, sprinting starts, golfing, and gymnastics, among other sports, have also been measured by dynamographic techniques. Figs. 3-7 and 3-8 illustrate some of the uses of a force platform.

The force platform, although reported in 1938 as one of the techniques for analyzing the gait of a cat walking on a treadmill, became the most exciting analysis technique of the sports world of the 1970s. The direct analysis of forces had not been studied in previous decades, and there was a need to know the nature of forces occurring during a movement. In addition to the implications for strength training and for general safety, the analysis of force-time histories (continuous force recordings with respect to time) provides a means to differentiate between mechanical and anatomic

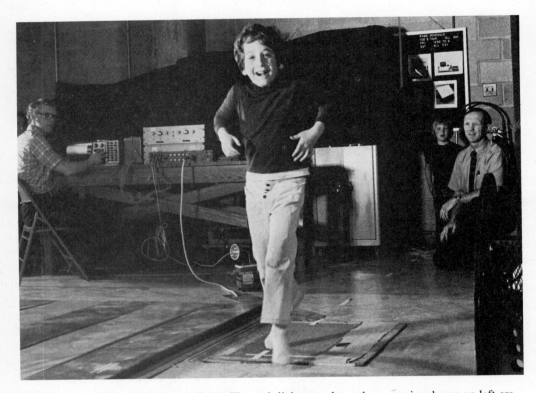

Fig. 3-7. Force platform is in a well. Oscillograph light recorder and accessories shown on left are used in fast action. Handicapped children were used as subjects in this study.

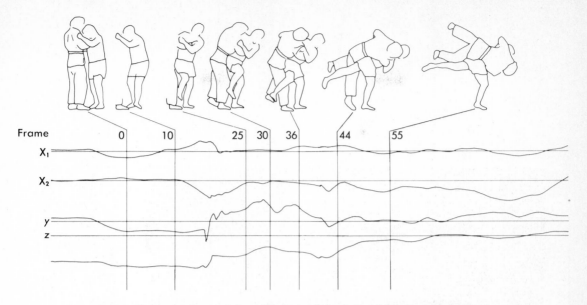

Fig. 3-8. Contourograms and three-dimensional force-time histories of judo throw.

factors. For example, Fig. 3-9 shows the incorrect application of force during a vertical jump, which produces greater velocity and a higher jump than in a mechanically correct jump. The reason for these results exists in the mass and muscle strength differences between the two performers. The performer in Fig. 3-9, *A,* did not have a muscle strength–body mass ratio sufficiently high to produce an adequate impulse (product of force and time of application of that force) and consequently a high velocity of projection. This is only one example of the many ways in which dynamography can assist the movement analyst toward a more complete understanding of movement.

OTHER TOOLS

There appears to be no limit to the numbers and types of instrumentation that can be developed and used for the analysis of human and animal movement. For example, laser technology provides a simplified means of recording velocities of objects (Figs. 3-10 and 3-11), as well as a hologram of the

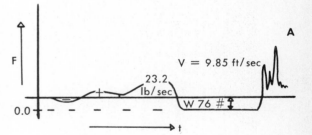

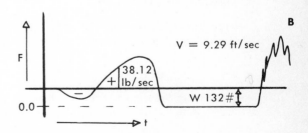

Fig. 3-9. Force-time histories of vertical jumps. Unskilled but lightweight jumper, **A,** produces greater impulse than skilled but overweight jumper, **B.**

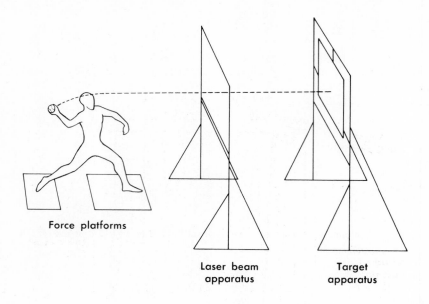

Force platforms

Laser beam
apparatus

Target
apparatus

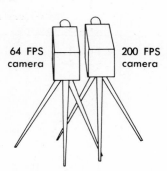

64 FPS
camera

200 FPS
camera

Fig. 3-10. Laser beam arrangement for determining velocity of thrown ball. (Drawing of experimental setup used by Jack Sanders in study at Indiana University in 1975.)

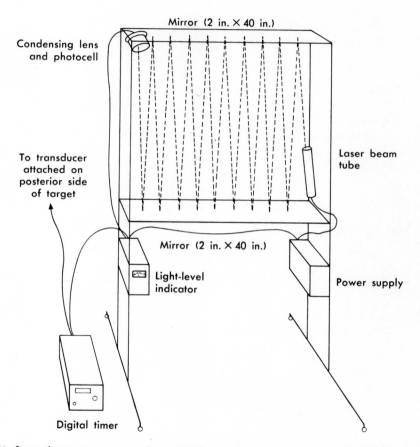

Fig. 3-11. Laser beam arrangement for determining velocity of thrown ball. (Drawing by Jack Sanders, showing apparatus used in his study at Indiana University in 1975.)

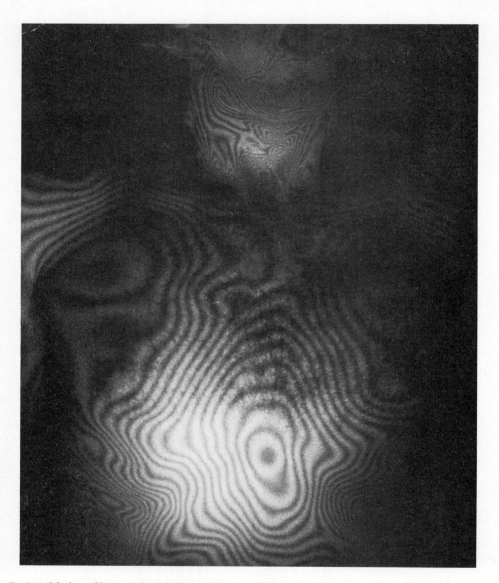

Fig. 3-12. Motion of human chest during exhalation. Hologram was made by ruby laser holography in which laser was double pulsed while subject exhaled rapidly into tube. Image seen is three-dimensional reconstruction of subject. Interpretation of photograph of hologram of subject requires mathematic analysis involving dark fringe lines in image, which reveals amount of movement by representing displacement of light wavelengths. Future use may include measurements of instantaneous surface velocity distributions in complex motions. (Courtesy S.M. Zivi TRW Instruments, Redondo Beach, Calif.)

human chest (Fig. 3-12). Many of these techniques, however, are not commonly used because of cost, lack of availability, lack of knowledge by kinesiologists, or too limited an application.

THEORETICAL TOOLS

Mathematic modeling of the anatomic characteristics of a living body can be combined with simulation techniques for the purpose of predicting performance achievements and developing new techniques of performance. Expertise in mathematics, anatomy, physics, and computers is required for bringing the use of these theoretic tools to fruition. More details will be given concerning these tools in Part Four.

Two of the basic tools of analysis of movement are mathematics and measurement. Movement parameters are measured in appropriate units of measurement. These measured values are then manipulated mathematically by placing them in equations requiring addition, subtraction, multiplication, and division. For quantitative analyses the reader may find it necessary to review basic mathematic procedures. In addition, basic trigonometric processes are valuable to the movement analyst. Therefore this basic information is included in Appendix B. Appendix A summarizes the International System of Units (SI), which is the system used in this book. Since many readers may be more familiar with the English system of measurement, a comparison of the two systems also is included in Appendix A.

MINI LABORATORY EXERCISES

Use several analysis techniques to obtain information about a jumping pattern. For example:

1. Observation: What can you see qualitatively and measure or estimate quantitatively?
2. Videography: What further data can you obtain that were not seen via the observation method? Did you discover errors in the observation data?

3. Force platform: How long was the force applied against the ground? What was the peak force? Does the pattern of the force-time curve suggest that the performance was a skilled one?

REFERENCES

Aristotle: Parts of animals, movements of animals, and progression of animals, Cambridge, Mass., 1945, Harvard University Press.

Basmajian, J.V.: Electromyographic analyses of basic movement patterns. In Wilmore, J.H., editor: Exercise and sports sciences reviews, vol. 1, New York, 1973, Academic Press, Inc.

Basmajian, J.V.: Muscles alive: their function revealed by electromyography, ed. 4, Baltimore, 1979, The Williams & Wilkins Co.

Duchenne, G.B.: Physiology of motion, Philadelphia, 1949, J.B Lippincott Co.

Hirt, S., Fries, E.C., and Hellebrandt, F.A.: Center of gravity of the human body, Arch. Phys. Ther. **25**:280, 1944.

Karpovich, P.V.: Swimming speed analyzed, Sci. Am. **142**:224, March, 1930.

Kluth, M.E.: The effect of starting block height on the racing dive, unpublished thesis, Pullman, 1971, Washington State University.

Muybridge, E.: The human figure in motion, New York, 1955, Dover Publications, Inc.

ADDITIONAL READINGS

Adrian, M.: Cinematographic, electromyographic, and electrogoniometric techniques for analyzing human movements. In Wilmore, J.H., editor: Exercise and sport sciences reviews, vol. 1, New York, 1973, Academic Press, Inc.

Amar, J.: The human motor, New York, 1972, Irvington Publishers, Inc.

Atwater, A.E.: Cinematographic analyses of human movement. In Wilmore, J.H., editor: Exercise and sports sciences reviews, vol. 1, New York, 1973, Academic Press, Inc., pp. 217-258.

Miller, D.I.: Modelling in biomechanics: an overview, Med. Sci. Sports **11**:115-122, 1971.

Miller, D.I., and Nelson, R.C.: Biomechanics of sport: a research approach, Philadelphia, 1973, Lea & Febiger.

Terauds, J., editor: Science in biomechanics cinematography, Del Mar, Calif., 1979, Academic Publishers.

Moving in a gravitational world

CHAPTER 4

The force of gravity

Plants, animals, and human beings respond according to their unique structure, and each structure can be and is modified by the environment in which it exists. Within the earth's environment, bodies are attracted to the earth at an acceleration rate of approximately 9.8 m/sec². This rate varies with respect to the distance of the body from the center of the earth, but any attempt to move the body upward requires muscular force in opposition to this attraction known as gravity. The required force is directly proportional to body mass, the quantity of matter the body possesses. The product of mass and acceleration of gravity is equal to body weight. The effectiveness and efficiency of upward movement is therefore determined to a major degree by the relationship of body weight to the force that the muscles of the body can produce, as well as to the speed of this force production.

Imagine the anatomic changes that would occur, particularly in muscle development, should human beings be compelled to move in another environment than on earth. At the sun, for example, body weight would be more than 30 times that of one's weight on earth. Without some major change in muscle morphology, human beings would be unable to move their bodies on the sun. Humans would weigh two and one-half times their body weight on earth if they lived on Jupiter. Contrast this with a weight of approximately 40% on Mars and 17% on the earth's moon. The astronauts had a great deal of difficulty walking on the surface of

the moon. Since their bodies kept rising upward, they had to use a short-step pattern with very low accelerations of the body parts. Atrophy of muscles, particularly those identified as antigravity muscles, would result from living on the moon.

According to physicists, although gravity is one of the minor forces in nature, gravity is one of the major forces with respect to movement. Every movement of a body part upward or downward is influenced by gravitational force—facilitating the downward movement and inhibiting or indirectly causing an upward movement. Since every volitional movement of body parts is rotatory, there will always exist a vertical component for every movement. Furthermore, since the force of gravity is a vertical vector (an arrow having a vector quantity, or magnitude of force, acting toward the center of the earth), it influences the efficiency of every posture or stance, as well as every movement. When muscle force is required to maintain a posture, the amount of force required is directly proportional to the efficiency of that posture. To determine whether or not muscles will need to contract, thereby exerting a counterforce to the gravitational force, one must resolve the gravitational force vectors acting on every particle of the body either into one force vector or into one force vector per body segment.

This single force vector acting on the body is called the gravitational line. This line passes through a point known as the balance point, center of weight, center of gravity, or center of mass. The position of the center of mass of a body is important in determining equilibrium and dynamic control. This chapter will investigate the erect posture and the relationship of the gravitational line to muscle force and body structure and then will present techniques for determining the position of the center of mass in a stationary body and in a moving body.

STANDING UPRIGHT

Human beings are bipeds whose upright posture makes them distinct from all other animals. Morton and Fuller say that "in his body form, in his completely erect bipedism and mental development, Man possesses characteristics that separate him undeniably from all other living creatures."* They are of the opinion that the physical differences that distinguish the human from other, closely related animal forms developed as a result of reaction to the force of gravity. To maintain an erect position human beings had to evolve certain skeletal and muscular changes. The human foot became the sole weight-bearing organ. Concerning the human foot arrangement, Morton and Fuller state:

(1) It permits the body center to occupy its central position over the area of ground contact so that the margin of postural security is equal forward and backward; (2) it places the direction of structural unbalance toward the front so that the muscular tension needed to maintain our erect posture is imposed entirely upon the large and powerful calf muscles; (3) the weaker anterior group of muscles is released from any active counterbalancing tension.*

In addition, they stress the value of the anteriorly unbalanced position of the body center in aiding

the initiation of forward movement. They also state that the only contact with the ground that a human being has is the bony architecture of two feet, and consequently the balance is on this small contact area.

Human lower limbs are more extended than are those of partially bipedal animals and are extended in line with the body. The human gluteus maximus as an extensor of the hip is unusually large and is counterbalanced by the large quadriceps femoris in front. The latter arrangement helps prevent the leg from flexing, which would cause a person to fall in moving forward as the foot strikes the ground.

The use of the arms and hands to support the body weight in the hanging position while the body was moved by a change in the position of the hands (called brachiation) enabled man's ancestors to develop changes in the arms and hands that produce free mobility in the shoulder girdle and wide movement in all directions in the shoulder joint. The upper limbs were lengthened and strengthened, and the movements of supination and pronation were developed in the forearms. The hand, including the digits and thumb, is common to certain related animal forms, but the human hand is the most flexible and dexterous.

To provide better balance, human beings developed one unique skeletal part, the human foot. Bony segments above the foot were altered, and among these was the pelvis, which gradually took a vertical, rather than a horizontal, position to support the weight of the torso better. To meet this function the pelvic bones shortened, thickened, and broadened. (For a detailed description of this evolutionary change, see Napier.) Howell says:

Man is a biped with a unique pelvis, and although neither cursorial (running) nor saltatorial (jumping) in a

---

*Morton, D.J., and Fuller, D.D.: Human locomotion and body form, Baltimore, 1952, The Williams & Wilkins Co.

strict sense, his adaptations should receive some attention. His pelvis has been shortened (craniocaudally) and
broadened. The ilium has expanded not only ventrally
but dorsally (thereby accentuating the greater sciatic
notch). The chief muscular stimuli concerned with the
shortening of the ilium seem undoubtedly to be the proper anchorage in the erect posture of the abdominal muscles and the broadening and shortening of the gluteus
medius complex; the iliacus is probably but little responsible. The position of the thigh in the upright posture has tended to reduce to zero the angle of the leverage of the hamstring muscles—a quandary that the
ischium has met by migrating dorsally, thus helping, but
to a rather poor degree, the functioning of the hamstring
muscles. As a result the ilioischiatic angle (of the axes of
these two elements) apparently is less than in any other
mammal. The pubis tends to follow the ischium dorsally.*

Since human lower limbs perform the functions
of both weight bearing and locomotion, structural
differences exist between the human and the lower
animals. Essentially the human being is less well
equipped to run, jump, or even stand than are other
animals. However, the upper limbs are free for
manipulation. Structural differences from the feet
to the pelvis provide for the weight-bearing and
locomotor functions. Similar differences, especially the lumbar curve, are present in the spinal
column and torso to adjust to the upright position.
The C-shaped curve of the spine in an infant develops into the anterior, posterior, or lateral S
curve of the adult. During the period of creeping
and progress into walking the spine undergoes
changes especially in the lumbar region to enable
the child to become an upright creature. Keith
states that the lumbar curve is seen only in the
human species.

Medawar states:

The "vertebral column" is not a column at all but is
more like a cantilever having the four legs as piers. The
vertebral column of a human being is no longer a simple
uninflected arc; it bends slightly forwards in the neck,
slightly backwards in the thoracic cage, forwards again

in the lumbar region, the small of the back, and backwards in the fused vertebrae that form the sacrum. That
is the mature pattern; in development, the neck flexure
appears somewhat before birth, and the lumbar flexure
between the ninth and eighteenth months of age.*

The center of gravity of the human body is elevated to a position high above and to the outer
borders of the feet, the supporting parts. This
unstable and potentially mobile structure must be
held in a standing position by continuous muscular
action because of the fact that it is a high vertical
structure with a small base.

Above the midline any body portion that is
moved to the rear or front to any great extent
makes the maintenance of balance more difficult.
Also a person whose body design is unusual, such
as large or tall, or who has a specific body part that
is unusually large or long may find that these conditions affect the ability to maintain an upright position. For example, a male with a heavy, tall
body and small feet will experience some difficulty
in standing and walking comfortably. His base is
not large enough to allow him to withstand as great
a displacement of force as he should. However,
Morton and Fuller believe that this instability is an
aid in the initiation of forward movement. Joseph
has said:

One may therefore conclude that in the posture of
standing at ease (military position) in most subjects,
stability at the ankle joints is maintained by the calf
muscles, mainly soleus, at the knee and hip joints by the
appropriate ligaments and at the vertebral joints by only
some parts of the sacrospinalis muscles. There are no
apparent differences between the sexes with regard to
the leg and thigh muscles. Movements such as swaying
at the ankle joints or flexion at the knee or hip joints or
flexion of the vertebral column result in activity in the
appropriate muscles, usually the extensors, which resist
the force of gravity.†

---

*Howell, A.B.: Speed in animals, Chicago, 1944, The Uni-
versity of Chicago Press.

*Medawar, P.W.: The uniqueness of the individual, New
York, 1958, Basic Books, Inc.,Publishers.
†Joseph, J.: Man's posture—electromyographic studies, Spring-
field, Ill., 1960, Charles C Thomas, Publisher.

In other words, not all muscles are used to maintain the standing position, as would be more likely in a vigorous movement such as running. The specific muscles used are rightly called *postural muscles*.

Hellebrandt has said that standing is really movement on a stationary base and that swaying is inseparable from the upright stance. Hellebrandt and others have shown that considerable sway occurs in forward, backward, and sideward directions. One of us (J.M.C.) has had his students measure the amount of sway that occurs during 5- and 10-minute periods of standing erect without moving (other than swaying) and with the feet placed close together. The longer the individual stands, the greater is the amplitude of sway. Usually after 15 minutes the individual will tend to faint and fall to the floor. One individual in a special experiment was able to stand erect for 25 minutes with his feet in a bucket of ice water. At the end of 25 minutes he fell to the floor and had to be revived. In speaking of a study of standing, Hellebrandt and Franseen state:

Weiner (1938) in South Africa combined the factors of exercise and a hot, humid environment in studying the ability to stand. He found that most of his adult male Bantu subjects could tolerate an hour of quiet standing after shoveling gravel for an equal period of time. When, in controlled experiment, the standing was undertaken in a cool room, no cases of collapse occurred.*

The muscles act as ''little hearts'' in helping push the blood back through the veins to the heart. When this action is lacking, the blood pools in the feet and the individual faints from lack of blood in the brain. Feet have increased in size as much as one and one-half shoe sizes after prolonged standing. A walk of one-half mile reduced the feet to normal size.

Concerning sway, Hellebrandt and Franseen have said:

There is general agreement that stance is steadied when the eyes are open and focused on a fixed point and least stable with the eyes closed. Distraction reduces sway. When the feet are together, the stance is unsettled. Turning the toes out to an angle of 45 degrees or separating the feet so as to equalize the coronal and sagittal diameters of support steadies the stance. Sway is much greater in the anteroposterior vertical orientation plane than in the transverse. Height and weight correlate poorly with stability. Thus the body may compensate in other ways for mechanically disadvantageous factors in physical build. Though kaleidoscopic at first sight, when carefully made, postural sway patterns are characteristic for each person and highly reproducible. There is lack of agreement chiefly as to whether stance training reduces postural instability or not, and whether fatigue is reflected as readily, as often implied, in an augmentation of sway.*

Joseph has listed several studies on sway. For example, one study showed that activity in the muscles of the calves of the legs was greater when subjects wore high-heeled shoes (2½ inches) than when they were barefoot. The increased muscular activity resulted from the unstable position created by the high-heeled shoes. Activity in the gastrocnemius muscle was increased the most.

The term *posture* has many meanings, depending on the person who is defining the term, as illustrated in the following discussion.

In 1889 Braune and Fischer described a posture in which a vertical line erected from the ankle intersected the axis of the knee joint, the axis of the hip joint, the axis of the shoulder joint, and the ear. This linear alignment of the body in an erect position presented a convenient posture from which to measure deviations, since all reference points fall along the same line. This posture, in which no part deviates from the vertical line, was named the *Normal-stellung,* or *normal standing posture.* Other postures, such as the relaxed and military, were also described, and deviations from normal posture were discussed. Normal posture does not correspond with the usual position of the body and can be maintained only momentarily. The usual

*Hellebrandt, F.A., and Franseen, E.B.: Physiological study of the vertical stance of man, Physiol. Rev. **23**:220, 1943.

*Hellebrandt, F.A., and Franseen, E.B.: Physiological study of the vertical stance of man, Physiol. Rev. **23**:220, 1943.

position of the body is a more relaxed posture. Although no attempt was made by Braune and Fischer to depict the normal standing as the ideal posture, such an interpretation became widespread. Many logical reasons have been given to support the contention that the normal posture of Braune and Fischer is the ideal one. Most of the reasons were based on the relationship of this posture to the healthy function of the internal organs. Posters showing this normal posture are displayed today on many schoolroom walls to depict a perfect standing position. Modifications are also seen in posture charts showing a similar ''normal'' sitting position—an unnatural but ''ideal'' position.

The statistical interpretation of normality is in terms of the frequency distribution of a population. In a healthy population the normal posture would be that assumed by the majority. Observations of people standing in line before ticket windows or on street corners reveal that practically no one is using the *Normal-stellung*. Instead, people shift from one position to another while standing or sitting. An investigator attempting to measure the usual postures of a population would be confronted with the task of erecting a frequency distribution of postures assumed by each person from day to day in various conditions of heat and cold, sickness and health, and sadness and joy. For women, as well as for men, a researcher would face the additional problem of fashion changes. After the model posture of each person has been determined, the frequency distribution for this population could then be erected. This statistical expression of normality of posture derived by the frequency of occurrence of one posture among others would necessarily include the range of differences and the amounts of deviations from the normal that could be expected from time to time. Thus the statistical normal posture cannot be a fixed value.

The physiologic concept of normality is that condition in which the organs and systems of the body function efficiently. Body postures affect physiologic functions. For one thing the energy requirements of different postures vary considerably. The rigid military posture requires about 20% more energy than the easy standing position. An extremely relaxed standing position requires about 10% less energy than an easy standing position. If one stands so as to be practically hanging on the ligaments (completely relaxed as much as possible), little more energy is used than in sitting or reclining. Hellebrandt and co-workers determined that the energy cost of standing is relatively small and that oxygen consumption during graded degrees of gravitational stress deviates insignificantly from the normal variations characteristic of recumbency.

Blood pressure rises when a person assumes a rigid, erect posture because of the muscular effort involved. The respiratory efficiency is difficult to assess in the resting state, since only a small part of the available lung tissues would provide ample area for the small requirement of gaseous exchange. Because of this excessive respiratory tissue the small gain in maximal diaphragmatic excursion and vital capacity resulting from changes in posture is inconsequential. Thus from the point of view of physiologic efficiency the rigid, erect posture is not the normal, since the efficiency of metabolic and circulatory systems is reduced.

Extreme curvature and poor alignment produce physiologic changes and are considered to be pathologic. Just how much deviation is possible without causing impairment of health and inefficient function of vital organs is a subject of discussion by several authors with some disagreement. Minor deviations do not appear to greatly affect the health and efficient function of the internal organs.

Erect posture is commonly associated with attitudes of readiness, self-confidence, and assurance. A relaxed or slouched posture may generally connote laziness and incompetence. For this reason the erect posture is the one most often aspired to and considered normal. Wells has stated that since relatively little is known about the upright posture, one should be careful of what one says about it. Hellebrandt and others have stated that one should not think of a standing posture as involving a rigid set of anatomic landmarks—lobe of ear, tip of acromion process, middle of trochanter, and head of fibula—in alignment. Certainly the erect posture gives a better appearance, since clothes fit better, the physique is shown to better advantage, and the face is held up so that attentiveness is indicated. Clothing models, stage and screen performers, and beauty contestants assume erect and stately postures to appear to the best advantage before an audience. However, exceptions have occurred in successful individuals. Superior intelligence and tremendous energy are sometimes housed in a body that is habitually slouched. Some great athletes assume a habitual posture of extreme relaxation.

Normal posture, then, is that which best suits one's own condition and the conditions of the environment. During attention to a stimulating situation the normal posture will be erect. In a condition of distress because of sad circumstances, normal posture will be characterized by a general sagging of all body parts. In extreme fatigue the normal posture will be that which conserves energy. The normal posture of physical attractiveness is one that displays the special qualities of the physique to the best advantage.

Metheny states her concept of posture as follows: "There is no single best posture for all individuals. Each person must take the body he has and make the best of it. For each person the best posture is that in which the body segments are balanced in the position of least strain and maximum support. This is an individual matter."* Goldthwaite and associates have stated, "There is not and cannot be one posture which is normal for all individuals and to which all individuals should conform."† Joseph points out that there is no single correct posture and that it is difficult to place anyone in an arbitrary grouping. Hellebrandt and associates drew the following conclusions from one of their studies:

*Metheney, E.: Body dynamics, New York, 1952, McGraw-Hill Book Co.
†Goldthwaite, J.E., et al.: Essentials of body mechanics in health and disease, ed. 5, Philadelphia, 1952, J.B. Lippincott Co.

(1) Gravitational stress patterns are highly individual. (2) Body alignment measured repeatedly during uninterrupted standing is variable. (3) There is no relation between the Wellesley posture score and the anteroposterior eccentricity of the center of gravity. (4) The evidence is contrary to theoretical expectation. It is suggested that the lack of association between the variables studied may be due to reliance on a posture criterion more related to esthetic than physiological concepts.*

CULTURAL DIFFERENCES IN POSTURE

Individuals, as well as family groups, various cultures, and age groups within cultures, show differences in standing and sitting postures. Although individual differences may be linked to many causes, even including attitudes and emotional states, the cultures and subcultures appear to develop postures distinct to their groups. The reasons probably are many but certainly include nutrition, climate, and training. Over 1000 different postures ranging from standing, squatting, kneeling, and sitting have been identified by Hewes. Although not common to the United States, at least a fourth of the population of the world habitually crouch in a low squat, both to rest and to work. In certain parts of Africa, India, Australia, and South America the "Nilotic stance" is a common resting position. This stance is a storklike posture in which the sole of one foot is planted against the support leg near the knee. Warm climate, bare feet, and unknown cultural reasons are likely reasons for adoption of this stance, as well as occupation or habit of carrying a long staff. Clothing affects styles of sitting for both men and women. However, clothing alone does not explain all posture differences.

MINI LABORATORY EXERCISES

1. Observe the postures depicted in Fig. 4-1 and determine which ones might indicate a characteristically rigid posture, which would tend to produce kyphosis (increased convex curvature of upper back), which would tend to produce lordosis (increased concavity of lumbar region), and which would tend to produce scoliosis (lateral curvature of the spine).

*Morton, D.J., and Fuller, D.D.: Human locomotion and body form, Baltimore, 1952, The Williams & Wilkins Co.

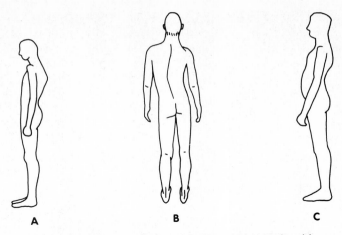

A   B   C

Fig. 4-1. Standing postures showing spinal column deformities.

2. Identify the muscles that would contract against gravity for each of the postures.

INDIVIDUAL DIFFERENCES IN STANCE

Among the various body types obese persons are likely to have the most erect posture as a result of the effort required to support excessive fatty tissue. Fat persons twist as they walk, and to reduce the amount of this turning they stiffen and take short steps. Persons with large abdomens often lean slightly backward to balance the weight in front. Some short, stocky people stand erect to make themselves appear taller and slimmer. Extremely thin individuals often lack the muscular strength needed to hold themselves erect. During the teen-age years many tall girls voluntarily slouch to appear more nearly the size of their shorter boy companions and thus spoil their attractiveness. Specialization in certain forms of hard work or strenuous athletic activity results in adaptations of posture. A coal miner carries the head and shoulders forward and the arms slightly bent in the position of work. The side horse specialist in gymnastics tends to become overly round shouldered and kyphotic if this activity is not balanced with others that exercise contralateral musculature. Postural

adaptations to specialized events may also be counteracted by a conscious effort to improve the carriage at all times when the person is not bent to the task.

Structural deformities cause postural compensations. A short leg produces scoliosis. This may be corrected by elevating the heel to lengthen the short leg. Pronated feet result in an anteriorly tilted pelvis and lordosis, which are corrected when the pronation is remedied.

Effect of pregnancy. The later weeks of pregnancy are marked by a large forward displacement of the center of gravity because of the combined weight of the embryo, its surrounding amniotic fluid, and the massive uterus. The resulting postural compensation is a slight backward lean and a backward shift of weight in the lumbar region. More weight is borne by the heels. The backward lean (although the center of gravity stays over the base) becomes more exaggerated as the pregnancy progresses. This adaptation occasionally corrects a customary slouch but usually causes increased lumbar stress.

Effect of shoe heel height. Julius Caesar is thought to have been the first to discover the advantage of elevating the heels. He observed that when heels were added to the sandals of his legions, the sol-

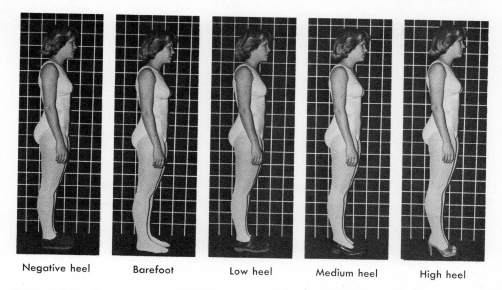

Negative heel   Barefoot   Low heel   Medium heel   High heel

Fig. 4-2. Effects of changes in elevation of heels on standing posture. Hip joint and background grid may be used to estimate gravitational line and center of gravity of body.

diers were able to march farther with less fatigue. When the calcaneus is elevated about 1.27 cm (0.5 in) above the level of the base of the ball of the foot, its shaft is brought to a tangent with the Achilles tendon, and thus the gastrocnemius and soleus muscles are able to exert a greater force in plantar flexion. If shoes without heels or with higher heels are worn after an individual has become accustomed to wearing heels of a certain height, the legs and feet become fatigued more quickly.

The ability of the human body to adjust to heel heights of 7.5 cm or greater is attested to by the skilled movements of women jitterbug dancers of the 1940s and disco dancers of the 1970s. Cowboy boots are worn by both women and men without mishap. Platform shoes, however, appeared to be the cause of numerous falling accidents. The high heel combined with the high sole may have caused a reduction in perceptual awareness of the position of the foot and delayed the kinesthetic and tactile responses to loss of balance, in addition to elevat-

ing the center of gravity of the body about 9 cm. Fig. 4-2 shows the changes in line of gravity and position of the center of gravity with different heel heights. Note that similar alignment of body parts, as well as knee angle and trunk position, can be achieved with any of these heel heights.

Standing at work. Continued standing may result in a pooling of blood and of other fluids in the feet, as well as lowering of the arches to such an extent that the foot may increase in size as much as one or two shoe sizes. Thus clerks, dentists, ticket takers, and barbers commonly wear shoes at work that are lacerated at the toe, ball, and top to allow for the expansion to take place. Probably in such work two pairs of shoes should be worn, one pair in the morning and a larger pair in the afternoon. A compromise in the form of loose-fitting shoes is sometimes made; however, this solution is poor because when no support is given, pronation occurs. A good shoe for standing is constructed so that most of the weight is borne on the outside of the foot, since this part of the foot is supported by strong

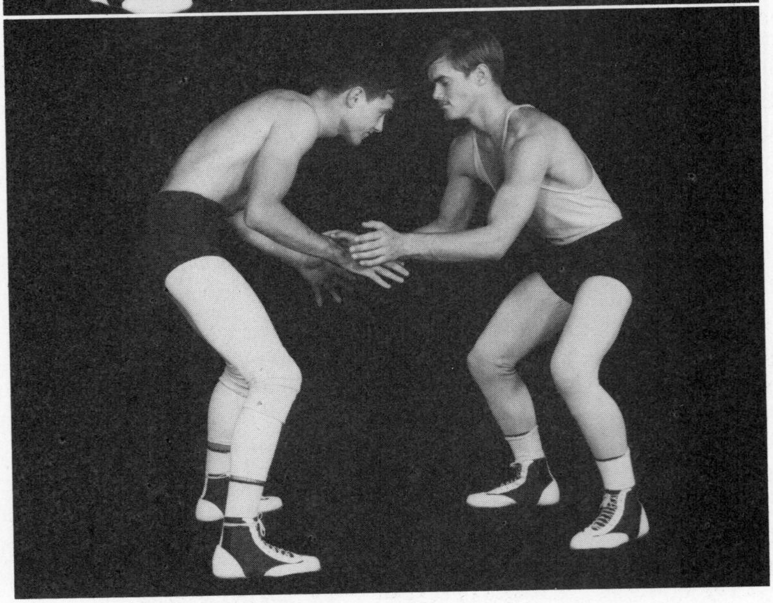

Fig. 4-3. Postures of readiness, **A**, Wrestlers are using staggered stances, which are best for moving rapidly forward or backward. **B**, Wrestlers are using parallel stances, which are best for moving right or left. (From Boring, W.J.: Science and skills of wrestling, St. Louis, 1975, The C.V. Mosby Co.)

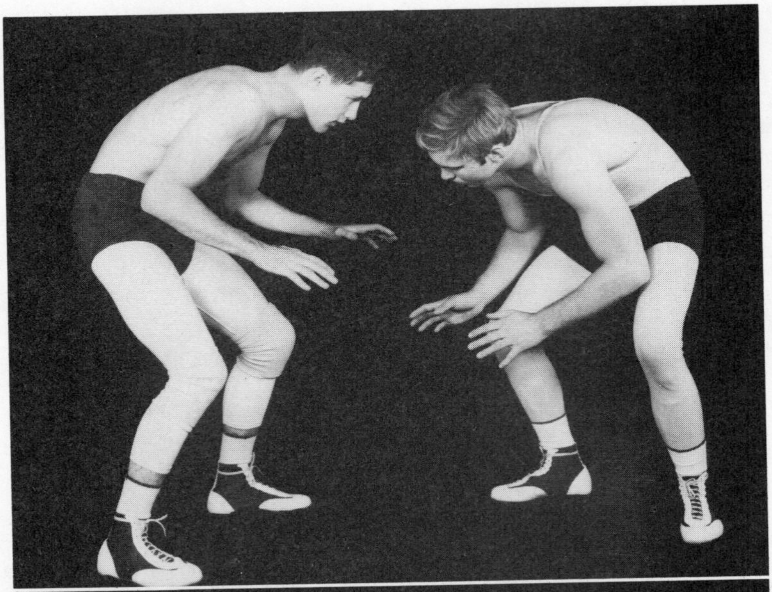

ligaments, whereas the inside of the foot is supported by long, thin muscles that are easily fatigued.

Posture of readiness. The standing posture is affected by a person's anticipation of forthcoming action. If no action is anticipated and the conditions of the external environment are unexciting, the response will be a relaxed posture. This is so well known that athletes can simulate a relaxed posture to deceive their opponents. In a game of basketball a player about to receive a pass can often deceive the defender by assuming a relaxed posture and passive countenance.

The posture of readiness when a rapid or strong movement is about to be performed is an alert one. The peak of attention is reached between 1 and 2 seconds after concentration is directed to the situation. The posture adapts to the condition; after the peak of attention is past, the posture either is relaxed or becomes unstable because of extreme tremor, resulting possibly from accommodation of the coordinating centers in the nervous system.

The position assumed during a state of readiness is in accord with the immediate tasks to be accomplished (Fig. 4-3). If the direction of movement is not known, the weight should be distributed over the surface of both feet. When the direction is known, the center of gravity should be shifted toward the anticipated direction. A slight flexion may occur at the ankle, causing the equilibrium of the body to be unstable and thus facilitating movement. The head, arm, and leg positions are also adjusted to the action to follow. The infielder in baseball leans forward and rises on the toes as the ball is pitched. The base runner taking a one-stride lead off the base will lean toward the next base and rise on the toes as the ball is pitched. In each instance the mechanical equilibrium of the body is disturbed and movement is commenced. The football quarterback crouches with the arms forward and the heels of the hands close together in a position of readiness to catch the ball. Such postures of readiness should not be held motionless for an extended length of time, since proprioceptor sensations, which govern the senses of position

and relationship of the body parts to objects in view, will be diminished and have to be reestablished before accurate movement can be accomplished. For this reason the golfer waggles the club near the ball while adjusting position in readiness for the swing. While poised for the pitch, the batter in baseball does the same thing to heighten the sensation of the position of the bat in relation to the body and to the path of the ball.

The causes of poor posture and the defects associated with pathologic handicaps should be the topic of discussion in books on adapted and corrective physical education. The discussion here has been centered only on the standing position of all human beings, normal and handicapped.

BALANCING ON HANDS

To keep the base of support wide when the handstand is being executed, the athlete spreads the fingers as wide as possible. The hands are turned slightly outward so that the fingers will be able to help counteract movements to the outside, and the thumbs are turned inward to maintain balance. A plumb line dropped through the center of gravity should fall at the base of the fingers to provide a supporting area from the heel of the hand to the tips of the fingers and thumb, through which the gravity plane can move without the performer's losing balance. This is especially true in the execution of the *one-armed handstand*. It is also important, in the performance of this move, to hold the parts of the body (arms, torso, and legs) in a relatively stationary position so that control is centered at the shoulder area, where the large muscles (deltoideus, triceps, pectoralis major, and latissimus dorsi) are able to exert their force.

CARRYING OBJECTS

Carrying an object increases the weight that must be supported by the feet and affects the positions of the gravity planes with reference to the body. If the carrier is to remain upright, these planes must be kept within the area of the supporting foot; segmental adjustments must be made. This is usually done by altering the trunk position.

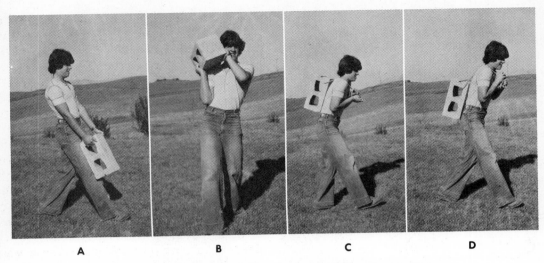

Fig. 4-4. Postural alignment while carrying load in various positions.

If the object is held in front of the body, the trunk will be inclined backward; if it is held in back, the trunk will be inclined forward; and if it is held to the side, the trunk will be inclined to the opposite side. The amount of inclination will be related to the weight, size, and distribution of weight of the object and to the height at which the object is carried. Note in Fig. 4-4 the differences in body position when carrying an identical weight, well distributed and not well distributed with respect to symmetry of the body (Chapter 6).

When loads are carried on the head, there is no inclination. Visitors to regions in which carrying objects on the head, especially among women, is common frequently comment on the excellent carriage of these people. Undoubtedly the additional weight high above the feet requires careful alignment of body segments.

Walking with a heavy load alters the stepping pattern. The center of gravity is not allowed to fall as far forward as it does in normal walking. With the load the step will be shortened, and the center of gravity will be held over the supporting foot for a longer time. It is interesting to note that when bulky packs of produce are loaded onto the backs

of Mexican Indian men by fellow workers, the carrier cannot sit down during the 16-km (10-mile) trip from the fields to market, because once the load is lowered he cannot lift it again without assistance.

PRINCIPLES OF EQUILIBRIUM

With respect to the various postures or static positions that have been presented, the following principles may be stated:

1. To maintain balance, humans, like all animals and inanimate objects, must keep the center of gravity in an area within and directly above the supporting base.
2. The larger the base, the greater the range in which the center of gravity can be moved without the body's falling.
3. The closer to the base the center of gravity is, the greater will be the angle of tilt necessary to move the center of gravity outside the base area. Thus the stability of the body is often said to be increased as the center of gravity is lowered.
4. The human body can use many body segments as a base—the feet, one foot, the

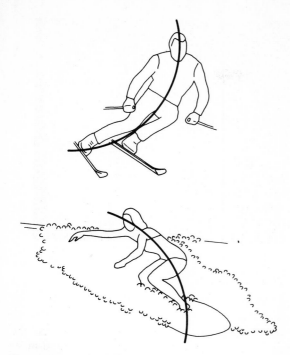

Fig. 4-5. Body lean during snow skiing and surfboarding.

hands, one finger (in the case of some acrobats), the head, the thighs, or the entire body.

5. The segments above the base can be adjusted to bring them into various positions. No general balance pattern exists, but whatever the base and the positions of the segments above it, the center of gravity must be kept over the base area if balance is to be maintained.

It is evident that each object a person carries is added to the weight of the human body in determining the center of gravity of the human-object system. In essence, the object becomes part of the human body, affecting the body's balance point and determining the position of the gravitational vector.

The principles stated above are applicable in situations in which movement does not exist.

These principles may or may not be valid for the dynamic situation, since movement itself introduces another force: ma, or Iα. The mass (m) of the body represents its resistance (inertia) to translation, which is multiplied by acceleration (a) to depict the force of a translating body. The I is the moment of inertia, or the resistance to rotation of a body. This resistance is multiplied by rotatory, or angular, acceleration (α) to depict the moment of force of a rotating body. Therefore the moving human body may be in "dynamic balance," that is, may not fall during instances in which the line of gravity falls outside the base of support. Note the lean of the bodies depicted in Fig. 4-5 during surfboarding and snow skiing. A further explanation of this phenomenon and of situations in which other forces are present will be considered in the next chapter.

DETERMINATION OF CENTER OF GRAVITY

The techniques presented in this section use the human being as the subject for the determination of the center of gravity of a body. Some modifications may be made in size of equipment, but the concepts are valid for all applications to living and inanimate objects. In activities such as horseback riding, the investigation of the center of gravity of the horse, the rider and the horse-rider system may prove useful in determining the positions of the rider that either interfere with the progress of the horse or enhance it.

A review of the concepts involved in the center of gravity is presented first, and then the determination of its location will be discussed.

All masses that are within the gravitational field of the earth are constantly subjected to a pull toward the earth's center; the greater the mass, the stronger will be the force of that pull. The force of gravitational attraction that the earth exerts on a body is called its *weight*. Gravitational force pulls downward on each point of a given body. The distribution of these points determines the position of the center of gravity of the body. If a board is suspended on a support, as in playground teeterboards, a downward pull is exerted on each side of the support. If the board mass on each side is equal in size and in distance from the support, the board will balance. If a child sits on one side of the balanced board, that side will be pushed downward, and the opposite side will move upward. In such unbalanced situations note that gravitational force, interestingly, is responsible for the upward as well as the downward movement. This upward movement caused by gravitational force will be shown later to be used by the body in many forms of locomotion. On the teeterboard a second child can take a position on the opposite side of the board, and if the distance from the board is adjusted, the board and the two children can be balanced. Within every mass is a point about which the gravitational forces on one side will equal those on the other. This balance point, determined in three planes of the mass, is the center of gravity.

Center of gravity in the transverse body plane

The point of balance in the human body has long interested investigators. The earliest of these employed the teeterboard to locate the transverse plane of that point. An Italian physicist, Borelli (1608-1679), placed a nude subject on a board in the prone position and then moved the board back and forth as it rested on a knife-edged support until the total mass balanced. He reported the balance plane to be one that cut the body "between the genitals and the pubis" Somewhere within this plane would lie the subject's center of gravity. Two German brothers, the Webers, in 1836 improved Borelli's method by first balancing the board and then sliding the subject back and forth until balance was obtained. They found the transverse plane of the center of gravity to be 56.8% of the height above the heel.

Half a century later (1889) the two Germans Braune and Fischer reported that the center-of-gravity plane was 54.8% of the height measured from the soles. Their conclusion was based on finding the point of balance in four fresh "normally built" cadavers that were frozen solid. The cadavers were first balanced on a knife-edge, and then a steel rod was driven into the cadaver at the determined plane. Each cadaver was suspended by the steel rod, and gravitational force moved the mass into a balanced position. When the body attained equilibrium, a plumb line was dropped from the point of suspension to locate the transverse plane of the center of gravity.

The most convenient method of locating the plane of the center of gravity is that proposed by the two Americans Reynolds and Lovett (1909). A board of a known length is supported at either end of a knife-edge. The knife-edges are placed on scales that can be adjusted to eliminate the weight of the board. The subject lies on the board, and the plane of the center of gravity is determined mathematically. It will be at a point on the board that can be determined by multiplying the weight on one scale by the distance from that knife-edge to the plane of the center of gravity. This product will equal that obtained by multiplying the weight on the second scale by the distance between the second knife-edge and the plane of the center of gravity:

$$w_1 d_1 = w_2 d_2$$

where w_1 equals the weight on scale 1, d_1 equals the distance from the line of gravity to w_1, w_2 equals the weight on scale 2, and d_2 equals the distance from the line of gravity to w_2. This equation can be reduced to one unknown by redefining d_2 as the distance between the knife-edge minus d_1. The use of this equation will be shown in the solution of the following problem:

PROBLEM: A subject weighing 660 N lies on a board, with the top of the head in line with the knife-edge on scale 1. The distance between the knife-edges is 1.50 m. The scale reading on the head scale 1 is 320 N; the other scale 2 reads 340 N. These values are placed appropriately into the previously presented equation, which in essence is the determination of the moments of force about the line of gravity.

SOLUTION:

$$320 \text{ N} \times d_1 = 340 \text{ N} (1.50 \text{ m} - d_1)$$
$$320 \text{ N} \times d_1 = 510 \text{ Nm} - 340 \text{ N} \times d_1$$
$$660 \text{ N} \times d_1 = 510 \text{ Nm}$$
$$d_1 = 0.773 \text{ m}$$

Since the head was even with the knife-edge, the distance from the top of the head to the transverse plane of the center of gravity is 77.3 cm. If the subject is 171 cm in height, the plane line of gravity is 45% of the height measured from the top of the head, and 55% of the height measured from the soles of the feet.

This procedure can be used when only one scale is available, since the reading on the second scale will always be the total weight minus the reading on the single scale (Fig. 4-6).

Using the scale method, other investigators have reported findings on the location of the transverse plane of the human center of gravity. Croskey and associates reported in 1922 that this plane is slightly higher in men than in women. The average height of the plane in men was 56.18% measured from the soles; the range of percentages was 55% to 58%. For women, the average was 55.44%; the range was 54% to 58%. Additional observations were made by Hellebrandt and co-workers, who found that in 357 college women the transverse plane averaged 55.17% of the height; the lowest observed was 53%, and the highest was 59%.

The most extensive study is that reported by Palmer, who located the transverse plane of the center of gravity in 1172 subjects—596 boys and 576 girls from birth to 20 years of age—and in 18 fetal cadavers. Palmer concluded that regardless of age or sex the plane can be estimated as follows:

0.557 height + 1.4 cm (0.551 in) from soles of feet

Since body segments differ in proportion to total height from birth to maturity, the plane of the center of gravity will lie in a different section of the body as age increases, but the proportion of height will be constant (Figs. 4-7 and 4-8).

Obviously a change in position of the limbs with reference to the prone torso will change the position of the center of gravity. If the arms are raised overhead or the hips flexed, the plane will move toward the head. Loss of body parts will also alter the position. Amputation of any part of the lower limb will raise the plane, and the height of the center of gravity will increase with the amount of

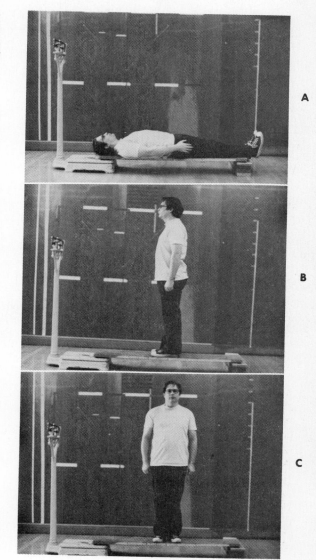

Fig. 4-6. Equipment for determining position of center of gravity of body in three cardinal planes.

body mass lost. The addition of a prosthetic appliance to replace the amputated limb will lower the center of gravity toward the normal position (Fig. 4-9).

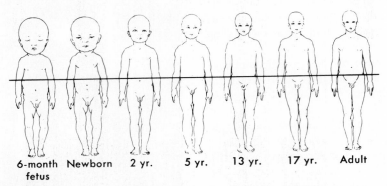

Fig. 4-7. Outline drawings of ventral aspects of body. Body lengths are scaled to reduce all figures to same height. Transverse plane of center of gravity is represented by transverse line. (From Palmer, C.E.: Child Dev. **15**:99, 1944.)

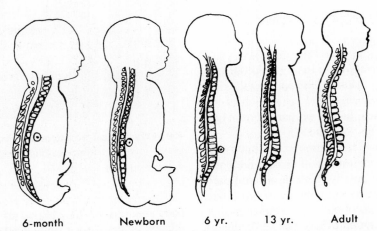

Fig. 4-8. Position of center of gravity with reference to spine at five different ages. (Modified from Palmer, C.E.: Child Dev. **15**:99, 1944.)

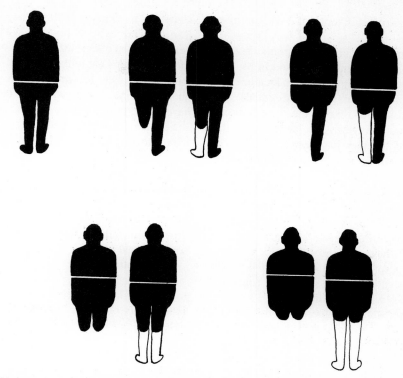

Fig. 4-9. Diagrammatic representation of influence of amputation of lower extremities on height of center of gravity and compensatory effect of prosthetic appliance. (From Hellebrandt, F.A.: J.A.M.A. **142:**1353, 1950.)

Center of gravity in frontal and sagittal body planes

In the preceding discussion the transverse plane of the center of gravity was located at a distance from the top of the head or from the soles of the feet. In balance and locomotor activities it is important to locate the gravity plane in the frontal and sagittal planes. If the Reynolds-Lovett method is used, the body must be stationary on the board, and some body point must be located with reference to the knife-edges. The transverse plane was determined by placing the top of the head in line with one of the knife-edges; if the frontal gravity plane is to be located while the subject is standing, some part of the foot will be taken as the reference point, and the distance of this part from one of the

knife-edges must be known. Since it is more convenient to stand near the middle of the board rather than near one end of it, a line on the board halfway between the knife-edges is convenient for measuring distance.

The same mathematic procedures described in the preceding section, which discussed the center of gravity in the transverse body plane, can be used to determine both the frontal gravity plane and the sagittal gravity plane (Fig. 4-6). Often it is desirable to locate the frontal plane with reference to the ankle joint. In this case if the ankle joint is 15 cm from the tip of the toes, the frontal plane is 4.5 cm in front of that joint. A perpendicular line passing through the foot at this point is often called the gravity line; in postural measures certain body landmarks are described in terms of deviation from this line.

When a person stands erect, the frontal gravity plane lies in front of the ankle joint and in back of the metatarsophalangeal joints. The location between these points differs with individuals and may differ from time to time in the same individual. This location between the ankles and the proximal end of the toes has been so frequently observed that it can be accepted as a human characteristic. Among the published reports are those of Cureton and Wickens, Hellebrandt, Fox and Young, and Brown. Over the years hundreds of students in our kinesiology classes have observed this phenomenon in themselves and in their classmates. Not only have they observed the location, but they have also seen that this plane is rarely stationary; it usually fluctuates, and the degree of fluctuation varies with the individual.

As the subject stands on the board for gravity-plane determination, the observer finds it difficult to make an exact scale reading because the dial needle fluctuates rapidly. The range of the needle varies with individuals but rarely exceeds 20 N. If one reading is desired, the best one to take is that about which the needle hovers; however, the extremes will also provide interesting information. The reason for the changes in scale readings is understood when one remembers that the body must balance on the small base provided by the upper surface of the talus at the ankle joint. Since the center of gravity of the body is ahead of the ankle joint, the body is unbalanced on this small surface. Gravitational force would tilt the body forward if no counterforce were present. The ankle extensors provide this force; the tension in these muscles must be sufficient to withstand gravitational pull if the erect position is to be maintained. Any slight change in any body part (solid, liquid, or gas) will change the distribution of weight; this will change the force of gravitational pull and consequently change the demand on the ankle extensors. The tension in the muscles may change also. Whatever the cause, the frontal plane is constantly shifting; yet it remains within the limits described.

Class observations in which students are asked to lean forward as far as possible without raising the heels and then backward as far as possible without lifting the toes (and without falling) rarely find that the gravity plane has moved back of the ankle or ahead of the proximal end of the toes. It does move beyond the normal limits for the individual.

Segmental alignment above the ankle is not a universal characteristic. Individuals differ in degree of pelvic tilt, in depth of lumbar, dorsal, and cervical curves, and in shoulder girdle and head position. All these factors will affect the distribution of weight. Yet when an individual stands in a habitual position, the frontal plane of the center of gravity will fall between the ankle and the metatarsophalangeal joints.

For location of the sagittal gravity plane, the subject stands on the board, with the right side toward one knife-edge and the left side toward the other. This plane has frequently been located to determine whether the subject is likely to carry more of the weight on one foot than on the other.

An arrangement for simultaneously determining the frontal and sagittal planes of the center of gravity has been presented by Waterland and Shambes. The subject takes a position on a base supported by three dial scales. Two photographs, a side and a front view, are taken by a synchronized shutter arrangement. The three scale readings shown in the photographs will equal the total weight of the subject. With these readings the positions of gravity lines in the frontal and sagittal planes can be calculated. These investigators have shown fluctuations of the gravity line in a "static" standing position. By placing on the supported board a paper on which the footprints of the subject were traced, they located the gravity line with reference to the feet (Fig. 4-10).

The triangular platform shown in Fig. 4-10 was used by Hasselkus to compare the postural sway of 10 women 21 to 30 years of age with 10 others 73 to 80 years of age. Greater sway was thought to be a possible indication of aging of the neuromuscular system. Each subject stood on the platform for three 18-second periods, during which cameras re-

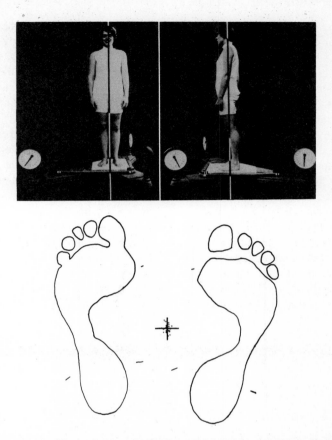

Fig. 4-10. Equipment used to determine gravity line in sagittal and frontal planes. Front and side view photographs are taken simultaneously; each view presents two of three dial scales. Gravity lines added to photographs after calculations represent mean of thirty determinations; each dot between feet represents one determination; center point of crossed lines represents mean of thirty determinations. (From Waterland, J.C., and Shambes, G.M.: Biplane center of gravity procedures, Percept. Mot. Skills **30:**511, 1970. Reprinted with permission of author and publisher.)

corded the scale readings every second. The area enclosed in the outer borders of the 54 calculated positions of gravity lines (such as + in Fig. 4-10) was expressed as a percentage of the functional base of support, a quadrilateral area enclosed in lines drawn along the lateral borders of the feet and across the back of the heels and connecting the heads of the first metatarsals. The older women's sway area covered an average of 43%, and the younger women's, an average of 23%. For all sub-

jects the position of the gravity line tended to be to the left and to the posterior of the geometric center of the functional base.

Center of gravity in moving body

Two methods, the scale and the segmental, have been used to determine the center of gravity in the moving body. Both methods require that the investigator "freeze" the moving body into static positions. This is done by selecting still photographs, frames of movie film, or posed positions determined by the observer and used to represent the sequencing of the movement. It is important to attempt to duplicate, exactly, the position of all body parts at each of the imposed stationary images of the movement. The position of the center of gravity in two planes can be found from each image.

Scale method. Triangular and rectangular boards utilizing two-four scales have been used in much the same way as the one-two scale method for determining the line of gravity in one plane. Davis devised a center-of-gravity board with three accompanying scales (Fig. 4-11). After the subjects had assumed various performer-position combinations, he determined (1) the center of gravity in the transverse and sagittal planes for the pike and stride positions and (2) the center of gravity in the

transverse and frontal planes for the normal position. Davis also photographed these performer-position combinations and utilized the segmental method for determining the center of gravity of each combination. His comparison of the two methods is presented in the discussion of the segmental method.

Segmental method. Another method of determining the location of the center of gravity in the moving body is the segmental method suggested by Dawson in 1935. This method is used when the performer is not present; only a photograph or movie film of the performance is available. Estimations of the weight of each body segment and the estimation of its center of gravity are utilized in the segmental method. Since the position of the center of gravity of the body is changed each time a body segment moves to assume a new position,

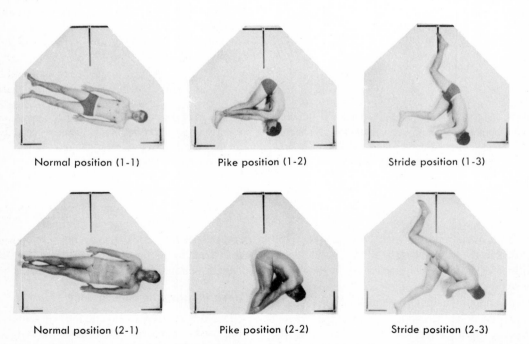

Normal position (1-1) Pike position (1-2) Stride position (1-3)

Normal position (2-1) Pike position (2-2) Stride position (2-3)

Fig. 4-11. Performer-position combinations assumed by two performers on center-of-gravity board. (From Davis, M.: Quality of data collected by the segmental analysis technique, unpublished doctoral dissertation, Indiana University, Sept., 1973.)

the effect of this new position must be ascertained. Over a century ago Braune and Fischer dissected cadavers and determined the weights of body segments and their centers of gravity. Other researchers also used cadaver data to provide input for use in the segmental method of determining the location of the center of gravity of a body. In 1955, Cleaveland, using 11 college men, determined these data on live subjects by means of a water submersion technique.

Marks on the body indicated the limits of each segment, and the body was lowered into a tank of water to each mark in succession. The weight of each segment was calculated by the weight lost and the amount of water displaced at each stage of submersion. The center of gravity of each segment was located at the point at which half the amount of weight was lost.

Kjeldsen and Morse have described significant differences in anthropometric measurements, including percentages of body segment weights, among women gymnasts, women nongymnasts, and men. To further elucidate differences, Hay presents an excellent compilation and discussion of the extensive data on segmental body weights and segmental centers of gravity. Partial listings of these differences are given in Tables 4-1 to 4-4. Note the similarities as well as the differences.

Limitations. Care must be taken when using the segmental method. A study by Davis on the validity, reliability, and objectivity of the segmental method revealed some of its limitations. The precision of the estimation of the center of gravity is significantly affected by the type of segmental data applied. Segmental data collected on men should not be used when analyzing the movements of women and children.

Davis also found the validity of the segmental method acceptable for use in kinematic analyses; however, he states that at present the method is not refined enough to be exact for kinetic analyses. When kinetic information is needed, it must come from equipment designed specifically for the purpose of measuring forces, such as force plates, accelerometers, and strain gauges.

Table 4-1. Weights of body segments relative to total body weight for women, expressed in percentages

Segment	Bernstein	Plagenhoef	Kjeldsen
Trunk		55.00	60.20
Upper arm	2.63	2.90	2.74
Forearm	1.82	1.55	1.61
Hand	0.64	0.50	0.51
Thigh	12.48	11.50	8.26
Calf (lower leg)	4.73	5.25	5.49
Foot	1.31	1.20	1.24

Table 4-2. Weights of body segments relative to total body weight for men, expressed in percentages*

Segment	Braune and Fischer	Cleaveland	Williams and Lissner	Dempster
Head and neck	7.06	7.03	7.9	
Trunk	42.70	48.30	51.1	49.4
Upper arm (2)	6.72	6.25	5.4	7.0
Forearm (2)	6.24	4.33	4.4	3.2
Hand (2)	(With forearm)	(With forearm)	(With forearm)	1.0
Thigh (2)	23.16	22.52	19.4	27.4
Calf (lower leg) (2)	14.12	11.52	19.4	9.4
Foot (2)	(With calf)	(With calf)	12.0	2.6

*Values for upper arm, forearm, hand, thigh, calf, and foot are for both segments in each case.

Table 4-3. Locations of centers of gravity of body segments for women, expressed as percentage of total segment length as measured from proximal end

Segment	Matsui	Bernstein
Head and neck	63	
Trunk	52	
Upper arm	46	48.40
Forearm	42	41.74
Hand	50	
Thigh	42	38.88
Calf	42	42.26
Foot	50	

Table 4-4. Locations of centers of gravity of body segments for men, expressed as percentage of total segment length as measured from proximal end

Segment	Cleaveland	Dempster	Matsui
Head and neck		(With trunk)	63
Trunk	53	60.4	52
Upper arm	42	43.6	46
Forearm	28	43.0	41
Hand	(With forearm)	50.6	50
Thigh	36	43.3	42
Calf	42	43.3	41
Foot	(With calf)	42.9	50

In Davis' study the reliability of the segmental method was high with intraclass correlations of $R_x = 0.9682$ and $R_y = 0.9443$ when the same center of gravity was identified from three repeated measurements.

In contrast, the objectivity of the segmental method was low. The reason for the inconsistency in measurements taken by several observers appeared to be related to individual interpretations of the locations of segmental end points. This was not a problem when testing the reliability. Therefore it might be misleading to analyze the position of the center of gravity of a person based on the data from a small sample of cadavers or live subjects. Further data from women, children, older persons, and physically disabled persons need to be acquired for a better understanding of the anatomic differences among people.

The segmental method is best used with data from the actual performer, at least submersing the limbs and estimating the trunk weight and center of gravity location. The segmental method, by means of the computer and without the errors of the scale method, allows the calculation of centers of gravity for many positions. Remember that the scale method requires that the person exactly duplicate the position of the movement.

Simplified version. A simplified version of the segmental method will be used to illustrate the basic theory underlying the method. Think of three children seated on a teeterboard and have each child represent a part of one human body. For example, child 1 would be the legs, child 2 would be the head and trunk, and child 3 would be the arms of a single human body. One child weighs 240 N* and is seated on the board 1.0 m from the fulcrum. Another child seated on the same side weighs 200 N and is 0.6 m from the fulcrum. The third child is seated on the opposite side, weighs 360 N, and is 0.8 m from the fulcrum. Since these body weights act as rotating forces, the effect of each force, multiplied by the distance from the fulcrum, is known as a moment of force. On the side where the heaviest child is seated, the moment will equal 360 N × 0.8 m, which is 288 Nm; on the side where the two lighter children are seated, it will be 240 N × 1.0 m + 200 N × 0.6 m, which equals 360 Nm.

The board will not be balanced with this arrangement. The board can be balanced by using one of two possible methods. First, the positions of

*One newton (unit of force) is that force which gives a mass of 1 kg an acceleration of 1 m/sec. The following formulas use the pound as the unit of measure: $1 \text{ N} = 10^5 \text{ dyn} = 0.2247$ pound; 1 pound $= 4.45 \text{ N} = 4.45 \times 10^5$ dyn.

the children may be changed. The child weighing 360 N might be moved to a position 1.0 m from the fulcrum, and the moment on that side of the board would then equal the 360 Nm moment of the opposite side. The second possibility would be to move the fulcrum. To determine the distance that the fulcrum should be moved, one would use the percentage weight of each child in relationship to the total weight of the three children to determine the force of each side:

$$
\begin{array}{llll}
\text{240 N:} & 0.30 & \times 1.0 \text{ m} = 0.30 \text{ m} \\
\text{200 N:} & 0.25 & \times 0.6 \text{ m} = \underline{0.15 \text{ m}} \\
& & \text{TOTAL} \quad 0.45 \text{ m} \\
\text{360 N:} & \underline{0.45} & \times 0.8 \text{ m} = 0.36 \text{ m} \\
\text{TOTAL} & 100\% \\
\end{array}
$$

The difference between 0.45 and 0.36, 0.09, shows the distance (in meters) that the fulcrum should be moved. The board is balanced by increasing the distance between the heaviest child and the fulcrum by 0.09 m; that between the fulcrum and each of the lighter children should be decreased 0.09 m. With these distances and the percentage weights, the moment values are as follows:

$$
\begin{array}{lll}
0.30 & \times 0.91 \text{ m} = 0.273 \text{ m} \\
0.25 & \times 0.51 \text{ m} = \underline{0.128 \text{ m}} \\
& \text{TOTAL} \quad 0.401 \text{ m} \\
0.45 & \times 0.89 \text{ m} = 0.401 \text{ m} \\
\text{TOTAL} & 100\% \\
\end{array}
$$

This proves that the center of gravity of the body (actually, only the line of gravity in one plane) is 0.09 m toward the head, which is represented by the lighter children. Thus what we did was consider one line of gravity, as represented by the fulcrum of the teeterboard, and reject it as not being the true balance point, or line of gravity, of the system. To find the position of the center of gravity of the total body, one may arbitrarily choose any line (which may or may not pass through some part of the body) as the line from which the position of the segmental centers of gravity will be measured. Moment of force values for each segment can be calculated (by the use of percentage weights). The

difference between the sums of the values on each side of the line will show the distance that the line should be moved to pass through the total-body center of gravity.

Information required. In using the segmental method for determining the location of the center of gravity of the body traced from a film of a boy throwing a ball (Fig. 4-12), the investigator must have the following information:

1. The percentage of total body weight of each segment (Tables 4-1 and 4-2)
2. The location of the center of gravity in each segment, usually reported as a percentage of the total segment length as measured from the proximal end of the segment (Tables 4-3 and 4-4)
3. The horizontal and vertical distance of each body segment center of gravity from a vertical and horizontal axis in the form of an *x*- and *y*-coordinate system as depicted in Fig. 4-12

The steps to follow in calculating the total-body center of gravity from a projected film image are as follows:

1. Project the image onto a piece of graph paper and trace the performer. (The standard Recordak viewer is ideal for this purpose.)
2. Establish a coordinate system on the graph paper in such a way that the origin is in the lower left-hand corner (Fig. 4-12). This confines all the data to the upper right quadrant, where all *x*- and *y*-coordinate values will be positive.
3. From the picture select two reference points that can be viewed in all the frames to be analyzed for a given performance and that are stationary objects—for example, the center of the dial on a wall clock or an electric wall socket.
4. Record the *x*- and *y*-coordinate values of the two reference points from the graph paper. In analysis of future frames of this same performance, these reference coordinate values must be exactly the same.

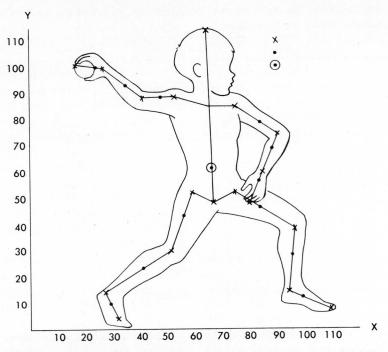

Fig. 4-12. Tracing from film of young child throwing ball, to illustrate points required to determine position of body center of gravity. **X** represents segmental end points; • marks segmental midpoints; ⊙ indicates determined body center of gravity.

5. Record the *x*- and *y*-coordinate values of each of the following segmental end points:
   a. Tragus of the ear
   b. Sternal notch
   c. Crotch
   d. Right shoulder
   e. Right elbow
   f. Right fingertips (distal point of right fingertips)
   g. Left shoulder
   h. Left elbow
   i. Left wrist
   j. Left fingertips (distal point of left fingertips)
   k. Right hip
   l. Right knee
   m. Right ankle
   n. Right toe
   o. Left hip
   p. Left knee
   q. Left ankle
   r. Left toe (distal point of left toes)
   These points are marked on Fig. 4-12.

6. Connect the segmental end points to form a stick figure.

7. Locate the center of gravity for each segment by the following procedure:
   a. Measure the segment lengths.
   b. Multiply this value by the appropriate percentage value from Table 4-3 or 4-4.
   c. Measure this amount from the proximal end of the segment. Mark this spot as the center of gravity for the segment; that is, if the trunk and head measure 10

Table 4-5. Segmental center of gravity locations, based on Fig. 4-12 and the coordinate values once segmental weight factors are considered

Segment	X-coordinate	X value weighted	Y-coordinate	Y value weighted
Head and neck	(With trunk)		(With trunk)	
Trunk	65.0	33.41	76.0	39.01
Upper arm (left)	81.5	2.45	81.0	2.43
Forearm (left)	88.0	1.41	69.5	1.11
Hand (left)	83.5	0.50	57.0	0.34
Thigh (left)	83.5	10.77	48.0	6.19
Calf (left)	95.5	4.58	30.0	1.44
Foot (left)	99.0	1.49	13.0	0.20
Upper arm (right)	48.0	1.44	89.0	2.67
Forearm (right)	35.0	0.56	93.0	1.49
Hand (right)	23.5	0.14	101.0	0.61
Thigh (right)	55.5	7.16	44.5	5.74
Calf (right)	41.0	1.97	24.0	1.15
Foot (right)	29.0	0.44	10.0	0.15
Total body		66.32		62.53

cm, then the center of gravity for this segment would be 0.604 × 10 = 6.04, or 6.04 cm from the crotch (using Dempster data on men [Table 4-2]).

   d. Repeat the procedure for all segments.

8. Record all the x- and y-coordinate values for each segment's center of gravity.
9. Multiply the x values for each segment's center of gravity by the percentage of the total body weight contributed by that segment (Table 4-3). Sum these values. This sum represents the location of the center of gravity of the total body in the x, or horizontal, plane.
10. Repeat step 9, using the y values for each segment's center of gravity.
11. The x- and y-coordinate total-body center of gravity can be located on the graph paper. Table 4-5 contains sample coordinate values on the image in Fig. 4-12.

Graphing the center of gravity. These measures and calculations illustrate a method by which the path of the body's center of gravity can be depicted in any skill. Such a procedure was used by Sparks, as seen in Fig. 4-13. To do so there must be a vertical and a horizontal reference line, neither of which has to pass through some part of the body, as did the lines in the illustration. The number of film frames necessary to determine the path will depend on whether the body is in flight or whether segments are changing position while the body is supported on a stationary base.

   Once the contact with the supporting surface has been broken and the body is in flight, the path of the center of gravity is determined by the velocity and direction imparted to it at takeoff and by gravitational pull. It is now a projectile and can be treated as such. The line of flight can be found by the method described in Appendix D. Once the body is in flight, no segmental movement will affect the path of the center of gravity. Therefore it is necessary to locate the position of the center of gravity at only two points (and the corresponding times). One point must always be the first frame in which contact has been broken—in which the body has just begun its flight. The second can be any frame before landing, but it is well to select a frame that is as far as possible from the first. The

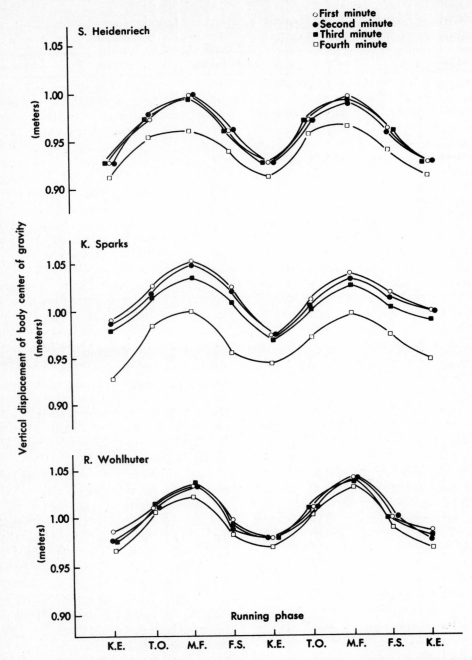

Fig. 4-13. Vertical displacement of body center of gravity of runners for each minute in 4-minute–mile run. All three runners show effect of fatigue during fourth minute. This was due to greater flexion at knees and general alteration of running style. *K.E.*, knees even; *T.O.*, toe off; *M.F.*, midflight; *F.S.*, foot strike. Stride for two phases is shown. (From Sparks, K.E.: Physiological and mechanical alterations due to fatigue while running a four-minute mile on treadmill, unpublished doctoral dissertation, Indiana University, May, 1975.)

frame selected will depend on the number of frames included in the film. The choice of the second frame is as far as possible from the first because there are always likely to be measurement errors; the longer the time and the distance that are measured, the smaller the percentage of error. Since the in-flight path of the center of gravity will be a parabolic curve, the question for that curve can be calculated from any two points on the curve. In this text when direction and velocity of body projections are reported, they have been determined by this method.

When the path of the center of gravity is depicted while the base is stationary and segments are moving, its position should be found in every film frame. In such situations the center of gravity is not a projectile, and movement of a segment will affect its path. To determine the path of the center of gravity in the takeoff phase of a standing broad jump, Johnson drew the vertical references line through the metatarsophalangeal joints and the horizontal line along the bottom of the toes. At the time the heels left the floor she found the center of gravity to be 72.6 cm (28.6 in) above the floor and 7.6 cm (3 in) ahead of the metatarsal joints. As the knees and hips flexed and the arms moved downward from the height of the backswing, the center of gravity moved downward and forward to a position 55.6 cm (21.9 in) above the floor and 26.4 cm (10.4 in) ahead of the metatarsophalangeal joints. (See Figs. 12-1 and 12-2.) At takeoff the center of gravity was 74.4 cm (29.3 in) above the floor and 57.9 cm (22.8 in) ahead of the metatarsophalangeal joints. Note that interestingly the center of gravity was ahead of the toes at the time the heels were raised—a further indication that gravitational pull, not muscle action, tilts the body (raising the heels). As the muscles act and move body segments, the position of the center of gravity is changed, so that it is outside the base of support, and the body falls forward, a fall that is controlled by the ankle extensors.

Calculations to determine the position of the center of gravity by this method involve a relatively long and involved process; yet understanding of the effect of segmental positions will be furthered by a limited number of determinations. If films are not available, various positions can be taken on the gravity board; for example, the subject either may stand on the board in a stride position with feet separated at a measured distance and trunk flexed at a measured angle or may lie on the board with upper and lower limbs held at measured angles to the trunk. Segmental calculations can then be compared with scale determinations.

For more extensive studies, work can be reduced by means of recently developed techniques. Motion analyzers and digitizers used in conjunction with computers (on-line or separate) can greatly increase the number of frames that may be feasibly analyzed in a given time.

(See *Kinesiology Review,* 1968, for article by Garrett, Widule, and Garrett. Also see Scheuchenzuber's center-of-gravity computer program, found in Appendix E, and Bates's program. The latter is more detailed, with several subroutines. Several graduate students have used it for analyzing their data in their doctoral dissertations.)

KINANTHROPOMETRY

Because of the diversity of physical (anatomic) characteristics of human beings, it is no wonder that researchers, teachers, coaches, physical therapists, and others concerned with education in and improvement of human movement have attempted to relate anatomic characteristics to movement performance achievements. A new scientific discipline has emerged to focus solely on the measurement of size, shape, proportion, composition, maturation, and gross function as related to such concerns as growth, exercise, performance, and nutrition. This discipline has been termed kinanthropometry and is closely aligned with ergometry, the measurement of work of muscles.

Some of the earliest measurements of morphology were done by Morpurgo in 1897, when he found hypertrophy in dogs that ran on treadmills. In that same century, Quételet formulated strength norms, determined secular trends in growth, and pioneered in human social statistics to form the

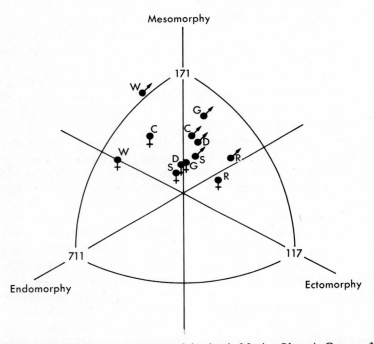

Fig. 4-14. Mean somatotypes of sports groups participating in Mexico Olympic Games. ♂, Male; ♀, female; *W,* weight throwers; *C,* canoeists; *G,* gymnasts; *S,* swimmers; *D,* divers; *R,* middle-distance runners. (Based on data presented by de Garay, A.L., Levine, L., and Carter, J.E.L.: Genetic and anthropological studies of Olympic athletes, New York, 1974, Academic Press, Inc.)

basis for some of the later work of kinanthropometrists. In this century physical educators have conducted numerous investigations into the relationship of selected physical characteristics and motor performances, including Olympic performances.

One of the more commonly used proportionality characteristics is the body typing called somatotyping. Since persons tend to observe the total body in rather general terms such as *skinny, fat,* and *muscular,* the somatotype has been very popular. The ectomorph is the linear or lean person, the endomorph is the person with excess adipose tissue, and the mesomorph is the person with a high proportion of muscle. Few persons exhibit only one of these attributes; most have a combination of all three. On a 7-point scale, the average person would be rated 4,4,4 (endo-, meso-, ecto-). Athletes tend to be more mesomorphic, except for the ectomorphs found in such events as long-distance running. Athletes also are usually taller than the normal population. In addition, numerous studies, more recently those using the Carter anthropometric somatotyping method, have shown clusters of each sports group in a unique place on the somatotype chart (Fig. 4-14). The uniqueness of each champion athletic group led countries such as East Germany to preselect and train young children for future national sports competition on the basis of anatomic characteristics.

Widths, lengths, girths, and other single anthropometric measurements do not correlate highly with any known skill. Ratios, indexes, and comparisons of one measurement with another have shown higher correlations with performance than did single measurements, but even these parameters do not provide more than a group predictability. A more complete approach is the use of a unisex phantom, or representation of a bilaterally symmetric average human body. More than 100 measurements are taken on a person to construct a profile of that person. The profile can then be compared with profiles at various times with respect to age, sports participation, nutrition, and other factors, as well as with profiles of other persons, including champion performers. When the unisex

phantom model was applied to data collected by Eiben (cited in Heath and Carter) on 125 women athletes participating in the European Track and Field Championships, 1966, the following differences among long jumpers, shot-putters, discus throwers, and the phantom were found:

1. The z score* of the long jumpers was more than $-1z$ with respect to breadth and girth measurements of the phantom's arm.
2. There was a difference of 1z between the long jumpers ($+0.73z$) and the shot-putters ($-0.31z$) on tibial height.
3. The shot-putters and discus throwers were more than $+2z$ above the phantom on chest depth and bitrochanteric width.
4. Thigh circumference z scores were near zero for the long jumpers, at $+1.2z$ for the discus throwers, and at $+2.07z$ for the shot-putters.
5. Body weight scores were similar to the thigh circumference scores.

From a biomechanical perspective, the athlete who is successful in projecting the body into space must be proportionally different from the one who projects objects. One must be cautious, however, not to confuse relationships with cause and effect. Just as Murpurgo found exercise to change the body, one cannot be sure how much the body is changed through participation and how much is inherited, and which proportion of each is vital to success in a motor skill. High correlations merely show relationships, that is, that one item is likely to occur with another item related positively to it. It has been shown that both bone and muscle hypertrophy with use. Tennis players, baseball pitchers, and other unilateral sports performers have heavier and larger limbs on one side of the body than on the other.

In the succeeding chapters certain anatomic characteristics that enhance, and certain anatomic characteristics that limit, certain movement performances will be described. In some cases the interaction and interdependency of factors prevent a complete separation of the pertinent anatomic

*A measure of variance.

characteristics from level of skill, motivation, and training.

MINI LABORATORY EXERCISES

1. On graph paper trace the outline (contourogram) of a performer from one frame of a movie film, mark the joints, and draw line segments between the joints. Using the segmental method described in this chapter, determine the center of gravity in two planes of the performer, as traced.
2. Using the scale method described in this chapter, determine the center of gravity in three planes of two human beings:
   a. In the anatomic position
   b. In a track starting position
   c. In a posture of your choice

REFERENCES

Bates, B.T.: The development of a computer program with application to a film analysis: the mechanics of female runners, unpublished dissertation, Indiana University, Aug., 1973.

Bernstein, N.: The coordination and regulation of movement, Oxford, 1967, Pergamon Press.

Braune, W., and Fischer, O.: Ueber den Schwerpunkt des menschlichen Korpers mit Rüchsicht auf die Austrustrung des deutschen Infanteristerm, Abh. D.K. Sachs Ges. Wiss. **15**:2, 1889.

Brown, G.M.: Relationship between body types and static posture of young adult women, Res. Q. Am. Assoc. Health Phys. Educ. **31**:403, 1960.

Carter, J.E.L.: The somatotypes of athletes: a review, Hum. Biol. **42**:535-569, 1970.

Cleaveland, H.G.: The determination of the center of gravity in segments of the human body, thesis, 1955, University of California at Los Angeles.

Croskey, M.I., et al.: The height of the center of gravity in man, Am. J. Physiol. **61**:171, 1922.

Cureton, T.K. Jr., and Wickens, J.S.: The center of gravity in the human body in the antero-posterior plane and its relation to posture, physical fitness, and athletic ability, Res. Q. Am. Assoc. Health Phys. Educ. **6**:(2) (supp.):93, 1935.

Davis, M.: Quality of data collected by the segmental analysis technique, unpublished doctoral dissertation, Bloomington, 1973, Indiana University.

Dawson, P.M.: The physiology of physical education, Baltimore, 1935, The Williams & Wilkins Co.

Dempster, W.T.: Space requirements of the seated operator, WADC Technical Rep., Washington, D.C., July, 1955, U.S. Department of Commerce.

Fox, M.G., and Young, O.G.: Placement of the gravity line in anteroposterior posture, Res. Q. Am. Assoc. Health Phys. Educ. **25**:277, 1954.

Garrett, R.E., Widule, C.J., and Garrett, G.E.: Computer-aided analysis of human motion, Kinesiology Review, p. 1, 1968.

Hasselkus, B.R.: Variations in the postural sway related to aging in women, thesis, University of Wisconsin, 1974.

Hay, J.G.: The center of gravity of the human body, Kinesiology, vol. III, 1973, American Association for Health, Physical Education, and Recreation.

Heath, B.J., and Carter, J.E.L.: A comparison of somatotype methods, Am. J. Phys. Anthropol. **24**:87, 1966.

Hellebrandt, F.A.: Standing as a geotrophic reflex, Am. J. Physiol. **121**:471, 1938.

Hellebrandt, F.A., Brogdon, E., and Tepper, R.H.: Posture and its cost, Am. J. Physiol. **129**:773, 1940.

Hellebrandt, F.A., and Franseen, E.B.: Physiological study of the vertical stance of man, Physiol. Rev. **23**:220, 1943.

Hellebrandt, F.A., Riddle, K.S., and Fries, E.C.: Influence of postural sway on stance photography, Physiotherapy Rev. **22**:88, 1942.

Hellebrandt, F.A., Tepper, R.H., Braun, G.L., and Elliott, M.C.: The location of the cardinal anatomical orientation planes passing through the center of weight in young adult women, Am. J. Physiol. **121**:465, 1938.

Hewes, G.W.: The anthropology of posture, Sci. Am. **196**: 122-128, Feb. 1957.

Howell, A.B.: Speed in animals, New York, 1965, Hafner Press.

Johnson, B.P.: An analysis of the mechanics of the takeoff in the standing broad jump, thesis, University of Wisconsin, 1958.

Joseph, J.: Man's posture—electromyographic studies, Springfield, Ill., 1960, Charles C Thomas, Publisher.

Keith, A.: Man's posture: its evolution and disorders. II. The evolution of the orthograde spine, Br. Med. J. **1**:499, 1923.

Kjeldsen, K., and Morse, C.: Research reports, vol. 3 (Adrian, M., and Brame, J., editors), Washington, D.C., 1977, American Association for Health, Physical Education, and Recreation.

Matsui, H.: Review of our researches, 1970-1973, Department of Physical Education, University of Nagoya (Japan).

Napier, J.: The antiquity of human walking, Sci. Am. **216**:56, April 1967.

Palmer, C.E.: Studies of the center of gravity in the human body, Child Dev. **15**:99, 1944.

Plagenhoef, S.: Patterns of human motion, Englewood Cliffs, N.J., 1971, Prentice-Hall, Inc.

Waterland, J.C., and Shambes, G.M.: Biplant center of gravity procedures, Percept. Mot. Skills **30**:511, 1970.

Wells, K.F.: What we don't know about posture, JOHPER **29**:31, May, 1958.

Williams, M., and Lissner, H.R.: Biomechanics of human motion, Philadelphia, 1962, W.B. Saunders Co.

ADDITIONAL READINGS

Bernstein, N.: The co-ordination and regulation of movements, Oxford, 1967, Pergamon Press, Ltd.

Clauser, C.E., McConville, J.I., and Young, J.W.: Weight, volume and center of mass of segments of the human body, Pub. No. AMRL-TR-69-70, Fairborn, Ohio, Aug. 1969, Wright-Patterson Air Force Base.

Gonyes, W.J.: Adaptive differences in the body proportions of large fields, Acta Anat. **96:**81-96, 1976.

Landry, F., and Orban, W.A.R.: Biomechanics of sports and kinanthropometry, Miami, 1978, Symposia Specialists.

Tanner, J.M.: The physique of the Olympic athlete, London, 1964, George Allen & Unwin, Ltd.

CHAPTER 5

Mechanical considerations

Before beginning a study of this section the reader should refer to Fig. 2-4. Keeping in mind the concepts shown in the model, one could describe the mechanical considerations in the analysis of motion in three parts: (1) forces and moments of force, (2) displacements with respect to time, and (3) impulse-momentum and work-energy. This organization is based on simplicity and on causal relationships. Forces and moments of force cause motion, which is identified as displacement with respect to time.

Enumeration of common forces and moments of force and an explanation of how forces cause motion are presented first. The reader should recognize some of these basic concepts because they were presented in Chapter 4. Next, a general description of displacements and time intervals of motion is presented to provide a basic understanding of what is known as the kinematics of motion. Since both the impulse-momentum and work-energy concepts provide a holistic understanding and a method of investigating movement of living things, discussions of these concepts are presented last.

The descriptions in this chapter will be general in nature but will include selected specific examples and applications. A complete understanding of these concepts will be possible after further description and application to the many activities described in the ensuing chapters. Reference to these concepts may also prove useful to the reader when studying the later chapters.

Classical mechanics, also known as newtonian mechanics, is the physical science that deals with movement or motion of material bodies of ordinary size moving at speeds that are slow compared to the speed of light. Therefore newtonian mechanics and laws, often referred to as Newton's three laws of motion, are applicable to the investigation of movement of humans, animals, birds, and fish, as well as machines built by humans. The mechanical considerations presented in this chapter are based on newtonian mechanics.

FORCES AND MOMENTS OF FORCE

As a force acts on a body, it is important to know its direction, since movement will occur in the direction of the force. Forces may act normal to the body (NF), as does a tail wind or a head wind; they may act parallel to the body (shearing or tangential force), as does friction; or they may act at any angle other than normal or tangential. Such forces are termed diagonal forces and can be resolved into normal and tangential components to facilitate analysis. In many instances the normal forces are vertical and the tangential forces are horizontal.

The vector resolution of one force into normal and tangential components typically can be done in one of two ways: the trigonometric method or the graphic method. These methods are explained in Fig. 5-1. The trigonometric method is based on the principle that in right triangles of various sizes but with identical angles, the ratio of one side of the

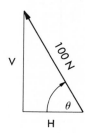
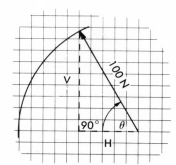

If magnitude (100 N)
and direction (θ)
are known, look
in trigonometry
table:

H = 100 N cosine θ

V = 100 N sine θ

If trigonometry table
is not available:

1. Draw vector of 100 N
magnitude at angle θ
with the horizontal

2. Construct right
triangle

3. Determine H and V
by measurement

Fig. 5-1. Trigonometric and graphic methods for resolution of vector components perpendicular to each other.

triangle to another side will always be the same. The graphic method involves more time in solving for the resultant force vector and may be less accurate, because of human error in measurement, than the trigonometric method.

The trigonometric information in Appendix B is useful for resolving any force acting on a body into normal and tangential components to better determine the effect of the force on the body. See Appendix B for further trigonometry concepts and for values of trigonometric functions.

If two or more forces act on the body, the forces must be added to determine the resultant direction of motion. Since forces are depicted as vectors, one method of determining the resultant effect is to resolve the forces into their components. All normal force vectors can then be added together; all forces with tangential vectors are added separately. The resultant effect can be determined by using either the graphic or the trigonometric method (tangent table).

The common external forces that act on human beings and animals are the force of gravity (weight), the ground reaction force, friction, water buoyancy, and drag and lift forces. In sports there are other forces, such as a person or an object, striking the person. In addition, there are internal forces, consisting primarily of muscle forces, reactive forces, and forces acting on the tissues of the body as a result of external or internal forces.

These forces will be discussed in the following sections, along with Newton's three laws of motion.

Relationship of Newton's three laws of motion to translation

Whether or not motion occurs is directly related to the magnitude of force. Newton's first law, the law of inertia, states that a body at rest will remain at rest until some force of sufficient magnitude to overcome its inertia acts on the body. This law also applies to bodies moving at a constant velocity. An explanation of this law will be made initially with respect to translatory motion in the vertical direction. The inertia of a body is known as its mass. Mass is measured in kilograms (newton-second^2/meter [Nsec^2/m]) in the International System of Units (SI), also known as the metric system, and mass is measured in slugs (pound-second^2/foot [lb-sec^2/ft]) in the English system. A small letter m is used to denote the existence of mass in equations.

Vertical motion. An upward movement can occur only if the force (F_y) acting on a mass is greater than the weight of the body (w). This can be proved by the application of Newton's second law, which states that the acceleration, and thereby the motion, of a body is directly related to the force acting on it and is inversely related to its mass. In equation form this principle is written as follows:

$$F_y = ma_y$$

where force (F) in the y direction equals the mass times the acceleration (ma) in the y direction.

In the case of more than one force, the symbol Σ is used with the above equation to indicate the "sum of all the forces." Stationary bodies standing on a floor have the acceleration of gravity acting downward on them. If a person stands on the ground, the ground exerts a force (measured in newtons [N]) equal to the force of gravity (w) but opposite in direction. This is in accordance with Newton's third law, called the law of interaction, or the law of action-reaction. The former title is preferred because the latter implies a difference in time between the actions (forces), when in fact the

reaction occurs simultaneously with the action. Given the situation, then, of a person's standing on the floor, since the two forces are acting in opposite y (vertical) directions, and since the forces are of equal magnitude, no movement will occur.

Linear motion in any direction. It is evident that linear acceleration will not occur and will not produce translation of the body if the $\Sigma F = 0$. Since movements occur in three planes, or in a three-dimensional world, the forces may be identified as F_x, F_y, and F_z, according to the Cartesian coordinate system* mentioned in Chapter 4. All these forces must equal zero for translational equilibrium to exist. If F_z and F_y equal zero, but $\Sigma F_x = 200$ N acting on the body, then a body weighing 490 N will be accelerated laterally in the direction of F_z at a rate of 4 m/sec^2. The process for determining this is as follows:

STEP 1: Always draw a free body diagram (FBD), that is, depict the body in some simple shape and draw all external forces acting on it. Draw the vectors to scale—large forces are longer than small forces (Fig. 5-2).

STEP 2: Determine in which of the directions—x, y, and z—the sum of the forces equals zero. NOTE: If diagonal forces exist, resolve these forces into F_x, F_y, F_z.

STEP 3: Determine which sum is not equal to zero and solve $\Sigma F = ma$.

$$\Sigma F_y = 0 \qquad \Sigma F_z = 0 \qquad \Sigma F_x \neq 0$$

$$\Sigma F_x = ma_x$$
$$F + R = ma_x$$
$$210 \text{ N} + (-10 \text{ N}) = \frac{490 \text{ N}}{9.8 \text{ m/sec}^2} \times a_x$$
$$200 \text{ N} = 50 \text{ N sec}^2/\text{m} \times a_x$$
$$4 \text{ m/sec}^2 = a_x$$

The acceleration is forward.

This basic law of motion, expressed as $F = ma$, indicates that a body will experience linear acceleration when the ΣF does not equal zero. For ex-

---

*A Cartesian coordinate is either of two coordinates used for locating a point on a plane being the distances of the point from each of two infinite, intersecting, straight-line axes of reference usually designated as x and y.

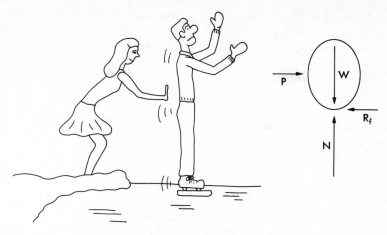

Fig. 5-2. Depiction of life situation by means of free body diagram. Forces acting on body are represented by force vectors. This method provides convenient identification of probable effects on body. (*P*, force of push; *W*, body weight; *N*, normal force; R_f, friction force.)

ample, during the act of jumping the reaction force is greater than body weight because the muscle force is causing the body to accelerate upward. By calculating the acceleration, one can use the preceding equation to determine the unknown reaction force. The difference between the body weight and the reaction force is equivalent to the effective muscle force. The greater the muscle force, the greater the acceleration, and therefore the greater the vertical distance of the jump. Furthermore, if two persons of different masses utilize equal amounts of muscle force, the person of lesser mass will be able to create greater acceleration than the person of greater mass. This is known as the inverse relationship of body mass to acceleration. Note these examples and the basic equation. F = ma summarizes only the external forces. Internal reactions, causing deformations of body tissues or resistance at joints and muscle forces, are not considered.

The force, R, represents the friction force that is always present whenever materials or bodies—solids, liquids, or gases—move with respect to each other. Since friction is an ever-present force during locomotion, as well as during all movements of living things, an understanding of the factors that determine the magnitude of the frictional force and the coefficient of friction for two interacting surfaces is vital to an analysis and understanding of movement.

Coefficient of friction. Friction is the resistance that opposes every effort to slide or roll one body over another. Friction may be a hindrance or a help in sports performance. Some general facts about friction include the following:

1. Static, or starting, friction is greater than moving, or sliding, friction.
2. Although many factors are involved, generally friction depends on the velocity, load, condition, and nature of the two surfaces that are interacting with each other.
3. In most practical sports situations friction tends not to depend much on the velocity of the sliding surfaces. However, starting friction is decidedly greater than sliding friction. Friction also usually decreases to some extent with increasing speed.
4. Friction depends on the nature and condition of the contacting surfaces because of the following:

a. Friction is less when the surfaces are smooth and hard.
b. With dry surfaces friction is approximately the same regardless of the size of the area of contact.
c. Friction is approximately proportional to the area of contact with well-lubricated surfaces.

The force needed to overcome friction is nearly proportional to the normal, or perpendicular, force with which the surfaces are pressed together, as follows:

$$\text{Coefficient of friction} = \frac{\text{Force of friction}}{\text{Normal force}}$$

Force of friction = Coefficient of friction × Normal force

Another way to present this is as a ratio, as follows: the force pressing the surfaces together is represented by N (normal force) and R (force needed to overcome friction): therefore $\frac{R}{N} = B$ where B is the coefficient of friction. The smaller B is, the less friction is created. On the other hand, the larger B is, the more the surfaces cling together, and the larger the force that will be required to cause slippage. Sometimes it is advantageous to produce surfaces that have a high coefficient of friction; at other times it is advantageous to do just the opposite.

Therefore the concept of optimal friction is an important one. One must select the two materials that will interact according to the needs of the situation and goals of the performance. Each situation has an optimal amount friction in which optimal performance can occur. Some coefficients of friction have been calculated for shoe-playing surfaces, but much of what is known about friction and the world of human and animal movement has been obtained through trial and error. Following are examples of player and equipment adaptation with respect to the element of friction:

1. Sprinters lean forward at the start of a race to reduce the friction that their feet make against the ground.
2. Ashes are put on automobile tires for driving on snow to increase friction so that sufficient traction against the snow can be secured.
3. In wet weather a small amount of silica sand placed on the hands of a football passer may enable him to throw the football more accurately because the coefficient of friction will be increased. However, wet, wrinkled socks inside a football player's shoes do the same thing and are likely to cause blisters.
4. Basketball players attempting to play on a floor that has been covered with wax for a dance may have to make the soles of their shoes irregular by cutting them with a knife so that there is sufficient friction between the soles and the floor surface to enable them to move.
5. Table tennis paddles that have a rough, irregular surface enable the players to put more spin on the ball because of the increased friction.
6. Surfaces such as the new, nonsmooth cement rings used for shot-putting and discus throwing prevent the performer from slipping too fast as he goes around and across the ring. Cleats and spikes on athletic shoes have the same effect. However, the placement of the cleats and spikes may affect the amount of friction created.

When the problem of slippage is too great and the surfaces cannot be changed, the performer will have to keep the center of gravity more nearly over the base of support. One will have to take short steps, should avoid too much body lean, and may have to drop the center of gravity as low as possible by squatting. In this way one will be able to remain in a playing posture and to perform at reasonable efficiency.

Because of the condition of a surface (for example, slick and wet), it is possible to "spin the wheels" too fast, and the coefficient of friction will be insufficient for the object, such as a car or a person, to move forward successfully. The two surfaces must be in contact with each other long enough for traction to take place. Moving at a slower speed enables this to occur.

Since frictional force is produced by the interaction of two materials, the coefficient of friction refers to this interaction, not to one material or the other. This coefficient of friction is equal to the tangent of the angle of slippage. If one surface can be tilted to produce an incline, the angle at which the second surface slips (slides) on this incline can be measured. The tangent of the angle can be determined by referring to Appendix B. This tangent value is equal to the coefficient of friction value. Frictional force is then determined by using the formula previously given, $R = B \times N$.

Frictional force may be determined directly by measuring, with a spring scale, the force required to cause one surface to slide on a second surface.

MINI LABORATORY EXERCISES

1. Place a rubber-cleated shoe with a weight inside on a wood surface and determine the frictional force and coefficient of friction by attaching a spring scale to the shoe and exerting a horizontal force on the scale. The highest value of the scale reading will be the limit of static friction. Note that the kinetic friction is slightly less than the static friction, which terminates as soon as slippage occurs. Calculate the coefficient of friction by

$$\frac{R \text{ (friction force)}}{N \text{ (weight)}}$$

2. Repeat the experiment using different surfaces.
3. Repeat the experiment using shoes with different soles.
4. If a spring scale is not available, place shoes on a board that can be tilted. Slowly increase the angle of inclination of the board until slippage occurs. The tangent of the angle at which the shoe slips is the coefficient of friction. To calculate the friction force, one must find the normal force by calculating $N =$ Weight $\times$ (Cosine of the angle of inclination).

Relationship of laws of motion to rotatory motion

When the newtonian laws of motion are applied to rotatory motion, moment of force is substituted for force, and moment of inertia is substituted for inertia in the following equation:

$$\Sigma F = ma$$

The equation becomes as follows, with the acceleration no longer linear but angular:

$$\Sigma M = I\alpha$$

where M = moment of force; I = moment of inertia; and alpha (α) = angular acceleration. Moment of force (M) is defined as the product of the force times its moment arm, that is, the shortest distance from the axis of rotation to the point of application of force. Moment of inertia (I) is defined as the rotatory inertia and is calculated by multiplying the mass by its radius from the axis of rotation (the radius is squared).

The determination of whether rotatory motion will occur is directly linked to the question of whether the point of application is other than through the center of gravity of the body. In the preceding examples of translation, the assumption was made that (1) the forces were acting through the center of gravity of the body or (2) any moments that might have existed were being ignored. In Fig. 5-3, however, the forces act at distances d_1 and d_2 from the turning point, which is both the center of gravity of the object and the axis of rotation of the object. The forces produce a turning effect, which is termed a moment or identified as torque. Since in Fig. 5-3 the sum of the forces is equal to zero, no translation occurs. If d_1 and d_2 did not exist—that is, if the force acted through the center of gravity of the object—it is evident that the sum of the moments would also be equal to zero, since the moment is calculated by multiplying the force by its perpendicular distance of application from the axis of rotation (center of gravity). Although the concept of moments of force is thoroughly discussed in Chapter 7, the fundamentals are presented in the following solution to Fig. 5-3.

If the moment of inertia of the object is determined to be 4 Nsec²-m, then the angular acceleration of the object will be 10 rad/sec². This is determined by the following equation and solution:

$$\Sigma M = I\alpha$$

$$40 \text{ Nm} = 4 \text{ Nsec}^2\text{-m} \times \alpha$$

$$\frac{40\ Nm}{4\ Nm/sec^2} = \alpha$$

$$10\ rad/sec^2 = \alpha$$

NOTE: Since the radian is a dimensionless unit, it is written after the value of alpha. One radian is equal to approximately 57 degrees, or 360 degrees divided by 2π. Thus 10 rad/sec² is equal to slightly more than 570 degrees/sec².

This example of two equal and opposite forces that act at equal distances from a point but produce the same direction of rotation is called a force couple. Since it has an internal reaction couple, the reaction force is not considered in this free body diagram of external forces. Such is the case in the majority of instances in which forces act on the human body. For example, in football the tackler may apply the force at the head, chest, center of gravity of the body (hips), thighs, or ankles of the ball carrier. If the force is at the crown of the head, the head is accelerated backward with rotatory motion, producing a reaction force at the atlas (rotatory point of head). Although there is little effect on the rest of the body, there is a high potential for neck or spinal cord or column injury. If the same force is applied at the chest, the ball carrier experiences rotation of the body above the lumbar region. Since the mass of these body parts is greater than the mass of the head, the acceleration is not as great as with the head. The reactive moment of force occurs in the vulnerable lumbar region of the spine, which again produces a risk of injury to the body. In both cases, since the feet are in contact with the ground, there may be little or no movement of the lower body. Application of this same amount of force through the center of gravity of the body will produce backward translation of the ball carrier, with no rotatory accelerations of body parts. If the force is greater than the mass of the ball carrier, the acceleration of the total body is linear. If the force is applied to the thighs or ankles, rotatory acceleration again occurs. In this case the feet are removed from contact with the ground, and the body rotates about its center of gravity. Free body diagrams of the forces and the

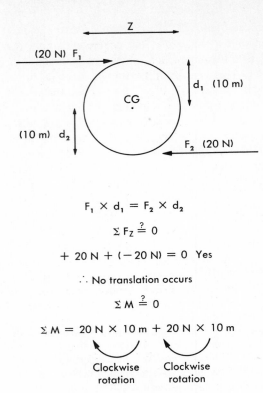

Fig. 5-3. Use of free body diagram to determine whether or not translation, rotation, or both translation and rotation would occur for given situation.

moments of force that produce rotatory accelerations in football are presented in Fig. 5-4.

Principles
1. Linear acceleration of a body will not occur unless the sum of the forces acting on a body is greater than zero.
2. Rotatory acceleration of a body will not occur unless the sum of the moments of force acting on the body is greater than zero.
3. As the force (or moment of force) acting on a body increases, the amount of acceleration of that body will also increase.

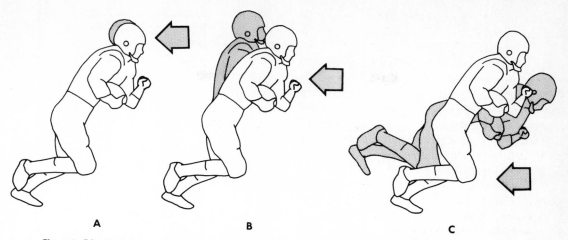

Fig. 5-4. Identical forces acting on different parts of body produce different moments of force. Straight-line vector shows point of application of force. Shaded body part shows resultant rotation of body parts caused by moment of force. Note that either the joint caudal to force or the center of gravity of entire body acts as axis of rotation for moment of force.

4. If the same force (or moment of force) acts on two body masses, the larger mass will accelerate the lesser amount.
5. It is the net result of all forces and all moments of force that must be added vectorially to determine whether or not acceleration is produced.
6. The direction and amount of acceleration can be measured by using the following formulas:

$$\Sigma F = ma \text{ and } \Sigma M = I\alpha$$

Changing the moment of inertia

A given force acting on a body to produce rotation can create varying magnitudes of angular acceleration merely by adjusting the body segments to create varying magnitudes of rotatory inertia. Since the moment of inertia is dependent on the distance of the center of gravity of the mass from the axis of rotation, this distance can be shortened by changing the angles at the joints. For example, angular acceleration is greatest when the leg is swinging forward and the angle at the knee is as small as possible. Conversely, the angular acceleration is least when the leg is swinging forward with no flexion at the knee.

This concept is important because nothing comparable occurs with linear motion. The mass is usually a constant when linear acceleration is being produced. The moment of inertia, however, can be changed, thus allowing a body part of constant mass to be rotated at a faster rate of speed even though the same amount of force is used at the same point.

Centripetal and centrifugal force

A unique force found in all rotatory movements is centripetal force. This force maintains the circular path of the body or body part. Centrifugal force is the equal and opposite force to centripetal force. A gymnast attempts to oppose the centrifugal force by chalking the hands or wearing palm gloves with built-in finger flexion when performing on a high bar or uneven parallel bars. High values for both centripetal and centrifugal force are recognized by numbness in distal segments during or after swinging movements and are recognized as pain in the proximal joint as a result of efforts to stabilize the joint during the swinging movement.

The calculation of centripetal force is derived, once again, from the basic equation $F = ma$. Since centripetal force (C_p) represents radial acceleration, the a can be written in terms of tangential velocity (V_t) or angular velocity (ω). The equation is as follows:

$$C_p = \frac{mV_t^2}{r} \text{ or } mr\omega^2$$

where r refers to the radius of the circle or arc.

V_t and ω are defined further in the section on displacements with respect to time. V_t is the linear velocity at the distal end of the segment that is moving. This velocity is in the direction tangent to the arc of movement. Further explanation of centripetal and centrifugal forces is presented in a later chapter in relation to specific activities.

Forces in air and water environments

As a body applies a force to, or interacts with, air or water, the particles of air or water are disturbed and experience a change in speed and direction in direct proportion to their resistance to the body. This resistance, which is in keeping with the law of interaction, produces what is termed a drag force. The amount of resistance of the fluid is dependent on its energy, which is influenced by pressure, velocity, and position with respect to the body encountered by air or water. The basis for the understanding of the human body's interacting

with the fluid, whether air or water, is Bernoulli's principle, which states that fluid pressure is decreased whenever speed of flow is increased.

Air and water flow past a symmetric object, such as a smooth ball, with a minimal disturbance in the flow pattern. Fig. 5-5 shows this laminar flow with little turbulence. Resistance may therefore be considered negligible, especially in an air medium; the fluid does little to alter the path of the object. Laminar flow will have different velocities, and the line of flow closest to the surface of the body will be the slowest. This difference in velocity will be dependent on the size of the shear stress, that is, the surface friction. For example, the skin of the dolphin offers an infinitesimal surface friction compared with human skin.

Contrast the laminar flow of Fig. 5-5 with the turbulent flow of Fig. 5-6. In Fig. 5-6, *A,* the object is asymmetric, and the flow separates from the object and produces eddies early in its flow past the object. This turbulence creates greater resistance to the movement of the object through the fluid—air

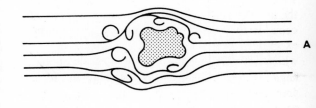

A

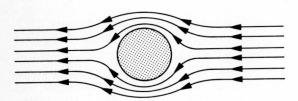

Fig. 5-5. Streamlined or laminar flow of fluid (or air) as a result of interaction with smooth-surfaced sphere.

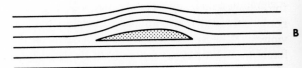

B

Fig. 5-6. A, Turbulent flow of fluid (or air) as a result of interaction with asymmetric, rough-surfaced, irregular object. **B,** Flow of fluid (or air) as a result of interaction with streamlined object.

or water. In fact, the eddies can create suction forces, which produce a backward force. Drag resistance is also increased in this situation as compared with that of Fig. 5-5. Drag is the force normal to the surface of the object on which the force is exerted. Thus the forward parts of the object encounter a resistance to forward travel. This resistance is known as drag force because it opposes motion.

Drag force exists with all bodies, of all shapes and sizes, traveling through air, water, or other fluid. Rough, deformed, or less streamlined bodies will experience greater resistance than will those bodies said to be "aerodynamically designed."

The lift force depicted in Fig. 5-6, *B,* involves an object shaped like an airplane wing and an effectively pitched hand of a skilled swimmer. In each case the flow of the fluid over one surface is faster, creating a low-pressure area, than over the other surface, for which there is a high-pressure area. Thus the airplane or a discus is lifted upward, and the swimmer may be moved forward or laterally depending on the position of the hand. This lift force always acts at right angles to the drag force, which is parallel to the direction of movement of the body or body part being analyzed. Both forces occur at all angles of tilt of this streamlined body except (1) at a 90-degree angle of rejection, in which only drag occurs, and (2) at a zero-degree angle, at which only lift occurs. Thus the 45-degree angle of incline of the body will experience equal amounts of lift and drag. The special effects of drag and lift forces will be discussed further in this chapter and also in Chapters 16, 17, 18, and 19.

Although special names have been given to the forces in air and water, they can be divided into normal and tangential forces and related to the previously described explanation of forces. Drag force can be considered a reaction force as a result of action of the body on the water. For example, as a rower pushes against the water with the oar blade, the water pushes back on the oar blade. This drag force prevents slippage, or movement backward of the oar, and causes the boat to move forward. Another normal force present in water has been termed the buoyancy force of water. This force supports a body in the water, causing the body to float if its density is less than that of water. This concept is explained in Chapter 18.

A further application of the principle of Bernoulli is noted in many ball-throwing, striking, and kicking activities. For example, in the case of a golf ball, backspin imparted to the ball by the golf club helps to create high- and low-pressure areas and thereby a drag-lift differential. This effect has also been called the Magnus effect, after a German engineer who is credited with first noting the curved path followed by a cannonball to which spin had been imparted before it became airborne. This rotation, seen in many projections of objects used in sports, usually is created by striking or otherwise exerting a force eccentric to the object. This creates rotation about an axis within the ball, and the ball veers right or left, up or down, or diagonally. This phenomenon is explained by the fact that as a body rotates, it tends to have the fluid next to it move with it, and the air or other fluid just beyond this so-called boundary layer is influenced. As the object travels through a medium such as air and meets the oncoming air, a high pressure is then developed on the side of the direction of the spin and a low pressure on the opposite side. The ultimate result is a curved, rather than a linear, path.

DISPLACEMENTS WITH RESPECT TO TIME

When movement occurs, the most readily identifiable parameter is displacement: how far the body or body part was moved and in which direction, whether linear or rotatory, the movement occured. Through the measurement of angles and distances, valuable information such as the following can be obtained:

1. Length of stride during walking: Is the stride too short or too long for efficient movement?
2. Direction of foot angle with direction of locomotion: Can the foot exert the muscular forces effectively with the measured angle?
3. Height of jump: Is the jump average, below

average, or above average according to achievement norms?

4. Direction of arm movement during throwing: Did the arm move toward the target?

5. Relationship of lean of trunk, position of legs, and other body parts: Are the distances and angles the same as those seen in highly skilled performances?

Displacement analysis is not enough because forces are ignored and therefore are an unknown quantity. For example, two balls may be thrown a distance of 9 m (30 ft), but one may take half the time to travel that distance than the other ball takes. Therefore using the following examples, one can conclude that one ball projection is effective whereas the other ball projection is not:

1. The faster ball, if thrown by a softball player to first base, will arrive to cause the batter–base runner to be ''out.''

2. The faster ball cannot be stopped by a soccer goalkeeper.

3. The faster ball cannot be intercepted by an opposing basketball player.

Displacement with respect to time is more important than displacement alone. Speed is the change in position (displacement) with respect to time if the displacement is not given a direction. If the direction is specified, the displacement with respect to time is called velocity. The equation for determining the magnitude of either is the same:

$$\text{Velocity} = \frac{\text{Change in position}}{\text{Change in time}} = \frac{\text{Displacement}}{\Delta \text{ time}}$$

Thus one may refer to the speed of a racehorse, a sprinter, or a sailboat as being a certain number of kilometers per hour or meters per second. The velocity would be in these same units but in the horizontal direction, at an angle of 20 degrees with the vertical, or in some other system denoting direction.

Angular velocities provide information concerning the ability to perform somersaults and move body parts fast enough for a given task. There is a basic relationship between linear and angular velocities, since the angular velocity (ω) can be re-

solved into two components. One component is parallel to the path in the arc at the instant of viewing. It is the tangenital velocity (V_t), since without the second component, radial velocity, the movement would continue on a tangent to the arc, in a straight line. The radial component is directed inward along the radius at each instant of time, to maintain the circular path of the limb. It is at right angles to the tangential component and could be considered normal to the movement. One relationship might be noted here:

$$V_t = r\omega$$

Given the same angular velocity, the tangential velocity will increase as the radius increases. This definition of V_t is very important in throwing, kicking, and striking activities and will be discussed in Chapters 14 and 15. It is also important in the swinging activities of gymnastics.

Knowing the speed or velocity of the movement does not provide information about the forces that created this speed or velocity. The rate of change in velocity, however, equals the acceleration of the body, from which one can calculate force: $F = ma$. The equation for determining the acceleration of a body is as follows:

$$\text{Acceleration} = \frac{\text{Change in velocity}}{\text{Change in time}}$$

Figs. 5-7 and 5-8 show the relationship of displacement, velocity, and acceleration with respect to angular and linear motion.

The following are known relationships concerning displacement, velocity, and acceleration, whether angular or linear:

1. When the amount of displacement increases from one time period to the next, the velocity increases.

2. When the displacement remains constant from one time period to the next, the velocity is constant and the acceleration is zero.

3. When there is a reversal of direction in displacement, the velocity will be zero at the instant of reversal.

Text continued on p. 83.

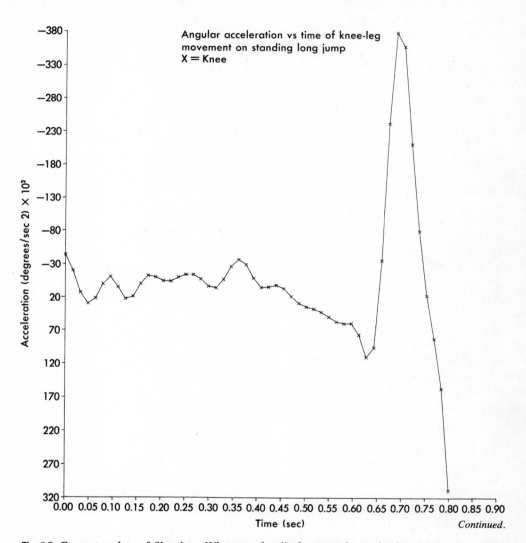

Fig. 5-7. Computer plots of film data. When angular displacement is maximal or minimal, angular velocity is zero. When angular displacement slope is greatest, angular velocity is maximal and angular acceleration is zero.

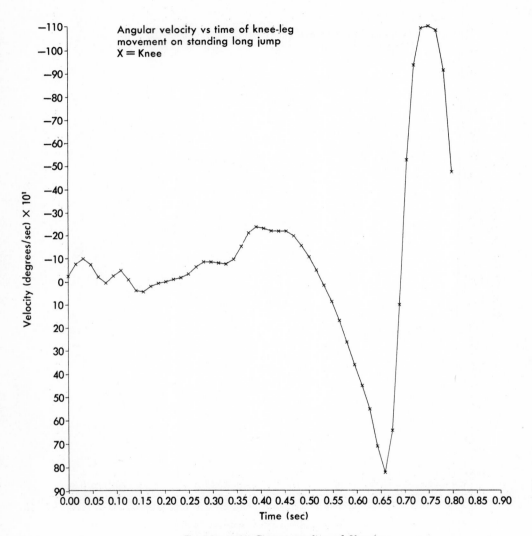

Fig. 5-7, cont'd. Computer plots of film data.

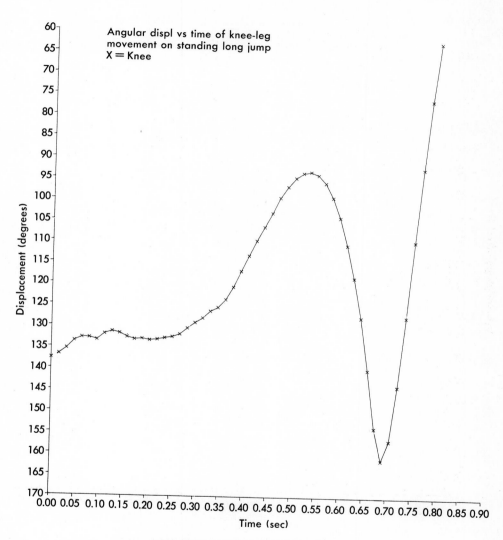

Fig. 5-7, cont'd. Computer plots of film data.

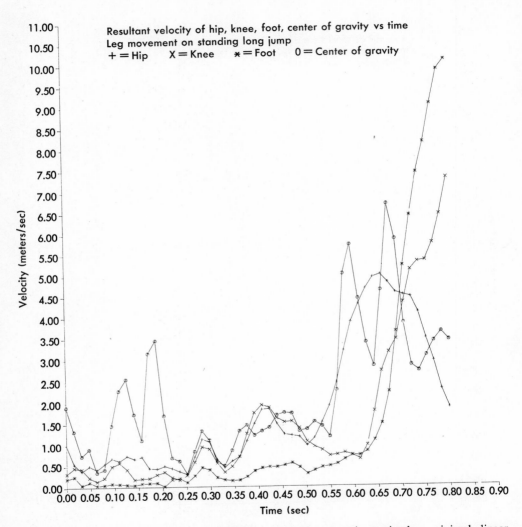

Fig. 5-8. Computer plots of film data. When linear displacement is maximal or minimal, linear velocity is zero. When linear displacement slope is greatest, linear velocity is maximal and linear acceleration is zero.

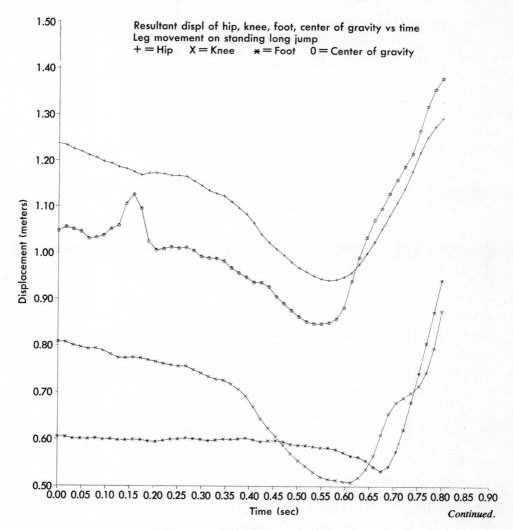

Fig. 5-8, cont'd. Computer plots of film data.

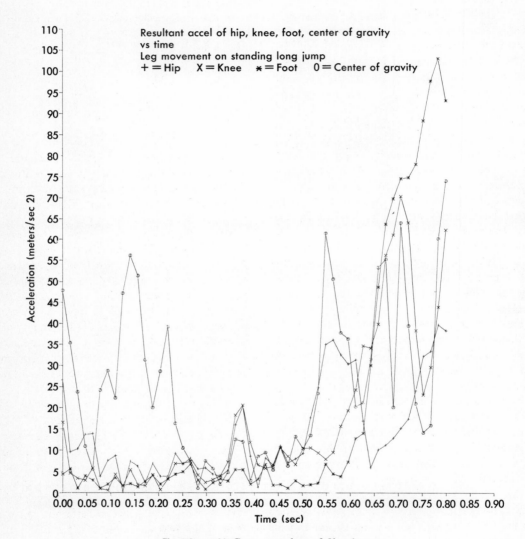

Fig. 5-8, cont'd. Computer plots of film data.

4. At the instant of maximal velocity, the acceleration is zero.

These relationships are seen readily in an analysis of running. The displacement of the body from the first stride to the fifth increases as the time for each stride becomes less. Thus the velocity increases, and since the velocity is not constant, positive acceleration occurs. At some point in time the length of stride and the velocity become constant; negative acceleration (deceleration) occurs until the acceleration ceases and becomes equal to zero. Minute changes probably occur in all forms of locomotion at the instant of foot plant and push-off, but these are being disregarded. The runner maintains this constant velocity, with zero acceleration, until the end of the race, at which time acceleration (change in velocity) occurs.

Although the total body kinematics just described for a runner may be defined easily, the same statement cannot be made with regard to the kinematics of the body segments. Accelerations and decelerations of the limbs continue to occur even when the total body moves at a constant velocity. Since limb accelerations are angular in nature and are derived from angular velocities, there are two components of angular acceleration that define α in linear terms: tangential and radial. Their directions are the same as those described for tangential and radial velocities.

Analysis of the kinematics of projectiles is easy if all forces are considered to be negligible except the force of gravity. The acceleration of any projectile then becomes the acceleration of gravity (9.8 m/sec² as an average value) in the vertical direction. A convenient equation for determining the kinematics of a projectile is $s = \frac{1}{2}at^2$, where s = distance in the vertical direction, a = the acceleration of gravity, and t = time. Although the formula $s = vt + \frac{1}{2}at^2$ can be applied more universally than $s = \frac{1}{2}at^2$, there is always some point during the flight of the projectile, whether a ball, a human body, an animal, or another object, at which the vertical velocity will equal zero and the descending flight pattern will begin. Thus the vertical velocity (vt) is equal to zero.

If the descent of the projected object is timed, the maximal vertical distance of projection may be calculated. For example, if a ball requires 1 second to fall to the ground from its highest elevation from the ground, this elevation is equal to 4.9 m.

When objects are projected horizontally, with zero vertical velocity, one can measure the height above the ground at the time of projection. Time is equal to the square root of $\frac{2a}{S}$, that is:

$$t = \sqrt{\frac{2a}{S}}$$

Then the velocity of the projectile in the horizontal direction can be determined, since the horizontal distance traveled, divided by the air time, will equal the horizontal velocity. The horizontal distance is easy to measure.

These displacements with respect to time provide insight into the kinetics of movement. As has been shown previously, an estimation of the forces acting on the body may be determined by measuring the acceleration of the body and multiplying this value by the mass of the body. If the force is known (measured by means of dynamographic devices), one can estimate the resulting acceleration of the body. Thus the outcome of the performance or the effectiveness of the muscle coordination may be assessed or predicted.

However, the force platform measures force with respect to time, not merely force. It is now necessary to approach the analysis of movement in a holistic manner and view force as an action occurring in a known period of time and through a known distance of application. Thus force itself exists as a temporal and spatial entity and should be viewed as such to more completely understand movement.

MINI LABORATORY EXERCISES

1. Select a smooth-surfaced plank 3 m long and set it on an incline.
2. Place a smooth-surfaced ball at the top of the incline and release the ball without applying force.

a. Using a stopwatch or an automatic timing device, record the number of seconds from release of ball until it rolls the 3 m.
b. Repeat the test until reliability is satisfactory.
c. Measure the angle of inclination of the plank.
d. Measure or calculate the height of descent of the ball. This can be determined trigonometrically by the following equation:

$$ht = \sin \theta \ (3 \text{ m})$$

which is the same as that explained in Appendix B: Opposite side = Sin θ (hypotenuse).
e. Using all these data, show that gravity is a constant force producing 9.8 m/sec². Remember the following equation:

$$s = \tfrac{1}{2}at^2$$

or

$$a = \frac{2s}{t^2}$$

f. Repeat the test, using two different angles of inclination of the board. The same results should occur.

IMPULSE-MOMENTUM

Although the external forces, such as gravity, that act on living bodies frequently possess constant magnitudes, rarely do any of the forces produced by the living body in motion have a constant magnitude. Each force acts for a period of time ranging from short to long in duration. Muscle forces required to maintain a static position may be of the same magnitude over a short period of time, but variation in muscle force during movement of a body segment almost always occurs. This variation is due to such factors as the angle at the joint, the speed of movement, the length of the muscle, and the position of the limb in space at each particular point in time. Furthermore, most human and animal movements require more than one contracting muscle or group of muscles. Therefore several forces are created when different body parts move in a prescribed sequence and with a specific speed. This utilization of several body parts in time is called coordination, which also may be referred to as a summation of forces, development of momentum, or creation of kinetic energy.

Summation of forces

The principle of summation of forces states that the force produced during movement of one body part will be added to the force produced by the next body segment, and so on until the final action. The most effective timing of these forces has not been investigated thoroughly for all movements of humans and animals. Evidence does suggest, however, that each force should occur at the time of maximal velocity of the preceding action. An investigation of velocity of motion is therefore necessary and can be approached through the following example:

A girl of elementary-school age creates muscle force for a short duration of time to accelerate her leg. The foot of her swinging leg contacts a soccer ball and applies force to the ball for a very short period of time. This causes the ball to accelerate, which creates velocity and displacement.

This physical phenomenon can be depicted as a cause-and-effect relation by using the equation $F = ma$ and modifying it to represent the force acting over a period of time (t):

$$Ft = mat$$

The product Ft is called impulse, or impulse of force, and its units are newton-seconds (Nsec). Since velocity equals at, the equation can be rewritten as follows:

$$Ft = mV$$

The product mV is termed linear momentum, and its units also are newton-seconds. This equation is known as the impulse-momentum equation. A given impulse will create a given momentum.

In actuality, the equation is more complex, since acceleration represents a change in velocity with respect to a change in time, not merely the relationship $a = \dfrac{V}{t}$. Readers acquainted with calculus will recognize the following rewriting of the equation as the integral Ft being equal to the change in momentum:

$$\int Ft = m_f V_f - m_i V_i$$

The subscript $_f$ refers to final momentum, and the subscript $_i$ refers to initial momentum. The integral

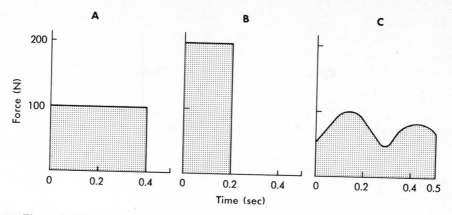

Fig. 5-9. Theoretical impulses of 40 Nsec but with different amounts of force and different durations of application of force. Most human and animal motion resembles variable magnitude of force application.

($\int$) merely means the area under a force-time curve. A force-time curve is a graphic representation of the amount of force occurring at each point in time over a selected period. Three such curves are depicted in Fig. 5-9. The areas of the rectangles of force-time can easily be determined by multiplying the length of time by the magnitude of force. In Fig. 5-9, *A,* the force was a constant 100 N for 0.4 second, whereas in Fig. 5-9, *B,* a greater force, but still constant, was applied for 0.2 second. The situation in Fig. 5-9, *C,* is the more common force-time curve seen with human and animal movements and is the more difficult area to measure. The areas of all three situations are identical and show that the person applied an impulse of 20 Nsec to the ball. Despite the difference in maximal force production, since the impulses are identical, the velocity of the ball will be identical for all three situations.

Therefore the product of force and time of application of the force will determine the amount of momentum that can be achieved. The human body makes a compromise between the development of maximal force and maximal time of application of force. If the person allows too much time, such as using a full squat position before jumping, maximal force cannot be achieved because the muscles are in a disadvantageous angle for exerting force upward. The time of execution of the propulsive action of leg extension will be too long. In long jumping, the jumper must have enough time on the takeoff board to complete the leg extension. Too short a time will be ineffective. Likewise, too long a time will cause the person to decrease the horizontal speed acquired during the run and therefore to decrease the force. Thus the ability to generate maximal impulse is dependent on anatomic considerations such as muscle strength, length of limbs, and position of limbs, as well as the ability to coordinate the movements (neurologic integration). Maximal impulse will be achieved by the best, or optimal, combination of force and time of application of force. Impulse creates velocity in a particular mass. Since a certain impulse will create a certain momentum, the greater the mass, the less will be the velocity. All the principles listed with respect to F = ma are applicable to the impulse-momentum equation.

Both the force platform and computerized cinematographic analysis have made it possible to analyze the impulse and momentum of performances and, from the point of view of safety, the impulse and momentum of impacts, or collisions.

Conservation of momentum

Linear momentum. Impacts, or collisions, of two bodies result in a change in momentum for each of the two bodies. This phenomenon has been called a transfer of momentum but is better defined as a conservation of momentum, which is simply a rephrasing of Newton's third law, the law of interaction (action-reaction). The law of conservation of momentum states that when two or more objects collide with each other, the total momentum after impact is equal to the total momentum before impact. For example, when a bowling ball traveling at 7 m/sec and weighing 98 N strikes a stationary pin weighing 9.8 N (these higher-than-normal weights are given for ease of subsequent computations), the momentum of the ball and of the pin after impact will be equal to the momentum of the ball and the pin before impact. The pin, being the lighter of the two masses, will have the greater velocity after impact, but the ball will not experience much loss of velocity after impact, since its mass is 10 times that of the pin. As an illustration, if the pin acquired a final velocity twice that of the "before-impact velocity" of the ball, the changes in momentums and ball velocity would be as follows:

Before impact   After impact

$$m_{b_1} V_{b_1} = m_{b_2} V_{b_2} + m_p V_p$$

$$\frac{98 \text{ N}}{9.8 \text{ m/sec}^2} \times 7 \text{ m/sec} = \frac{98 \text{ N}}{9.8 \text{ m/sec}^2} \times V_{b_2} + \frac{9.8 \text{ N}}{9.8 \text{ m/sec}^2} \times 14 \text{ m/sec}$$

$$70 \text{ Nsec} = 10 \text{ Nsec}^2/\text{m} \times V_{b_2} + 14 \text{ Nsec}$$
$$56 \text{ Nsec} = 10 \text{ Nsec}^2/\text{m} \times V_{b_2}$$
$$5.6 \text{ m/sec} = V_{\text{ball after impact}}$$

The ball velocity decreased by 1.4 m/sec, whereas the pin velocity increased 14 m/sec. The momentum of the ball was 70 Nsec before impact and 56 Nsec after impact.

Since velocity is a vector, the assumption was made that the collision of the bowling ball and pin was a head-on collision and that all velocities were additive, that is, along the same line. If the impact had been at an angle, the momentums would have been resolved into two components (planar motion) or into three components (three-dimensional motion) to calculate the angles of deflection of both objects after impact. Because of the conservation-of-momentum principle, both objects will be deflected from their original line of motion because the impact will have a component parallel (shear force) to the objects, as well as perpendicular (normal) to the objects.

Success in the sports of billiards, racquetball, handball, and squash, as well as other games in which balls rebound from surfaces, rely on the performer's ability to judge both the ball's angle of rebound and its speed of rebound. Although trial and error, as well as experience, may be prime factors in acquiring such judgment, the ability to solve the conservation-of-momentum equations and to explain the concept may provide the analyst with a means of shortening the trial-and-error method. The necessary skills will be thoroughly treated in Chapter 15. In addition, any spin force, friction force, and deformation of the two bodies during impact will introduce factors that will affect the measured velocities after impact. The bowling ball–bowling pin impact was as nearly a perfectly elastic situation as can be seen in any sport. An elastic situation is one in which no momentum is dissipated in heat energy, energy to deform the materials, or other forms of energy. The effect of not so perfectly elastic situations, such as when two human bodies collide or a tennis ball collides with a racquet, will be discussed in the work-energy section of this chapter.

Angular momentum. Moments of force also act over a time period. The created momentum from the product moment of impulse (Mt) is termed angular momentum and is written as I_ω. The moment of inertia (I), or the resistance to rotation or turning, is measured as the mass of the object multiplied by the radius, squared, of the rotating body. The ω is equal to angular velocity. Since mass rarely changes within a movement, the importance of the radius in the determination of I is primary.

The same principles of linear momentum are applicable to angular momentum. The special case of conservation of angular momentum needs to be considered because this phenomenon often is seen in the angular motion of dancers, skaters, divers, gymnasts, jumpers, and other persons involved in airborne athletics, as well as in any person or animal using rotatory movements. For example, a diver will tuck in the arms and legs, an action that concentrates the mass closer to the axis of rotation and thus decreases the moment of inertia of the body about this axis. Since angular momentum can be altered only by external couples or eccentric (off-center) forces, and since the tucking of body parts is due to internal forces, angular momentum is not affected and will not change. Thus angular velocity increases to maintain the constant angular momentum and to allow the diver to execute a turn in a shorter time. The dive can therefore be completed well above water level to provide for a nearly vertical and controlled entry into the water. In another example the ballet dancer and ice skater will start a slow spinning motion with the arms held horizontally and then will bring the arms quickly to the chest area to increase the angular velocity of the spin. The reverse action with the arms will be used to slow the spin and initiate another movement.

Thus athletes, by changing the length of their body segments to redistribute their masses, are able to cause changes in their angular velocities (ω) because of the conservation-of-angular-momentum principle. The momentum remains the same, but the overall movement appears different to the viewer and to the performer because of the change in ω. These changes in ω produced by movement of body parts will vary with the body segment involved, as well as with different individuals. For example, the leg has a greater mass than the arm; consequently movement of the leg will produce a greater change in ω. Long-limbed and heavy-boned individuals will be able to produce greater changes in ω than will individuals with short limbs or lightweight distal segments. If a person attempts to perform rotatory movements with weights either held in the hands or strapped to different body parts, a more dramatic change in angular velocity will be noted with a redistribu-

tion of these weights than without weights, since there will be a greater change in the moment of inertia.

Principles

1. Greater impulses of force produce greater changes in momentum and greater final velocities.
2. For the same impulse, the greater the mass, the less will be the final velocity, since the momentum remains constant.
3. Given the same force, an increase in time of application of force will impart greater velocity to a body. In striking activities this may be possible and is referred to as "hitting through the ball."
4. Maximal impulse can be created by maximizing the force, by maximizing the time of application of force, or by combining optimal force with optimal time. The latter strategy usually is preferred for movements involving locomotion or jumping.
5. Momentum is conserved in the collision of two or more objects; large masses will have low final velocities compared to small masses.
6. Angular momentum is conserved within a body by an increase in the angular velocity as a result of a decrease in the moment of inertia, and vice versa.
7. Since a moving body possesses momentum, an impulse of force will be required to stop or reduce the speed of the body.
8. A body in motion would require no force to keep it moving in a vacuum. Since, however, friction or some other resistance always exists to some extent to reduce the velocity of a body in motion, equal and opposite impulses of force are required to counteract these resistances and thus maintain the momentum of the body. These impulses are minute compared to the impulse required to develop the existing momentum.
9. To capitalize on the momentum of one's body or body part, one must make each subsequent application of an impulse of force

before the momentum has been reduced appreciably by resistances such as friction. Skilled swimmers apply this principle, as do other persons displaying what is termed rhythm, grace, and coordination.

MINI LABORATORY EXERCISES

1. Using a twist board, piano stool, or revolving chair, turn a person on the device. Time the number of revolutions for the following positions:
   a. Arms held at sides while standing
   b. Arms held at sides while standing; move arms to shoulder level while standing
   c. Order of step b reversed
   d. Weight placed in the hands and steps b and c repeated
   e. Twice the weight used in step d placed in the hands, and steps b and c repeated
   f. Other positions of your choice selected
2. Estimate the changes in the moment of inertia (I) by calculating the angular velocity (ω). Remember that the angular velocity must be expressed in radians:

$$\frac{360 \text{ (revolutions per second)}}{(2 \pi)}$$

3. Draw conclusions concerning angular momentum and movement of body parts.

WORK-ENERGY

The work-energy approach views the kinetics of motion from a different perspective than did the impulse-momentum approach. The product of force and of the distance over which this force acts represents the work done by the force on an object. Thus the concern is with the distance rather than with the time of force application. When work is done, a change in energy results. Potential energy is the capacity to do work, but no motion exists. Kinetic energy (KE) is the net result of work. The work-energy equation is as follows:

$$\int Fd = \tfrac{1}{2}mV_f^2 \times \tfrac{1}{2}mV_i^2$$

and the units are newton-meters (joules).

The work-energy approach is useful in analyzing weight lifting and for analyzing and ranking movement tasks with respect to mechanical work

and power. Collisions in which deformations are an important component of the interaction of two bodies, as in trampoline bouncing, also are better for analyzing from a work-energy approach than from an impulse-momentum, or simple F = ma, approach.

The work-energy approach is as applicable to rotatory motion as it is to linear motion, and one can explain the principle of conservation of energy in much the same way as the conservation-of-momentum principle. Conservation of mechanical energy does not always occur, however, since friction is a nonconservative force. Heat energy always results in situations in which friction exists.

Although applications will be discussed in Part Three, one of the most revealing applications of the work-energy concept concerns the downward swing of an object, for example, a gymnast on the uneven parallel bars. Fig. 5-10 shows a taller person and a shorter person beginning a downward swing from a horizontal position. The taller person will take longer to reach the vertical position because gravity is a constant force accelerating the body downward. Since the center of gravity of the body of the taller person must drop 1.3 m to reach the bottom of the swing, the shorter person will reach the bottom sooner. Work done by the taller person will be 1.3 m × Body weight, and 1.0 m × Body weight for the shorter person. Potential energy exists at the start of the movement; therefore initial ½mV² = 0. Since the final kinetic energy is equal to the work done, if both persons were of equal mass, the taller person would experience greater downward velocity during the swing than would the shorter person.

MINI LABORATORY EXERCISES

1. Place a ball on the floor, holding your hand in a position to push the ball forward.
2. Maintain contact with the ball for 10 cm, pushing with a constant force.
   a. Note the apparent speed of the ball.
   b. Record the distance the ball travels and the time of travel.
   c. Calculate the velocity of the ball.

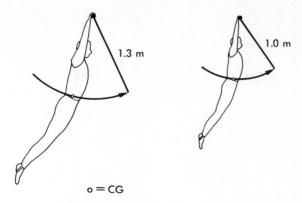

Fig. 5-10. Free body diagram showing differences in arcs of swing and vertical drops of center of gravity *(CG)* of two persons of different stature. If both body weights are equal, or if taller person has greater body weight than shorter person, taller person will do more work and develop greater kinetic energy than shorter person. Vertical drop (radius) × Weight = Work.

3. Repeat step 2 but apply the force for a distance of 20 cm.
4. Weigh the ball.
   a. Calculate its mass: $\dfrac{N}{9.8 \text{ m/sec}^2} = \dfrac{\text{Weight}}{\text{Gravity}}$
   b. Calculate the kinetic energy for each situation: $\frac{1}{2}mV^2$
   c. Calculate the force: $F\dfrac{KE}{d \text{ (in meters)}}$
5. Interpret the data: What was the effect of doubling the distance of force application? Did you hold the force constant?

Potential and kinetic energy of collisions

Characteristics of elasticity. When two objects collide, the forces exerted on both objects tend to deform both objects. The property that enables a body to recover its original shape or volume is referred to as elasticity and is measured as the ratio of stress to strain, called Young's modulus of elasticity. Stress refers to the amount of force per unit area of collision, and strain is the amount of distortion (deformation) with respect to original size.

A scrutiny of the elastic properties of certain types of materials may be interesting and may have value in furthering one's understanding of the kinetics of collisions. Rubber, for example, is not perfectly elastic and therefore does not return to its original shape if distorted to the maximum. In fact, high-tempered steel and spring brass are much more elastic than is rubber. All gases act as perfectly elastic substances; for example, gas is used in pneumatic tires. Liquids are also perfectly elastic but difficult to compress. The inside of the best golf balls has a liquid core. In the place-kick the toe of the shoe of the kicker often distorts the ball as much as one third of its original shape. The baseball is temporarily flattened against the bat as much as one fourth. A golf ball may be distorted as much as one tenth or more and a tennis ball up to one half of its original shape.

Deformations are noted in shafts of long-handled implements such as rakes and hockey sticks but are not so noticeable in shafts of hammers, shovels, hoes, and short-handled implements. Some plastic used in the manufacture of sports and game equipment for children of elementary-school age may deform readily but may not easily regain their original shape. When used as striking implements these plastics are ineffective because the striking implement deforms to a greater extent than does the object to be struck. Therefore the ball does not acquire sufficient velocity for the child to experience success.

The characteristics of elasticity explain why a

small boy can hit a tennis ball farther than a baseball. The tennis ball can be compressed to the point at which it is considerably distorted. The strings of the racquet also are distorted (stretched). Potential energy is acquired. The ball and racquet remain together for a greater time (achieve greater impulse—Ft) and for a longer distance (achieve greater work—Fd), and therefore the mass of the ball will not deflect the racquet backward to any measurable extent. The work done by the boy on the baseball, however, will not be sufficient to distort it and ''carry'' the ball. The greater mass of the ball also will resist the movement more than did the tennis ball. Golf instructors recommend that some women and small men not purchase an expensive golf ball because they will not be able to compress an expensive ball (because of its liquid center) to the same degree that they can a cheaper ball, which has only a rubber center.

Coefficient of elasticity. The coefficient of elasticity is a number that has been derived to represent the characteristics of a collision between two objects. It does not measure the elastic properties of either material, but the interaction of the two materials. This coefficient of elasticity of two objects colliding with each other can be determined by the following experiment:

1. Drop a ball from a known height.
2. Measure the height of the rebound.
3. Calculate the coefficient of elasticity (e) by the following relationship:

$$e = \sqrt{\frac{\text{Height of rebound}}{\text{Height dropped}}}$$

A second method is to measure the velocity (V) of the rebounding object before and after impact. The energy lost during the collision will be represented by the loss in velocity. The equation is as follows:

$$e = \frac{\text{V after impact}}{\text{V before impact}}$$

Racquetball, handball, and squash players increase the coefficient of elasticity (also called coefficient of restitution) between the ball and the

rebounding surfaces by heating the ball. ''Never play with a cold ball'' is an adage to be followed, since the ball will not rebound as far, as fast, or as consistently as will a ''hot ball.'' Different playing surfaces will also alter the rebound of balls. Plagenhoef has studied the characteristics of balls interacting with different surfaces in terms of both coefficient of friction and coefficient of elasticity and has found a variety of values for the same ball under different conditions, including the speed of the ball as it enters the collision.

Handball players sometimes follow a procedure that has a bearing on this discussion. They soak a ''stale'' handball in hot water. The heat causes a rearrangement of molecules inside the handball, which will then bounce for a while as much as when it was new. Handball players also sometimes soak their hands in hot water to help prevent bruises. The fluid in the hands is brought to the surface and helps the skin to withstand blows.

The concept of stored energy because of easily deformed materials used for landing surfaces is an important one, especially in springboard diving and in trampolining. The material has the potential to do work on the performer by virtue of the distance through which the material has been deformed. As the material is regaining its original shape, the potential energy of the system is transformed into kinetic energy and the person rebounds from the surface. Divers change the fulcrum of the diving board and thus change the distance through which the board will deform. The result is more or less kinetic energy and a corresponding change in the height of the dive.

MINI LABORATORY EXERCISES

1. Determine coefficients of elasticity for balls interacting with various surfaces. Use the following equation:

$$e = \sqrt{\frac{\text{Height of rebound}}{\text{Height of drop}}}$$

2. Test environment factors such as the following:
   a. Heated ball
   b. Cold ball

c. Underinflated ball
d. Ball with attached padding

REFERENCE

Plagenhoef, S.C.: Patterns of human movement: a cinematographic analysis, Englewood Cliffs, N.J., 1971, Prentice-Hall, Inc.

ADDITIONAL READINGS

Daish, C.B.: The physics of ball games, London, 1972, English Universities Press.
Dempster, W.T.: Free-body diagrams as an approach to the mechanics of human posture and motion. In Evans, F.G., editor: Biomechanical studies of the musculoskeletal system, Springfield, Ill., 1961, Charles C Thomas, Publisher.
Hooper, B.G.: The mechanics of human movement, New York, 1973, American Elsevier Publishing Co., Inc.
Merzkirch, W.: Making fluid flows visible, Am. Sci. **67:**330-336, May-June 1979.
Terauds, J., and Dales, G.G., editors: Science in athletics, Del Mar, Calif., 1979, Academic Publishers.
Tricker, R.A., and Tricker, B.J.K.: The science of movement, New York, 1967, American Elsevier Publishing Co., Inc.

CHAPTER 6

Anatomic considerations: structure and forces

Human beings, animals, fish, and birds do not choose their structure; each structure is inherited. Within limits, structure can be modified by environment, exercise, and nutrition. Therefore movements may be modified, since movements are dependent on structure. Movements, however, have limitations imposed by inheritance of the structure of bone, muscle, joints, and nerve patterns. Thus structure influences function, and function influences structure. It is important to understand this interrelationship because movements are produced by forces, and forces act on the body structures. This chapter will describe the structure of bones, joints, and muscles to provide a basis for the understanding of Chapter 7, which describes the foundation of movement: the muscle-bone lever systems. In addition, the effect of forces on bone will be presented to show how this particular structure can be modified.

THE SKELETON

Skeletons of modern terrestrial forms have many similarities. Differences exist in the number of bones and in the types of articulations between the bones that limit the types of locomotion and manipulation possible by any given species. The human skeleton has more than 200 bones, 126 forming the appendicular skeleton. The appendicular skeletons of hoofed quadrupeds, however, have

fewer bones, and therefore quadrupeds lack versatility in manipulation skills. On the other hand, the lack of a clavicle in the cat allows it to "leap" farther than would be possible with a clavicle limiting the flexion of its forelimbs.

Bones articulate with other bones to produce joints, which may be classified according to the following six major types that are important to movement analysis:

1. The gliding joint (arthrodia), in which either the bones glide over one another or one or more bones glide over another bone, is best illustrated by the articulating surfaces of the vertebrae and the tarsal and carpal bones. Most of the movement between any two surfaces is extremely small but may be large in respect to a total segment, such as the whole foot. Each small movement is added to the next one to achieve a wide range of movement.

2. The hinge joint (ginglymus), in which one surface is round, with a knoblike end that fits into another, concave surface, and the action is hingelike and usually in only one plane about a single axis, is exemplified by the elbow joint as it moves in flexion and extension.

3. The ball-and-socket joint (enarthrosis) has the capacity to move in many planes and

many axes. Many actions, such as extension, flexion, circumduction, rotation, abduction, and adduction, are accomplished by this type of joint.

4. The condyloid joint (ovoid joint) has movement similar to the ball-and-socket joint but ocurring in only two planes, forward and backward and from side to side. The articulations between the carpal bones of the wrist and the metacarpals of the fingers are examples of this joint.
5. The saddle joint, in which flexion, extension, abduction, and circumduction may be accomplished, is an unusual joint found only in the thumb and in the articulation between the carpal and metacarpal joints.
6. The pivot joint (trochoides) permits movement in one plane about one axis. An example of the movement accomplished by this joint is rotation of the radius in the forearm.

The joints listed above are diarthrodial joints: they possess a ligamentous capsule that encases the joint and the synovial fluid, which lubricates the joint and regulates the pressure within the capsule. Two other types of joints, synarthrodial and amphiarthrodial, are not discussed because they allow negligible or no movement.

Although the types of movements are predetermined by the structure of the joint, the range of motion (ROM) is determined not only by the structure of the joint but by such factors as use, disease, injury, and extensibility of muscles, tendons, and ligaments and by the size of more distal body parts involved in the change of angle at the joint.

The arrangement and number of muscles, ligaments, and tendons surrounding a joint influence its ROM. These tissues are lengthened through use, and ROM increases with respect to the direction of lengthening. Thus, if movement is practiced in the flexion mode but never in the extension mode, ROM of flexion will increase, whereas ROM of extension will show a decrease. Likewise, an injury that separates (tears) the medial collateral ligament at the knee will show an increased abduction capability but no change in adduction.

Although very young persons appear to be more flexible (have a greater ROM) than any other age group, there are no data to show any other age-related changes in flexibility. Likewise, sex differences per se are also nonexistent. Differences that appear as a result of comparisons of age or sex groups can be attributed to primary causes, such as physical activity patterns, participation in specific sports, and habitual postures of work. For example, gymnasts have greater hyperextension at the elbow; baseball pitchers have greater ROM at the wrist; and hurdlers have greater flexion at the hip than do members of an average population. Conversely, persons whose occupations involve constant sitting usually show a decrease in horizontal extension (also termed horizontal abduction) at the shoulder. The ROM also may be reduced after participation in a weight training program designed to cause hypertrophy of the biceps brachii. In the case of extreme development of the biceps brachii, the ROM may be limited to 90 degrees of flexion at the elbow, whereas the norm shows 120 degrees of flexion before the tissues of the upper arm and forearm contact each other and prevent further change in angle at the joint.

Tendinitis, bursitis, calcium deposits in the muscle, osteoarthritis, and other disorders produce pain and resistance to movement at a joint. Therefore the ROM will be decreased, or it may be normal but executed at a slower-than-normal speed. Often the contralateral (opposite) limb may be used as a comparison of ROM that has been lost as a result of one of these disorders.

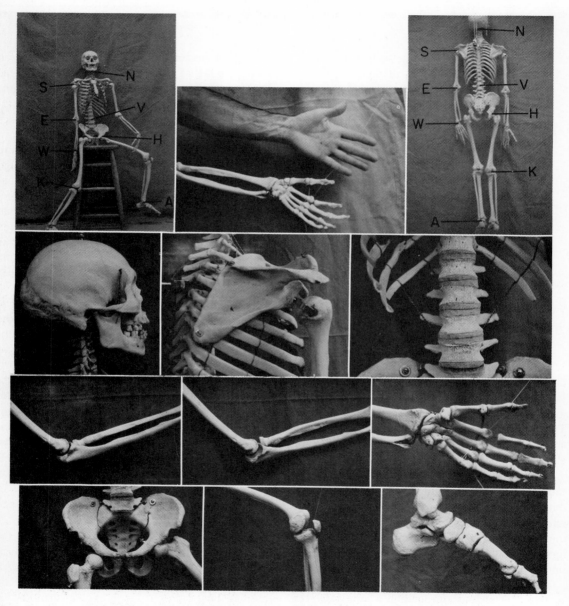

Fig. 6-1. Joints of human skeleton. (Letters shown reflect first letter of each joint.)

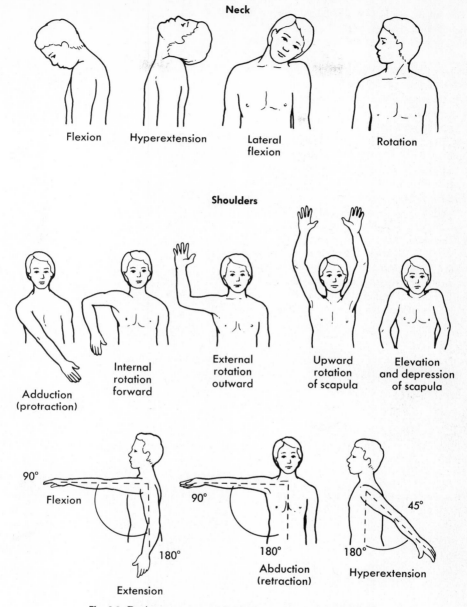

Fig. 6-2. Basic movements of skeleton: neck and shoulders.

MINI LABORATORY EXERCISES

The shapes at the ends of the bones forming the joint determine, to a large measure, the type of joint. The muscle and ligamentous structure about the joint primarily determine the range of motion possible for each of the planes of motion.

1. Observe in Fig. 6-1 the joints of the human skeleton and identify the joints with respect to the six types.
2. List the anatomic movements for each of the joints.
   a. Flexion—action of two adjacent segments approaching one another
   b. Extension—action away from flexion

c. Hyperextension—a segment extended beyond its normal starting position in extension

d. Adduction—movement toward the midline of the body

e. Abduction—movement in the frontal plane away from the midline of the body

f. Circumduction—movement of a segment in a conelike or circular motion

g. Rotation—movement of a segment in a rotatory action about its own longitudinal axis; outward rotation of the forearm so that the palm of the hand is turned upward, called *supination;* inward rotation of the forearm, called *pronation;* eversion and inversion—movements of the foot outward and inward; elevation and depression—movements of the shoulder girdle occurring in the sternoclavicular joint

3. Measure the ROM of several persons at one or more joints. Use a goniometer to read the angle at the joint when it is at each of its terminal angles, such as maximal flexion and maximal extension at the joint.

4. Study the drawings of the basic movements at the joints, Figs. 6-2 to 6-4.

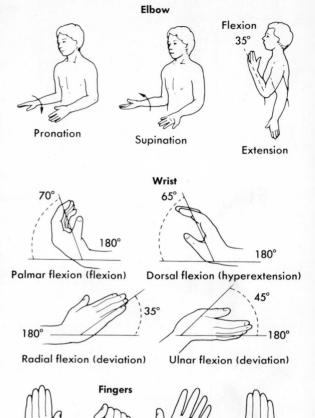

Fig. 6-3. Basic movements of skeleton: elbow, wrist, fingers, and trunk.

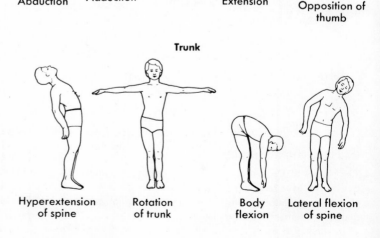

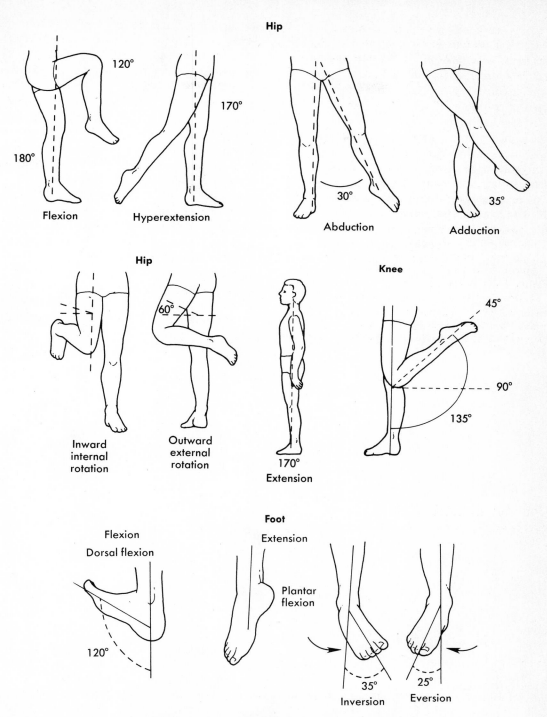

Fig. 6-4. Basic movements of skeleton: hip, knee, and foot.

Bones

Bones constitute the rigid structure of the body that must withstand all the muscle, tendon, and ligament forces, as well as the force of gravity and external forces resulting from blows, falls, or other types of collisions. Each bone has an outer, compact layer and an inner, cancellous (spongy) layer. The compact layer (cortex) usually is thicker in the cylindrical or long bones forming the appendages than in flat bones, which tend to have large muscle masses attached to them. The cancellous layer consists of a network of trabeculae enclosing spaces filled with blood vessels and marrow. Bone in general, and the long bones in particular, since long bones have a central cavity, acquire maximal rigidity with minimal weight of material. Bones are approximately 32 times stronger than muscles.

There are two major forces acting on bones: gravity and muscles. Gravity is always present and acting on bone. When muscles contract, forces are exerted on the bones. Stress is defined as the force per unit area acting on the bone. The bone reacts with an equal internal resistance to the force. There are two stresses that act axially (along the longitudinal axis), tending to elongate or to compress a bone. Elongation is produced by a force that acts to pull the bone apart, and the stress is termed tension (Fig. 6-5). The bone also becomes narrower as it elongates. The opposite occurs with compression, which is the type of stress produced by a force that tends to shorten and widen the bone. Pure compression and pure tension occur only if the force, also called a load, acts directly along the long axis; otherwise a bending moment occurs, causing tension in some portions of the bone and compression in other portions. In addition, some portions may have no stress placed on them. When a material is stressed in a fashion that causes one part to slide over another because of a blow, this stress is termed shear. Examples of various kinds of stress are given in Fig. 6-5, bone being the stressed material.

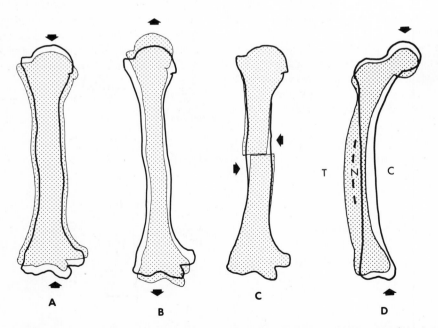

Fig. 6-5. Forces acting on bone to produce stress. **A,** Tensile stress. **B,** Compressive stress. **C,** Shearing stress. **D,** Bending moment.

A person in the upright position will experience compression on the skeletal system because of gravity. For example, the weight of the upper body rests on the knee, producing compression at that joint. The alignment of the bones, however, is such that true compression does not exist. Note in Fig. 6-5 how the weight of the upper body on the hip does not act through the long axis of the femur but produces a bending moment. The placement of the feet also will determine how the line of gravity acts through the bones. Muscle forces also act to produce stresses in bone, in addition to causing them to move. Usually a bending moment that produces both compression on the concave side of the bone and tension on the convex side of the bone is the result of muscle action.

The interplay of muscles acting on a single bone is complex and interesting as one studies the effect of muscle force on bone. Comparison of the shape of the humerus with that of the femur, for example, can be made by drawing the muscle force vectors and the gravitational line of bone weight. These diagrams (Fig. 6-5) clearly identify the potential for a curved femur, as compared with a straight humerus.

Thus the result of forces acting on materials is deformation. If the deformation tolerances of the material are exceeded, breakage will occur. The deformation per unit length is termed *strain*.

Many materials of the body have a linearly elas-

tic characteristic; that is, they deform a measurable rate for each increment of stress up to or approaching the breaking point of the material.

The hardness, compressive strength, and rigidity of bone are due to its mineral content. The tensile strength and elasticity of bone—that is, its ability to revert to original form after deformation—is due to collagen. Young bone is mainly collagenous. With age the collagen content is reduced and bone mineral is increased to constitute 60% to 70% of adult bone. The main minerals are calcium and phosphate. Water, primarily in a bound state, constitutes 25% to 30% of adult bone. During old age the mineral content of bone is reduced, and breaking strength decreases as a result of further loss of collagen, causing the bone to become brittle. Fig. 6-6 shows the changes in this deformation-strength relationship with age.

Bone modeling theories

Several theories have been proposed to link bone structure and function to external forces acting on bone. The early work of Wolf* and others has shown a mathematic relationship between trabecular direction of bone cells and the lines of stress placed on the bone. In particular, the head and neck of the femur have been studied exten-

---

*Cited in Brunnstrom, S.: Clinical kinesiology, Philadelphia, 1962, F.A. Davis Co.

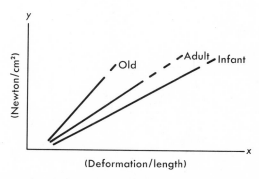

Fig. 6-6. Changes in stress and strain characteristics of bone with age. Stress is measured on *y*-axis, and strain on *x*-axis.

sively, and unique directions of the trabeculae in the neck, in the shaft, and at the greater trochanter have been shown.

There are four types of bone cells: osteoblasts, osteocytes, osteoclasts, and undifferentiated mesenchymal cells. The osteoblasts form new bone, and the osteoclasts resorb bone. Osteocytes are osteoblasts that have become trapped within intercellular material. Under appropriate stimuli the mesenchymal cells give rise to either osteoblasts or osteoclasts.

The osteocytes and collagen are oriented in two ways: randomly and lamellarly. Lamellar bone alternates, by a 90-degree shift, the orientation of fibers. This arrangement adds strength and prevents a fracture line from extending without encountering great resistance. A spiral arrangement of lamellae around a haversian canal is called an osteon unit.

These facts and numerous x-ray films of the architecture of bone by Hall have given rise to

what has been described by Evans as "the bone-cell response theory." Fig. 6-7 depicts this theory in its simplest form. As stress is placed on a bone site, the osteoblast activity is increased and new bone cells are formed at that site. Conversely, at nonstress sites osteoclast activity predominates and bone cells are resorbed. Thus bone remodeling occurs in direct response to loads placed on the bone.

Although diet and other factors also influence bone growth and bone remodeling, the stresses placed on bone are a major consideration, as evidenced by analysis of normal growth of bones in children; bone responses to treatment, immobilization, and changes in environment (outer space); and the effects of sports and physical work on bone.

Normal growth of bones in children. The bones of infants are mostly cartilaginous and deform readily. Their breakage is rare, and one considers the bones to be very elastic. As the upright position is achieved, the spinal column, which is C shaped at

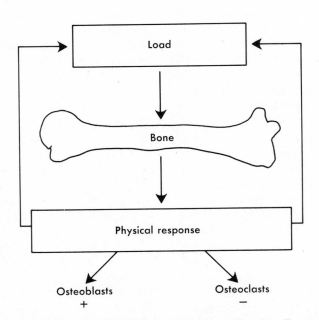

Fig. 6-7. Theoretical representation of bone-cell response theory. (Based on Evans, F.G.: Stress and strain in bones, Springfield, Ill., 1957, Charles C Thomas, Publisher.)

birth, begins to acquire the characteristic S-shaped appearance seen in the adult. The weight of the head, the position of the ribs anteriorly to the column, and the movement of the arms and tilting of the pelvis to a functional sitting position—all produce forces that remodel the shape of the spinal column. One might state that no two spinal columns are alike; that is, hereditary, nutritional, and specific postures that cause forces to act along certain lines with respect to the spinal column result in differing degrees of curvature in the cervical, thoracic, lumbar, and sacral regions.

Once the child begins to walk, a bowlegged appearance is noted. Since the bones of the legs also tend to deform with body weight, the amount and permanency of bowleggedness will depend on the calcium content in the bones, the laying down of new bone in response to the bending moment caused by the upright posture, and other factors. Permanent bowleggedness and other bone deformities will affect movement patterns and the ability to perform certain types of movements.

An extreme remodeling of the fibula has been reported in a boy born without a tibia. The fibula was made to bear the body weight. After the boy learned to walk, a second x-ray film was made, and the fibula had taken on the shape of a tibia similar to any tibia shown in any anatomy book.

Ridges, tuberosities, and other protuberances existing at the site of muscle or tendon attachments are a direct response to the tensile stress at the site. The size of these bony landmarks might well be an indication of early muscle use and strength. The strength of the bone can be exceeded, and instances of sports injuries to young children have included avulsions, that is, bone pieces separated from the rest of the bone. Such an injury occurs at the site of a muscle attachment when the muscles have become too strong too early in relation to bone strength.

A common site of injury to long bones is at the epiphyseal plate. This plate is a cartilage ring separating the long shaft of the bone from the bulbous end. Until this cartilage ossifies, it represents a weakness in the otherwise ossified bone and is a probable site for dislocation during instances of trauma to the bone. This cartilage normally ossifies after puberty, usually before the age of 21 years but at different ages with respect to the specific bones.

Bone responses to treatment, immobilization, and changes in environment. When slight tensile stress is placed on a fractured bone, the bone heals faster and becomes stronger than it does without this stress. Conversely, a bone that is immobilized begins to atrophy, bone cells are resorbed, and the bone loses strength. The influence of gravity as a stressor was recognized when the astronauts returned from trips to outer space, where the strong gravitational force of the earth was not present. The loss in mineral content—that is, the strength substances of bone—was measurable. This destruction of bone is of major concern to the kinesiologist because increasing possibilities of living or traveling other than on the earth and within its atmosphere have become realities.

Effects of sports and physical work on bone. Persons participating in unilateral sports such as tennis, baseball (especially a baseball pitcher), and racquetball typically show asymmetric development of bones. The tennis arm shows hypertrophied bones as well as muscles. The bones and muscles of the jumping leg of a high jumper also are hypertrophied. A male high jumper whose performance caliber was in the 2 m (7 ft) range was able to jump twice as high leading with the left leg as with the right leg. Indirect measurements of bone and muscle were made by measuring the girth of the thigh and the diameter of the shank and knee. Differences between these anthropometric measurements of the legs corresponded to the differences between the jumping performances.

Thus bones may be strong or weak, depending on the stresses placed on them. Muscles pulling against weak bones have been the cause of bone fractures, especially in baseball pitching, javelin throwing, and the throwing of hand grenades. These fractures are due to torsion on the bone. Torsion involves a twisting or turning of the bone with one end fixed and constitutes primarily a shearing stress on the bone.

Although data concerning ethnic or racial influences on bone density are not conclusive, blacks have been found to have denser and therefore stronger bones than whites. Men, both whites and blacks, have denser bones than women. The effect of exercise cannot be ruled out as a factor in these differences, since many of the population samples consisted of active, low-income blacks and more affluent, sedentary whites. One study in South Africa indicated that the diet was an important influence on bone density. Affluent blacks floated in water as easily as did whites, whereas the less affluent blacks showed the generally accepted characteristics of low fat, dense bones, and decreased ability to float. Caution is advised when attempting to link a cause and effect to bone strength and ethnic grouping.

Bones are strongest in compression, next strongest in tension, and least strong in shear. When a bending moment occurs, the fracture occurs on the tensile side. Take a piece of wood (pencil, ruler, or stick), hold it at each end, and bend it. Notice where the stress fracture appears initially. The same phenomenon is true for ligaments, tendons, and muscles. Although figures are not available on human tolerances in life, the limits of bone strength (ability to withstand stress) have been estimated from cadavers. For example, in the femur the limits are as follows: compression, 1406 to 2109 N/cm² (20,000 to 30,000 psi); tension, 703 to 1406 N/cm² (10,000 to 20,000 psi); and shear, 281 N/cm² (4000 psi). Naturally these values differ for each bone and each person. Increased physical exercise can increase the strength of bones.

The bones are weakest at the growth plate (epiphyseal line) before ossification. Thus contact sports offer one of the greatest risks of bone fractures to children. The latter decades of life also are a high-risk time with respect to bone fractures. If osteoporosis, or loss of bone minerals, occurs, fractures may occur with forces no greater than those experienced during normal activities of daily living.

Since bones serve to protect body organs, act as part of the movement system, and support body weight of terrestrial species, damage to the bones because of their inability to cope with the forces acting on them is of vital concern to all kinesiologists and teachers of movement.

MUSCLES

Muscles, ligaments, and tendons produce their own forces and, in turn, may be stressed as a result of collisions to the body, shearing forces to the bone, and tensile forces greater than the tolerances of the muscles. The muscles of the body produce stresses on many body parts other than bone, such as skin, organs, and connective tissue. When muscles allow the inhalation and exhalation of air, the airflow produces stresses on the walls of the airways. Similarly, the cardiac muscle initiates the blood flow, which causes arterial, capillary, and venous wall stresses.

Ligaments primarily contract to restrict movement at the joint, and tendons transmit the forces of the muscle to the bone. Since muscles are the prime producers of movement, the remainder of this chapter will be devoted to a description of the muscles, the nature of muscle tension development, and the roles muscles play in the schema of movement.

Approximately 435 voluntary muscles are found in the human body. Schottelius and Schottelius state that the importance of the body musculature is readily appreciated when one learns that it constitutes 43% of the body weight, contains more than one third of all the body proteins, and contributes about one half of the metabolic activity of the resting body. Simple and complex activities are involved when the muscles are activated against the bones to which they are attached, causing the bony levers to move. Coordination and organization of these muscles are necessary when movement takes place. This often involves not only individual muscles or a group of them but also constituent parts of muscles, as Fulton has pointed out.

When a muscle contracts, its attachments are normally drawn toward each other. This contraction exerts a tension on whatever is attached to the ends of the muscle. If the muscle fibers are pulling against the tendons or ligaments attached to bones, the muscle will tend to draw the bones closer together.

Types of muscle

The three kinds of muscles—cardiac, smooth, and skeletal (striated)—vary in accordance with their function. Cardiac and smooth muscles have similar functions, and both surround hollow organs. Cardiac muscle is that of the heart. It has some characteristics in common with skeletal muscles and is classified as striated. However, single muscle fibers such as those noted in skeletal and smooth muscle are not obvious in cardiac muscle. Smooth muscle is found in blood vessels, the digestive tract, and certain other organs of the viscera. Cardiac and smooth muscles contract slowly, rhythmically, and involuntarily. Skeletal muscles are different. They are activated voluntarily as well as reflexively, and their fibers contract with great rapidity. Huxley has stated that striated muscles can shorten at speeds of up to 10 times their resting length in a second. Skeletal muscles are usually attached to bone and cartilage. Under an ordinary light microscope these muscles are seen to be crossed by striations, whereas the smooth muscles have none. Most of the discussion in this chapter is concentrated on skeletal muscle and its function.

Characteristics of fibers of skeletal muscle

Skeletal (striated) muscle fibers are so named because they are found principally in the muscles moving the skeletal framework. Skeletal muscle is also attached to cartilage and is characterized by the cross-striated arrangement within the fibers. Functional characteristics of striated muscle are rapidity and volitional control. Whereas the contraction of cardiac and smooth muscle is mainly

reflexive, the striated muscles can be contracted by voluntarily initiated motor nerve impulses.

The individual unit of a skeletal muscle is the long, slender muscle fiber; depending on arrangement within the muscle, it will vary from 1 mm to 30 cm in length. The biceps muscle has some 600,000 fibers. Elftman has estimated that 250 million muscle fibers are present in the human body. Each fiber has an elastic connective tissue covering with slender extensions attached to bones.

Huxley states:

Striated muscles are made up of muscle fibers each of which has a diameter of between 10 and 100 microns. [A micron is a thousandth of a millimeter.] The fibers may run the whole length of the muscle and joint with the tendons at its ends. About 20% of the weight of a muscle fiber is represented by protein; the rest is water, plus a small amount of salts and of substances utilized in metabolism. Around each fiber is an electrically polarized membrane the inside of which is about a tenth of a volt negative with respect to the outside.*

A muscle consists of many thousands of *fibers* arranged parallel to each other (Fig. 6-8). Each fiber is covered with a connective tissue, or membrane, called *endomysium*. These fibers are arranged together in bundles, 20 to 100 in number, called *primary* bundles. These bundles are often called *fasciculi* and are grouped by connective tissue called *perimysium*. Several bundles wrapped together with perimysium form *secondary* bundles, and several of these bound together form *tertiary* bundles. The entire muscle is covered with connective tissue called *epimysium,* which holds the bundles together as a unit.

The connective tissue makes up the framework of the muscle and becomes the area of attachment either by a tendon or by itself directly to the bony levels. The blood is housed in the capillary beds, which are single-celled, layered structures embedded in the endomysium. Anson states, ''The

---

*Huxley, H.F.: The contraction of muscle, Sci. Am. **199**:67, Nov., 1958.

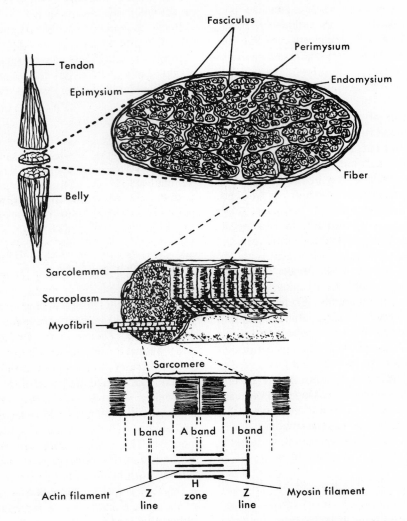

Fig. 6-8. Details of muscle structure. (Adapted from Crouch, J.E.: Functional human anatomy, Philadelphia, 1965, Lea & Febiger, and from Langley, L.L., Telford, I.R., and Christensen, J.B.: Dynamic anatomy and physiology, ed. 3, New York, 1969, McGraw-Hill Book Co.)

connective tissue sheaths, the larger intramuscular septa and the tendons of the muscles are richly supplied.''*

Each muscle fiber is cylindric in shape and tapers toward the ends. Its component parts are myofibrils, sarcoplasm, and sarcolemma (Fig. 6-8).

1. The *myofibrils,* also called *fibrils* or *sarcostyles,* are arranged in columns of several hundred to several thousand in each muscle fiber.
2. The *sacroplasm* comprises about half the muscle fiber and is the fluid within which the contractile part of the muscle moves.
3. The *sarcolemma* is the membrane that conducts the action potential through the fiber. The endomysium is the covering on the outside of the sarcolemma.

Technically the endomysium acts as the insulator, whereas the sarcolemma functions as a vehicle through which the action potential is carried to all sarcomeres. The sarcolemma also acts to hold the sarcoplasm in place.

The myofibril is the contractile structure of the muscle and is composed of long, thin elements. Myofibrils are arranged longitudinally parallel and are cross striated. The repeated variations in density, that is, the amount of proteins along the myofibrils, cause this appearance. A myofibril is 0.5 to 1 μm in diameter. Each myofibril is composed of 400 to 2000 tiny filaments arranged parallel to the length of the myofibril, and each consists of light and dark bands. Mautner has stated:

A more lucid picture of these structures is obtained by observation in polarized light, where only substances that have the property of anisotropism, or birefringence, may be seen to glow. Skeletal muscle possesses this quality. The dark or dense band glows in polarized light, and therefore is called the anisotropic or A band. In polarized light, the light band becomes the dark band and is called the I or isotropic band.†

*Anson, B.J.: Morris' human anatomy, New York, 1966, Mc-Graw-Hill Book Co.
†Mautner, H.E.: The relationship of function to the microscopic structure of striated muscle: a review, Arch. Phys. Med. Rehabil. **37:**286, 1956.

The proximal end of skeletal muscle is usually attached to a heavier bone than is the distal end. Therefore, when the muscle contracts, the distal bone is the one more likely to move. The effect of contraction on the lever depends on the position of the attachment and also on the length of the muscle fibers and their arrangement within the muscle.

There are two main types of arrangement of muscle fibers: *fusiform* and *penniform.* In the fusiform arrangement the muscle fibers are distributed in longitudinal fashion in the muscle, allowing for maximal ROM. The sartorius is a good example of fusiform muscle. Its long, slender fibers are stretched between two heavy tendons. It is the longest muscle in the body and has the greatest ROM in contraction. The sartorius in a man of average size will shorten about 20 cm (8 in) during the full action of flexing the hip and knee joints and turning the thigh outward. This great ROM is achieved at the sacrifice of strength. In addition, the parallel arrangement of muscle fibers permits such muscles to move over small distances with great speed.

The penniform arrangement of muscle fibers is similar to that of the barbs of a feather. A tendon is in the position of the quill of a feather. Variations in the penniform arrangement include *demipennate, bipennate, multipennate,* and *circumpennate.* Some of these arrangements are illustrated in Fig. 6-9. In demipennate muscles, such as the adductor magnus, the fibers are arranged diagonally between two tendons and look like a feather cut in two along the quill. Pennate muscles possess a feather-shaped fiber arrangement and include the flexor digitorum longus, peroneus tertius, and flexor pollicis longus. Fibers of bipennate muscles are double feather shaped, as in the vasti medialis and lateralis. Multipennate arrangements of muscle fibers are found in the broad muscles, such as the deltoideus and the pectoralis major. Circumpennate fiber arrangements are noted in circular muscles, such as the orbicularis oris and the levator ani.

The diagonal pulling position of the penniform muscles allows a greater number of fibers to act in

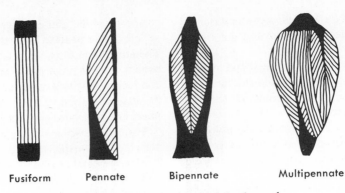

Fusiform   Pennate   Bipennate   Multipennate

Fig. 6-9. Fiber arrangement in skeletal muscle.

a given mass, but there is a loss in the ROM because these fibers are shorter. As a rule a long sheath of tendon extends nearly the entire length of penniform muscles. In the peroneus longus the tendinous sheath is 46 cm (18 in) long, whereas the longest muscle fibers measure only 2.5 cm (1 in). The greater number of fibers available for action in the penniform muscles allows only a limited ROM of the muscle but provides great strength.

The action of the muscle is such that its fibers always contract in a straight line; thus a three-part muscle may actually have discrete and different actions because of the manner in which its fibers are laid. This is evident in large muscles, such as the deltoideus. However, those muscles with tendinous extensions, such as those to the hand and foot, as they cross the wrist or ankle to connect with each finger digit or toe phalanx, are able to pull at a changed angle to contract in a straight line. Furthermore, in fusiform as compared to multipennate arrangement, the muscle has the advantage of long fibers but has a narrow origin and insertion. The reverse is true in the multipennate muscle—with broad origin and insertion, there are muscle fibers running parallel to the contracting ones.

Stimulation of muscle fiber

The conduction of an electrochemical impulse along the sarcolemma of a muscle fiber causes suf-

ficient shift of ions within the fiber to bring about the formation of an actomyosin complex. Mautner has commented on the importance of the elastic properties of the sarcolemma and its collagenous fibrils in muscle contraction. He contends that the stretching of elastic fibers constitutes a creation of mechanical energy by the chemical process of contraction. He continues, "Implications of these springlike structures are that a bouncing or recoil effect upon reversal of motion exists, making the reversal smoother and faster."*

In the stimulation of a nerve an action potential either travels over the entire neuron or does not travel at all. This is known as the all-or-none law. However, the force of contraction of a muscle fiber may vary in accordance with its contractile state—appropriate nutrients present, fibers not fatigued, and other such conditions. As to the compliance of muscle fibers to the all-or-none law, one should note that "all" must be recognized as subject to a quantitative variation in interpretation. A muscle fiber may also obey the all-or-none response, but a muscle may not, since it is graded in its response. Muscles may not have a refractory period. It could be called an *all-or-something response,* since the force of contraction may vary. Not only does an

---

*Mautner, H.E.: The relationship of function to the microscopic structure of striated muscle: a review, Arch. Phys. Med. Rehabil. **37:**286, 1956.

entire muscle display a graded response, but the same phenomenon can also be exhibited by individual fibers.

One might ask the following questions: (1) Do muscle fibers always obey the all-or-none law? The variation comes in what *all* means. If the stimulus is insufficient, it will be *nothing,* not *something.* (2) Can a muscle fire a second time without a refractory period? Yes, it may be reliably stated that such is the case. (3) Does myelination really come in degrees of thickness? The measure of thickness of myelin sheath has been given as 180 Å. The sheath is described as *lamellar,* and it is suggested that there may be about 100 layers in a mature sheath. It appears that myelination does occur in degrees of thickness.

Afferent nerve fibers are the avenue of communication between the muscle proprioceptors and the central nervous system. The spindles are one type of muscle proprioceptors and are evenly distributed in striated muscle. Mautner has said, "Any pull or stretch exerted on the intrafusal fiber and the spindle will be transmitted via the heavily myelinated nerve fiber, the two motoneurons, and the monosynaptic reflex arc to the muscle fibers, producing a reflex shortening, the myotatic reflex."* This is considered to be the fastest reflex contraction because only one synapse is involved, heavy myelination is present, and a relatively high conduction velocity is possible. The process escapes cortical control for a short time. The small efferent nerve reacts to produce the needed amount of increased discharge volley because of the stretch. This small-nerve and spindle control is considered to be the most important in the control of the maintenance of postural attitudes. When any muscle is placed in a state of readiness, a pull of only 0.05 mm is needed to activate the annulospiral ending and cause the myotatic reflex to function. Mautner has stated: "Tonus, locostation, and locomotion, which are similar in principle, all be-

ing load against gravity, depend on this myotatic reflex. Tonus restores lost balance between agonist and antagonist fiber, locostation maintains standing by restoring somewhat larger loss of balance, and locomotion regains much more obvious loss of balance."* Lifting a heavy load produces a summation of myotatic reflexes for the production of strength. The same would be true for an all-out effort in several sports.

Mautner has called adenosine triphosphate (ATP) the master substance in human muscular activity. If this is true, then the myotatic reflex should be the master switch and the muscle spindle the master key.

Some muscles give the appearance of being redder in color than others because in some fibers the sarcoplasm contains relatively more myoglobin than in others. Myoglobin, which is a pigment in muscle similar to hemoglobin, has a greater affinity for oxygen and also dissociates oxygen five times faster than does hemoglobin. The redder muscles are supplied with a red pigment that may serve to store oxygen. They are therefore more suited for performing long, sustained, slow (static) pulls. Thus it is not surprising to find that postural muscles are darker red than are many others. Whiter muscles tend to tire more quickly when subjected to sustained loads over a prolonged time. They are, however, peculiarly adapted to performing fast contractions. A comparison of the muscles of domestic fowl with those of wildfowl illustrates this point. Muscles in the wings and breast as well as in the legs of a wildfowl are usually composed of many red fibers, whereas a domestic bird has more pale fibers in the muscles of the breast and wings from lack of use. In the human body the soleus, as well as most extensor muscles, has a higher percentage of red pigment than do the gastrocnemius and most flexor muscles. The gastrocnemius is fast acting and initiates an action quickly; the soleus moves to sustain the action. The extensor muscles have the task of maintaining

---

*Mautner, H.E.: The relationship of function to the microscopic structure of striated muscle: a review, Arch. Phys. Med. Rehabil. **37:**286, 1956.

*Mautner, H.E.: The relationship of function to the microscopic structure of striated muscle: a review, Arch. Phys. Med. Rehabil. **37:**286, 1956.

posture, whereas the flexors initiate action. In human muscle, however, the distinction between red and white fibers is not as clear as in muscle of fowl and domesticated birds.

Weiner explains the difference between the finely coordinated function of the central portion of the eye, particularly its concentration on visual information, and the function of the periphery of the eye. In the central portion there is often a one-to-one relationship between a motor neuron and the muscle fibers (one-to-one relationship between the rods and cones and the fibers of the optic nerve). On the periphery of the eye the relationship is one optic nerve fiber to ten or more end organs of muscle fibers. Thus the middle of the eye is used to discriminate carefully on movement, and the peripheral fibers are used as pickup mechanisms for centering and focusing, which are necessary in determining the details of an action. A somewhat similar arrangement exists between a motor neuron and the muscle fibers of the fingers as compared to those of postural muscle. In the finger muscles the ratio of muscle fibers to each motor neuron is less than in postural muscles. Thus finger muscles can perform more finely coordinated movements.

Muscle tension

The approximately 75 pairs of muscles that are directly involved in moving the levers to maintain posture or in activating movement of all or a part of the body are capable of doing a great deal of mechanical work. Schottelius and Schottelius commented on the work of a muscle by saying that the amount of mechanical work done by a muscle is determined by multiplying the newtons of the load lifted by the height to which the load is lifted as measured in millimeters (or meters); the result expresses the work in newton-meters. It is possible for a muscle to contract when no mechanical work is involved. If a load is too heavy and is not lifted, the muscle has then accomplished no mechanical work; all the expended energy appears as heat and would have to be measured by the amount of oxygen consumed. The *optimal* load for a muscle to lift is one in which maximal work can be accomplished each time the muscle contracts. On the other hand, if the muscle can barely lift the load and develops the maximal tension that it can generate in doing so, it lifts the *maximal* load. It has been stated that no muscle can do sustained work when the load that it lifts is greater than one third to one half of its total capacity.

It is generally believed that a given muscle's strength is directly proportional to its physiologic cross section. This means that the cross section is measured in such a way that it is perpendicular to all the fibers of the muscle and not at an angle, as is often the case in an anatomic cross-section measurement. Thus penniform muscles are deemed to be stronger than quadrilateral ones. Evans states, "The force which a muscle can exert when it contracts depends upon the number, length, and arrangement of its fibers, the geometric relations of the muscle fibers to the tendon, the angle of insertion of the tendon on the bone, and the distance the tendon inserts from the joint axis about which movements occur."[*]

The tension that can be exerted by a muscle becomes less as the muscle becomes shortened. It has been postulated by some writers that this decrease results from internal friction; since a muscle does not liberate more heat as it rapidly shortens, however, this does not appear to be the case. Huxley has said:

When the muscle shortens, it exerts less tension: the tension decreases as the speed of shortening increases. One might suspect that the decrease of tension is due to the internal viscosity or friction in the muscle, but it is not. If it were, a muscle shortening rapidly would liberate more heat than one shortening slowly over the same distance, and this effect is not observed.[†]

Hill has shown that a muscle while shortening does liberate more heat but only in proportion to the distance that it shortens and not to the speed. When a muscle is stretched between two bones in such a fashion that it is elongated, this elongation

---

[*]Evans, F.G.: Biomechanical implications of anatomy. In Cooper, J.M., editor: Selected topics in biomechanics, Chicago, 1971, The Athletic Institute.
[†]Huxley, H.E.: The contraction of muscle, Sci. Am. **199:**67, Nov. 1958.

gives the muscle an advantage, in that the range of contraction is large before tension is significantly reduced. Huxley says:

Such muscles can exert a tension of about 3 kilograms for each square centimeter of their cross section—some 42 pounds per square inch. They exert maximum tension when held at constant length, so that the speed of shortening is zero. Even though a muscle in this state does no external work, it needs energy to maintain its contraction; and since the energy can do no work, it must be dissipated as heat. This so-called "maintenance heat" slightly warms the muscle.*

Huxley has further said that striated muscles can shorten at speeds that are equal to 10 times their

*Huxley, H.E.: The contraction of muscle, Sci. Am. **199**:67, Nov. 1958.

resting length in a second. They can also relax in a fraction of a second. This is because each fiber of a muscle is surrounded by an electrically polarized membrane that contains one tenth of a volt negative with respect to the outside portion. When an impulse travels down a nerve to the motor endplate, which is in contact with the muscle fiber, it depolarizes the membrane, and a substance (probably calcium) is released throughout the fiber. Then the process of liberation of energy takes place as mentioned previously, and the fiber contracts.

The behavior of a muscle in regard to shortening and lengthening has been investigated by Fick. He distinguishes between five lengths of a muscle, as shown in Fig. 6-10. The amplitude of a muscle is the range from maximal contraction to maximal

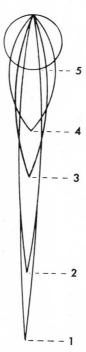

Fig. 6-10. Length of skeletal muscle in five different conditions. *1,* Maximum resting length after insertion has been severed; *2,* maximum length of intact muscle when elongated by pull of muscles on opposite side (according to Weber-Fick law, twice the length of condition shown in *4*); *3,* natural length of noninnervated muscle; *4,* maximum shortening of intact muscle in extreme flexion (usually half the length of condition shown in *2*); *5,* length of maximally stimulated muscle after insertion has been severed (one fourth to one sixth the length of condition shown in *2*).

stretch. A muscle works through a range somewhat less than its total amplitude, and its greatest contractile power is in the elongated phase.

A muscle that shortens (when contracting) to a greater extent than another has the advantage of contracting through a great distance but would lack strength in lifting a limb. The classic long-fiber muscle is the sartorius, which is reported to be able to contract a maximum of 57% of its resting length. Normally muscles with short fibers contract considerably less than this—some even less than one-third their length.

Graduation of contraction. Since an electrically polarized membrane surrounds each fiber, Huxley states:

> If the membrane is temporarily depolarized, the muscle fiber contracts; it is by this means that the activity of muscle is controlled by the nervous system. An impulse traveling down a motor nerve is transmitted to the muscle membrane at the motor "endplate"; then a wave of depolarization (the "action potential") sweeps down the muscle fiber and in some unknown way causes a single twitch.*

He further reports that even when a frog muscle was cooled to the point of freezing, the depolariza-

---

*Huxley, H.E.: The contraction of muscle, Sci. Am. **199**:67, Nov. 1958.

tion of the muscle membrane caused it to be activated into action within 0.04 second. The smallest unit of muscular movement is therefore the twitch. A weak contraction is one in which only a few fibers are involved. In *postural tonus* a few fibers are contracting all the time in an alternating fashion. As the volleys of impulses to the muscle through the motor nerve fibers are increased, new fibers are stimulated and thus brought into contraction. The extent of the effort is determined by the number of fibers sent into contraction.

Measurement of the increase in the number of active muscle fibers is only one way in which contraction may be graded in strength. The interval between repeated stimuli and the frequency of the responses account for changes in tension. As the interval is shortened and the responses become more frequent, the muscle tension is increased (Fig. 6-11).

A muscle fiber that receives a second stimulus while still responding to the first contracts to a greater degree than if it is responding to a single stimulation. If the interval between the first and second stimulus is as brief as 25 to 50 m/sec, the resulting summation of contraction may triple the tension of a single twitch.

A continuous series of rapidly repeated stimuli sent to a muscle evokes a prolonged contraction,

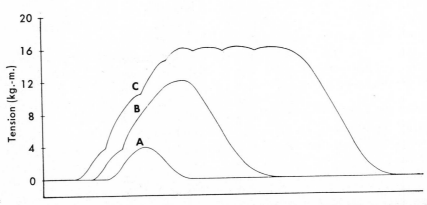

Fig. 6-11. Response of skeletal muscle to successive excitations. *A*, Single twitch; *B*, summation; *C*, tetanus.

with tension as much as four times as great as that of a simple twitch. The stimuli may arrive in such rapid succession that the muscle remains in contraction as long as the stimulation continues or until the muscle becomes fatigued.

Types of muscle contraction. Muscle contraction can be classified generally in three types: concentric, eccentric, and static. *Concentric* contraction occurs when a muscle develops sufficient tension to overcome a resistance and shortens. A body lever is moved in opposition to a given resistance. When an individual picks up an object such as a book, some of the muscles of the arm, such as the biceps brachii, shorten as the book is moved (for example, to a table). *Eccentric* contraction occurs when the resistance is not overcome, but the muscle lengthens during the action. Eccentric contractions may occur when muscles are used to oppose a movement but not to stop it, as in the action of the biceps brachii in lowering the arm gradually, whether the weight is greater than can be lifted or a light object is being slowly placed on the floor. The main characteristic is that the muscle lengthens during the action. Both concentric and eccentric contractions are called *isotonic* because the muscle changes length during the movement.

A *static* contraction occurs when a muscle that develops tension is unable to move the load and does not change length. The effort exerted by the muscle is insufficient to move one of the body levers. This condition may occur when the load is too heavy or when opposing muscles contract in opposition to each other, thus preventing movement. This fixation of a muscle's action into a static contraction is termed *isometric* because the muscle develops tension without changing length.

Classification of muscles according to function

For action to take place the muscles of the body develop teamwork through training and practice. However, individually they can do only two things—develop tension to various degrees or relax in various manners.

Since a muscle either develops increased tension within itself or relaxes (in varying degrees), it per- forms various roles as action of the skeletal levers takes place. The shape, arrangement, size, and location, including whether it is a one- or two-joint muscle, the length and nature of the tendons at the origin or insertion or both, the type and mechanical advantage(s) of the bone(s) to which it is attached, and the insertion's angle with and distance from the fulcrum of the action bones are all factors in determining how the muscle functions in moving its bony lever. Some method of classifying these roles and functions of muscles and giving them names is needed by the student of kinesiology. However, muscles are normally classified with regard to their direction of pull on the joint and the subsequent skeletal movement. Such actions as extension, flexion, adduction, abduction, and lateral and medial rotation are classified according to the direction of the movement produced in the limb. In the following pages descriptive terms are used in a more or less arbitrary manner to defend and describe these roles and functions.

It has been mentioned previously that muscles seldom operate singly; rather, they act in cooperation with one or more other muscles or as members of a team (sometimes involving most of the major muscles of the body) in a variety of combinations and patterns. Muscular contraction is not always for the purpose of causing the levers to move. It may involve contraction to help steady or support the lever, to stabilize a body part, or even to neutralize the undesired action of some other muscles. Primarily, then, muscles are *movers, stabilizers,* and *neutralizers*.

Mover, or agonist. A muscle that is known to be the principal mover or one of the principal movers of a lever is called a *mover*. This muscle, which contracts concentrically, may be directly responsible, along with one or more other muscles, for movement of a lever. The muscle is known as a *prime mover* when it has or shares primary responsibility for a joint action. When a muscle aids the prime mover in its action, it is known as an *assistant mover*. The biceps brachii is known as a prime mover of both the elbow in flexion and the forearm in supination. In addition, because of the position of its two-headed origin on the scapula, it aids in action of the shoulder joint. For example, the long head of the biceps brachii, although not often involved in shoulder abduction, becomes involved under certain circumstances. Brunnstrom claims that patients have been taught by therapists to use this muscle to abduct the shoulder when the deltoideus and supraspinatus have been paralyzed.

Although, as previously stated, a contracting muscle usually moves the lighter of the bones to which it is attached, when the feet (or the hands) are fixed and supporting the body weight, the proximal (heavier) segment is moved. This is called *reversed action*. When the foot is on the ground in running and jumping, contraction of the ankle extensors moves the leg, not the foot; contraction of the knee extensors moves the thigh, not the leg. When the hands are supporting the body weight in a hanging position, contraction of the elbow flexors moves the upper arm, rather than the forearm.

Stabilizer, fixator, or supporter. A muscle that steadies, fixes, or anchors a bone or body part against contracting muscles is known as a *fixator*, or *supporter*. The support may also be used to combat the pull of gravity and the effects of momentum and interaction. For action to take place, one end of a muscle must be free to move and the other end firmly anchored.

A stabilizing muscle is rarely in static contraction, because the part being stabilized is in motion. Actually the anchoring part may be gradually moved to direct or guide the moving part as it performs its task.

The hip flexors stabilize when the rectus abdominis and other muscles flex the thoracic and lumbar spine (from the supine position). On the other hand, the abdominal muscles and lumbar spine extensors stabilize when the thigh is being extended by the gluteus maximus, hamstrings, and adductor magnus (especially when the knee is extended and the thigh is flexed beyond a 45-degree angle). However, when the foot is fixed and supports the weight, knee action extends the thigh (reversed muscle action). The parallel pull along the long

axis of the bone that is accomplished by certain muscles makes them better suited for stabilizing a joint than others. Thus shunt muscles are considered better stabilizers than spurt muscles. This arrangement is convenient because the slower, stronger muscles help support the limbs, whereas the weaker, faster ones produce the limb movement.

Antagonist. A muscle that acts as an *antagonist* is one that in contracting tends to produce movement opposite to that of the mover. In extension, the extensors are the movers and the flexors are the antagonists. After studies of muscle action, Elftman concluded that antagonists play a strong role in walking and running. In such actions when the limbs are about to complete a movement, the pull of the antagonists aids in the deceleration of the limb.

Neutralizer. A muscle that acts to prevent an undesired action of a mover is called a *neutralizer*. Rasch and Burke use this term to avoid the difficulty with the term *synergist*. If a muscle both extends and adducts but the performer wishes to extend only, the abductors are activated to prevent adduction. They are neutralizers preventing the undesired action of the agonist.

Synergist. Authors have presented many different meanings of the term *synergist*. Morris has stated that writers in this field show little agreement, but the term continues to be used. Some call a muscle that functions as a neutralizer a *synergist*, and others use this term to mean a muscle that aids and abets the action of other muscles. Wright classifies muscles in this category as true synergists and helping synergists. The *true* synergist is a muscle that acts to prevent an undesired action of an agonist but has no effect on its desired action. The *helping* synergist is one that helps another muscle to move a lever in a desired way and at the same time prevents an undesired action.

Classification of movement

Studies of the electrical activity and the changes in tension in the various muscles involved in a voluntary movement have illustrated that a close cooperation exists between anatomically antagonistic muscles. The adjustment of the time relations and the magnitude of the responses to degrees of resistance and velocity of movement are infinitely variable. Nevertheless, rather fixed patterns of responses to different movements have encouraged systems of classification of movement. Some of these systems have been reviewed and summarized by Hill. A classification along these lines is as follows: (1) slow tension movements, (2) rapid tension movements, and (3) rapid ballistic movements.

Slow tension movements. Slow movements of body parts and objects that offer great resistance are phasic in character. A phasic movement is indicated by moderate to strong cocontraction of antagonists. The cocontraction serves to fix the joints involved in the action and to aid in accurate positioning of the body part or object being moved.

In the slow, controlled forms of movement the antagonistic muscle groups are continuously contracted against each other, giving rise to tension. Tremors occur when antagonistic muscles are in contraction and balanced against each other in fixation.

Voluntary movement has been observed by Travis and Hunter to be a continuation of a tremor without interruption of the tremor rhythm. The elementary unit of a slow, controlled movement is the *tremor*. If a short movement is attempted, its amplitude is determined by that of the tremor. Ability to make movements more and more minute is limited not by sensory methods of control but by the fundamental tremor element. Stetson and McDill have determined that the magnification of the visual field does not improve the delicacy of minute movement.

Slow, controlled movements result from a slight increase in the algebraic sum of the number of muscle fibers contracting the positive muscle as against the number of fibers contracting in the antagonist muscle group. The limb moves in the direction of the group exerting the stronger pull, and tension of the two groups of antagonistic muscles is continually readjusted.

Rapid tension movements. A movement in which tension is present in all the opposing muscle groups throughout the motion may be considered a movement of translation superimposed on fixation. Rapid shaking may develop from tremors of fixation, with one group of contracting muscles suddenly initiating the movement, followed by contraction of the antagonistic group to stop the movement. Control of these faster movements cannot be attained more often than 10 times in a second, since modifying the course of a movement is possible only at the tremor terminations and not at other points in the movement. If the tremor cycles average 10 each second, then no modification of the movement could occur in less than one tenth of a second. This limitation is imposed on the maximal rate of tapping. If the rate of tremor is 10 a second, then the rate of tapping cannot exceed that value. Travis has shown that a majority of movements of the faster type synchronize with the tremor cycle.

Rapid ballistic movements. A ballistic movement, begun by a rapid initial contraction of the prime mover, proceeds relatively unhindered by antagonistic contractions and is followed by a relaxation of the protagonist while the movement is still in progress. During a movement such as throwing a baseball, the antagonist progressively decreases in activity during the throw, indicating cocontraction. In comparison with the activity of the prime movers, however, the tension in the antagonists is slight during the ballistic type of movement. There is some question whether true ballistic movements occur in sport skills.

One of the greatest differences between skilled and unskilled movements centers around changing tension movements to ballistic movements. Attempts to make ballistic movements with muscles that are already fixed are fatiguing. Tension in one group of muscles necessitates an increase in the intensity of contraction of other sets. The spread of intensity results in rigidity, which is wasteful and restrictive.

In a ballistic movement such as a golf swing the moving limb swings rapidly about a joint, and the movement is terminated by co-contraction of the opposing muscles and the loss of momentum. If a movement is arrested by a strong contraction of the antagonistic group of muscles and as a result moves in the opposite direction, the movement is said to be *oscillatory*. Movements of great amplitude are more economical than those of small amplitude because of the intensity and continuity of muscular activity required to stop and start each phase of oscillation. A fast, shallow kick in swimming requires more effort to gain the same propulsive force than a slower, deeper kick requires. Hubbard has stated that fast action of a limb involves muscular contraction that acts as an impulse (Ft, some force for some time). A limb once set in action by an impulse will continue to move by virtue of its own momentum until acted on by an outside force. The muscle, having developed energy in the limb, then tends to relax.

MINI LABORATORY EXERCISES

1. Palpate the muscles of the arm and back while a person performs an isometric contraction against resistance to flexion at the elbow. Describe your findings and explain them with respect to muscle function.
2. Ask this same person to lift a heavy weight, using flexion at the elbow. Palpate the muscles and compare your findings with those in step 1.
3. Have a person perform a half or full squat, first with the trunk in an erect position and then with the trunk in a flexed position. Palpate the thigh muscles during the descending and ascending movements under these two conditions. Discuss your findings with respect to muscle function.

REFERENCES

Brunnstrom, S.: Comparative strengths of muscles with similar functions, Phys. Ther. **26**:59, 1946.

Elftman, H.: The force exerted on the ground in walking, Arbeitsphysiologie **10**:485, 1938.

Elftman, H.: The function of the arms in walking, Hum. Biol. **11**:4, 1939.

Elftman, H.: The work done by muscles in running, Am. J. Physiol. **129**:672, 1940.

Evans, F.G.: Stress and strain in bones, Springfield, Ill., 1957, Charles C Thomas, Publisher.

Evans, F.G.: Biomechanical implications of anatomy. In Cooper, J.M., editor: Selected topics in biomechanics, Chicago, 1971, The Athletic Institute.

Fulton, J.F., editor: Textbook of physiology, Philadelphia, 1955, W.B. Saunders Co.

Hall, C.B., and others: Normal human locomotion (film series), La Grange, Ill., Associated Sterling Films.

Hill, A.V.: Living machinery, New York, 1927, Harcourt Brace Jovanovich, Inc.

Hill, A.V.: Muscular movement in man, New York, 1927, McGraw-Hill Book Co.

Hill, A.V.: The mechanics of voluntary muscle, Lancet **2**:947, 1951.

Hubbard, A.W.: Homokinetics: muscular function in human movement. In Johnson, W., editor: Science and medicine of exercise and sports, New York, 1960, Harper & Row, Publishers.

Huxley, H.E.: The contraction of muscle, Sci. Am. **199**:67, Nov., 1958.

Mautner, H.E.: The relationship of function to the microscopic structure of striated muscle: a review, Arch. Phys. Med. Rehabil. **37**:286, 1956.

Morris, R.: Coordination of muscles in action: correlation of basic sciences with kinesiology, New York, 1955, American Physical Therapy Association.

Rasch, P.J., and Burke, R.K.: Kinesiology and applied anatomy, Philadelphia, 1963, Lea & Febiger.

Schotellius, B.A., and Schotellius, D.D.: Textbook of physiology, ed. 18, St. Louis, 1978, The C.V. Mosby Co.

Stetson, R.H., and McDill, J.A.: Mechanism of different types of movements, Psychol. Monogr. **32**:18, 1923.

Travis, L.E.: The relation of voluntary movements to tremors, J. Exp. Psychol. **12**:515, 1929.

Travis, L.E., and Hunter, T.A.: Muscular rhythms and action currents, Am. J. Physiol. **81**:355, 1927.

Weiner, N.: Cybernetics, Garden City, N.Y., 1953, Doubleday & Co., Inc.

Wright, W.: Muscle function, New York, 1928, Paul B. Hoeber, Inc.

ADDITIONAL READINGS

Adrian, M.J.: Flexibility in the aging adult. In Smith, E.L., editor: Exercise and aging. In press.

Barham, J.N., and Wooten, E.P.: Structural kinesiology, New York, 1973, Macmillan Publishing Co., Inc.

Basmajian, J.V.: Muscles alive: their functions revealed by electromyography, ed. 4, Baltimore, 1979, The Williams & Wilkins Co.

Basmajian, J.V.: Electromyographic analyses of basic movement patterns. In Wilmore, J., editor: Exercise and sports sciences, vol. 1, New York, 1973, Academic Press, Inc.

Basmajian, J.V., and Macconaill, M.A.: Muscles and movement: a basis for human kinesiology, Huntington, N.Y., 1977, R.E. Krieger Publishing Co., Inc.

Butler, D.L., Grood, E.S., Noyes, F.R., and Zernicke, R.F.: Biomechanics of ligaments and tendons. In Hutton, R., editor: Review of exercise and sports sciences, vol. 6, Philadelphia, 1979, The Franklin Institute Press.

Evans, F.G.: Biomechanical studies of the musculoskeletal system, Springfield, Ill., 1961, Charles C Thomas, Publisher.

Frankel, V.H., and Burstein, A.H.: Orthopaedic biomechanics, Philadelphia, 1970, Lea & Febiger.

Frost, H.M.: The laws of bone structure, Springfield, Ill., 1957, Charles C Thomas, Publisher.

Frost, H.M.: An introduction to biomechanics, Springfield, Ill., 1967, Charles C Thomas, Publisher.

Holland, G.J.: The physiology of flexibility: a review of the literature, Kinesiol. Rev., pp. 49-61, 1968.

Leighton, J.R.: Flexibility characteristics of three specialized skill groups of champion athletes, Arch. Phys. Med. Rehabil. **38:**580, 1957.

CHAPTER 7

Muscle-bone lever systems

Early kinesiologists likened the movement apparatus of living bodies to a lever system. Bones were the levers that were rotated by means of muscles and external forces. Anatomically, each animal and human is born with muscle attachments at particular sites. During body growth and development the muscles increase in strength, the bones become larger and longer, particularly in the case of the appendages, and the weights of the body segments change. Therefore the effectiveness of the lever system will also change. During extremely rapid growth periods, such as during puberty in humans, the lever system may seem unwieldy and unfamiliar to the person. The individual must learn again how to use the body. This was evident among the top Olympic-caliber female gymnasts who were champions at age 14 and appeared less skilled 1 or 2 years later because of changes in distribution of segmental weights and because of longer levers.

This chapter is designed to explain lever systems and their functions; to show application of effective and efficient use of the muscle-bone lever systems; and to provide a method for analyzing those lever systems which are operating at a given instant.

ELEMENTS OF A LEVER

A lever is a machine, a device, for transmitting energy: it is able to do work when energy is transmitted through it. In the human body, energy derived from muscular contraction is transmitted by the bones to move body segments. These segments may transmit energy to external objects more advantageously than is possible without a lever system.

The lever is commonly defined as a rigid bar that revolves about an axis or a fulcrum. In the body the location of the axis or the fulcrum is readily identified as a line (axis) passing through, or a point (fulcrum) within, the joint in which the movement occurs. Since these joints have widths, and since the bones forming a joint have one or more contact points, such as condyles, the concept of an axis of rotation is more reasonable than that of a fulcrum.

Identification of the rigid bar may be more difficult if the word *bar* suggests a straight mass whose length is considerably greater than its width or thickness. The word *rigid*, too, may present difficulties if it suggests an undivided, continuous mass. One should realize that exteral levers can vary in shape and in structure. A hammer can be used as a lever in both driving in and pulling out a nail. Yet the hammer is neither a straight bar nor does it need be an undivided mass; the head need only be securely attached to the handle. Even the common crowbar, often cited as an example of an external lever, although usually one continuous mass, could be an effective device for transmitting energy if it consisted of two or more segments bound together firmly enough to withstand the forces to which it might be subjected.

The student of kinesiology (biomechanics) must

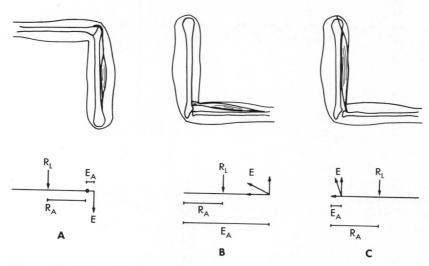

Fig. 7-1. Types of lever systems. **A,** First class—axis lies between effort *(E)* and resistance *(R)*. **B,** Second class—resistance lies between axis and effort. **C,** Third class—effort lies between axis and resistance. (*EA,* Effort arm; *RA,* resistance arm.)

realize that body levers may vary in shape from the traditional rigid bar. One or more bones may be bound together by muscles firmly enough for them to function as a single mass. For example, the bones of the upper and lower arms can be held together by muscles crossing the elbow joint; the bones of the entire arm, the shoulder girdle, the vertebrae, and the pelvis can be held together by muscles crossing all intervening joints. These variations from the common concept of external levers may suggest that lever identification in human movement is difficult. It will be simplified if the forces acting on the lever are classified as effort and resistance forces and the types of lever systems are classified according to the spatial relationships of the effort and resistance forces and the axis. There are two basic types of lever systems: (1) the type in which the forces act at points on both sides

of the axis, as in a teeterboard, and (2) the type in which the forces act only on one side of the axis, as in a door that rotates about its hinges. This latter type is usually subdivided into two types, depending on which of the opposing forces, effort or resistance, is closer to the axis.

These three types of lever systems are depicted in Fig. 7-1. Note that the lever with the space arrangement E-A-R is referred to as a first-class lever system. The second-class lever system has the arrangement E-R-A, and the third-class system has the arrangement R-E-A, in which the lever is viewed from the distal end to the proximal end. The elements of the lever systems are enumerated as follows:

1. The *axis* is depicted as a real or imaginary line passing through the joint and about which the rigid mass of the limb (lever) rotates. The axis will

always be perpendicular to the plane of movement of the lever.

2. The *point of application of effort* is the point at which the contracting muscle is attached to the moving bone.

3. The *effort* is that force acting at its application site and is represented by a vector. The vector is always the muscle—that which creates the movement volitionally.

4. The *effort arm* is the moment arm for the effort, that is, that distance from the axis to the site of muscle attachment. All the parts of the rigid mass of the lever between the axis and the point of application of effort compose the effort arm. However, the measurement of the effort arm is the perpendicular distance from the axis to the effort, not the curvature or other conformation distance along the bone.

5. The *point of application of resistance* is the point at which the external object, or the center of gravity of the mass of the lever, is applied.

6. The *resistance* is that force acting at its application site which is represented as a vector having the opposite direction to that of the effort. In the case of the first-class lever system, the direction is the same, but the effect on the lever is opposite. For example, if the effort direction and site of application cause clockwise rotation, the resistance would cause counterclockwise rotation.

7. The *resistance arm* is the moment arm for the resistance, that is, that distance from the axis to the resistance vector. All the parts of the rigid mass of the lever lying between these two points compose the resistance arm. Again, the measurement of the resistance arm is the perpendicular distance from the axis to the resistance vector. Thus all three lines—axis, resistance vector, and resistance arm—are mutually perpendicular. Note that in Fig. 7-1 all the axes are horizontal, the resistance and effort vectors are vertical, and the moment arms (resistance and effort) are horizontal but at right angles to the axes.

In descriptions of body levers the points E and R will not be precisely located. The attachment of a muscle will necessarily cover more than one point,

or there will be two or more muscles involved in the lever system. An average position must be selected arbitrarily. Likewise, R may also cover more than one point, and usually there are at least two resistances; one is the weight of the segment, and the other is an external object. The axis, too, may cause some problems in analysis, since the axis may be a line of intersection of the body and an external object, such as the foot with the floor or the hands with the vaulting horse. This lack of precision should not hinder the understanding of the lever action in the body nor the utilization of the basic concepts concerning lever systems in the analysis of human and animal movements.

Function of bony levers

As previously stated, the bony lever, together with the forces acting on this lever, is known as a lever system. If bone and muscle were isolated from the body, the lever system would resemble that depicted in Fig. 7-2. Muscle M attaches to bone V and H. The action of the muscle is one of shortening. The result of this muscle shortening may be movement (rotation) of bone V and bone H, of only bone V, of only bone H, or of neither bone. If bone H is the distal bone, it is the bone more likely to move, since its mass is apt to be less than that of the more proximal bone V. Furthermore, since the distal end of bone H is free to move, the resistance of the lever to movement is minimal. The more proximal attachment of bone V to another body segment adds additional mass to bone V; therefore bone V will probably remain stationary. Examples of these three movement possibilities are shown in Fig. 7-3.

When both bones move, the lever system actually becomes two lever systems, the muscle being the common force for each system. An analysis of the bone-muscle lever system is easiest if done on a planar level with two opposing forces. In reality, a complete analysis necessitates the investigation of moments of force in a world of three-dimensional forces. Referring again to Fig. 7-1, *A,* one can see that the muscle movement of force is equal in magnitude and opposite in direction to the mo-

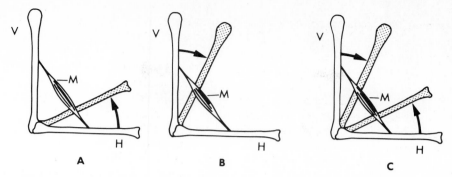

Fig. 7-2. Effects of muscle *(M)* contraction on lever system. **A,** Produces movement of distal bone *(H)*. **B,** Produces movement of proximal bone *(V)*. **C,** Produces movement of both bones *(V* and *H)*.

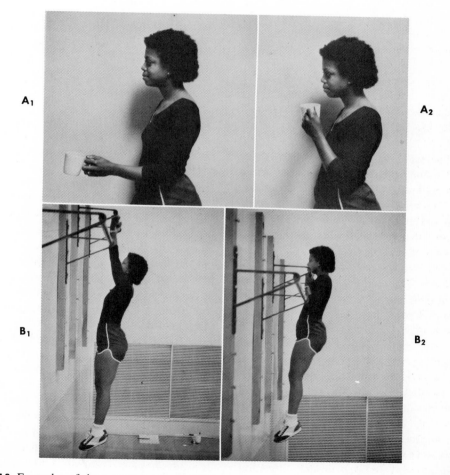

Fig. 7-3. Examples of three movement possibilities as a result of contraction of biceps brachii. **A,** Distal segment moves. **B,** Proximal segment moves because distal end is fixed.

Continued.

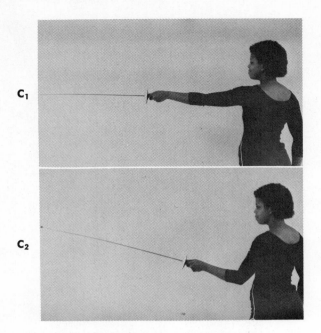

C_1

C_2

Fig. 7-3, cont'd. C, Both proximal and distal segments move.

ment of resistance created by the weight of the forearm, since no rotatory movement is occurring. The attachment of the triceps brachii can be estimated to be 15 mm from the elbow joint, whereas the center of gravity of the body segment is approximately 195 mm from the elbow joint. Therefore the muscle force must be 13 times that of the weight of the body segment (remember that the moments of force must be equal in magnitude). The muscle force is calculated by means of the moment-of-force equation, which states that the product of the force acting perpendicular to a lever and its perpendicular distance (moment arm) from the axis of rotation equals the moment of force about the axis. Note that the line of the muscle vector, the distance from the muscle insertion to the joint, and the axis of rotation are mutually perpendicular to each other. Referring to the Cartesian coordinate system, y = muscle, x = moment arm, and z = axis. Note that the gravitational vector also is vertical, or in the y direction, its moment arm is x, and the moment of force,

again, is about the z-axis but in the counterclockwise direction.

An example of the important concept of "mutual perpendicularity" is given in Fig. 7-4, which shows a comparison of the resistance moments produced in each of three options in holding a softball or baseball bat in the ready position for a pitched ball. In all options the wrists represent the axis of rotation, and the resistance arm is measured as the horizontal line (distance) from the extended line of the joint to the line of gravity of the bat. Note how the moment arm *(RA)* increases as the bat position changes from a nearly vertical position to a nearly horizontal position. The longer and heavier the bat, the more muscle force will be required of the relatively small muscles acting at the wrist. Is it any wonder that the characteristic adjustment that batters make when their muscles are not strong enough for the task is to space the hands 15 to 25 cm apart? With this adjustment the batter has introduced a first-class lever system into the ready position. The hand closest to the end exerts

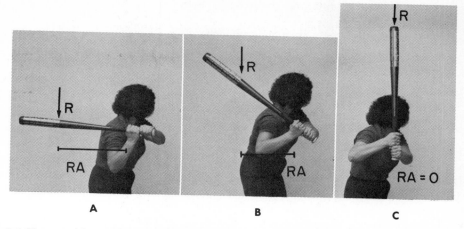

Fig. 7-4. Three positions of bat during stance phase of batting. Resistance arms *(RA)* and resistance vectors *(R)* are depicted for ease of comparison of moments of force acting on wrists.

an opposite force to that of the weight of the bat, while the other hand, which lies between these two forces, acts as the balance point, or fulcrum. The mechanical advantage of the lever system is thus enhanced. The batter now uses the stronger muscles acting at the shoulder and elbow, as well as the weight of the upper arm, rather than relying on the muscles that cross the wrist.

Components of muscle force

Muscles rarely exert forces that are solely perpendicular (90 degrees) to the longitudinal axis of the bone; usually the muscles pull at angles of less than 90 degrees. Furthermore, the angle of pull changes as the angle at the joint changes. The force vector for the muscle, then, is diagonal to the longitudinal axis of the bone and can be resolved into its two components by using the graphic, or trigonometric, method described in Chapter 5.

Muscles, then, provide both a force that is capable of moving the bone and a force that acts on the joint. In most instances the force acting on the joint acts to increase the integrity of that joint. This force is termed a stabilizing component, since it tends to draw the moving bone into the joint, that is, into a closely packed position. This force, which acts along the bone and has no moment of

force, is also referred to as a reaction force, or tangential force. The movement component of force acts at right angles to both the axis and the bone and is termed a normal force. When the bone to be moved is in a horizontal position, the movement component is a vertical force and the stabilizing component is a horizontal force.

There are instances in which the usual stabilizing force becomes a dislocating force; that is, it acts to pull the bone (lever) away from the second bone forming the joint. This occurs whenever the angle of pull of the muscle exceeds 90 degrees.

The stabilizing component of muscle force is important when the person or animal must exert great isometric forces or move at high speeds. These high speeds create great centrifugal forces, which act to pull the lever away from the joint. Dislocation would result if this stabilizing component and other assisting muscles did not exist.

Muscles possessing a larger stabilizing component than moving component are called shunt muscles. The angle of muscle pull is less than 45 degrees. Muscles having a larger moving component than stabilizing component are called spurt muscles, and their angles of pull are greater than 45 degrees. Although this classification is convenient, some muscles can act as shunt muscles with respect to their action on the distal bone and as spurt muscles with respect to the proximal bone. For example, in most activities of daily living, sports, and work, the brachioradialis functions as a shunt muscle. During the act of chinning, this muscle acts as a spurt muscle as it moves the proximal bone. Therefore this classification is useful if one remembers to identify the moving bone and the point of attachment of the muscle on that bone.

An important fact to remember is that the angle of the muscle with respect to the bone is a changing angle; therefore the amount of stabilizing and movement force also changes (Fig. 7-5). A mathematic calculation of the forces acting in two static limb positions in which an object is held is given in Fig. 7-6. Note the use of trigonometry to measure the perpendicular moment arms of the resistance and the perpendicular component of the effort vector.

If the joint permits movement in a certain plane, the ability of the person to produce movement in that plane will depend on the following:

1. Number of muscles capable of moving the body part in that plane
2. Force of each muscle and its angle of pull, cross section, and distance from the axis (joint)
3. Number of objects resisting the movement
4. Weight of body part being moved and the distance of its center of gravity from the joint
5. Weight of external objects attached to or held by the body part and their distances from the joint

Thus it is the ratio of the moment of force produced by the muscles to the moment of force produced by the resistances that determines whether or not movement will occur when muscles contract. The formula is as follows:

$$\frac{R \times RA}{E \times EA}$$

- If the ratio is equal to 1, no movement occurs.
- If the ratio is equal to greater than 1, the resistance produces the movement.
- If the ratio is equal to less than 1, the muscles produce the movement.

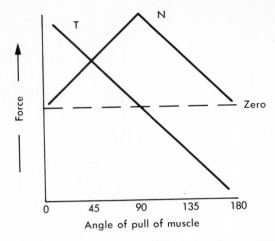

Fig. 7-5. Relationship of stabilization and movement components of muscular force. (*N*, Movement force [normal or perpendicular to bone]; *T*, stabilization force [parallel to bone, either toward or away from joint].) Below zero: for angles greater than 90 degrees, stabilizing force becomes dislocating force.

These calculations of muscle moments to produce movement presuppose that the body part is stationary and that the body part is accelerated from zero to an undefined acceleration. When a body part is moving, the movement itself is a force (*Iα*) because it maintains the object in its path and speed of rotation. Muscle force required to stop the motion is equal to the force of the motion plus the resistance moments of force previously described. This relationship is logical because a moment of force greater than the resistance moment was required to cause a certain amount of movement measured in units of acceleration. These types of calculations can be achieved by means of movie film analysis. Dillman was one of the first to estimate moments of force of muscles, which cause both acceleration and deceleration of a body part, during movement. This type of research is relatively new and undeveloped.

Single-muscle levers

The reader is encouraged to measure the moment arms and angles of muscle pull and to esti-

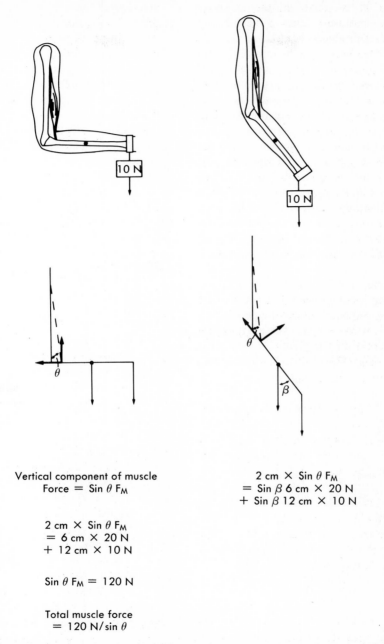

Vertical component of muscle
Force $=$ Sin θ F$_M$

2 cm $\times$ Sin θ F$_M$
$= 6$ cm $\times$ 20 N
$+ 12$ cm $\times$ 10 N

Sin θ F$_M$ $= 120$ N

Total muscle force
$= 120$ N/sin θ

2 cm $\times$ Sin θ F$_M$
$=$ Sin β 6 cm $\times$ 20 N
$+$ Sin β 12 cm $\times$ 10 N

Fig. 7-6. Free body diagrams for mathematic determination of amount of muscle force required to hold object in one of two different positions.

mate the amount of muscle force required to initiate movement as presented in the following
analyses of single-muscle lever systems. Any
muscle force that produces a moment of force
greater than the resistance moment will produce
movement.

Single-muscle levers in sagittal plane

Action of biceps brachii in forearm flexion. The
action of the biceps brachii is illustrated in Fig.
7-7, in which the muscle is shown supporting a
weight-resting in the hand. The drawing might also
be visualized as a "flash" representation of a
phase of upward movement of the weight. If the
movement starts with the upper arm and forearm at
the side, and if the upper arm is held in that position as the forearm moves forward and upward, the
forearm moves through the sagittal plane. The axis
of movement will be a line that is perpendicular to
the plane of movement and, in this situation, that
passes through the elbow joint. This line will lie in
the transverse and frontal planes, since a line may
lie in two planes, and both of them are perpendicular to the plane of movement—the sagittal. The
rigid bar includes the ulna and radius and the bones
of the wrist and hand. The effort arm is that section

of the radius and ulna that lies between A and the
attachment of the muscle (approximately 3 cm in
length). The resistance arm includes the bony mass
extending from A to the center of the weight, including the total length of the radius and ulna, the
wrist and metacarpals, and a portion of the proximal phalanges, approximately 20 cm in length.
The lever is not a simple, continuous mass but
consists of several bones bound together by muscles, tendons, and ligaments. The weight of the
forearm and hand is not included in this analysis.
The arrangement is A-E-R, a third-class lever.

Since it is known that if the weight is to be
supported, the length of A-E times the amount of
muscular force must equal the length of A-R times
the weight of the supported object, it can be seen
that the amount of muscular force must be more
than six times the weight of the object. If the object
is to be moved, the force must be even greater.

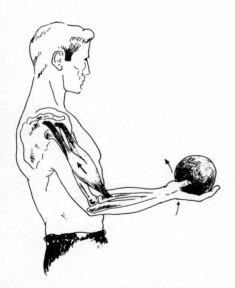

Fig. 7-7. Action of biceps brachii in forearm flexion.

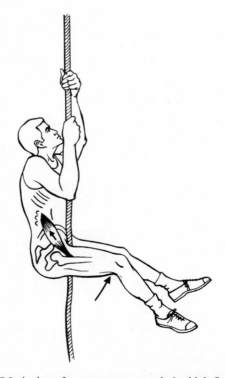

Fig. 7-8. Action of greater psoas muscle in thigh flexion.

Note that in identifying the lever elements one needs to consider only the muscle attachment to the moving segment. It is the point at which energy is applied to the lever. The muscle must have another point of attachment, but that attachment is not part of the lever, although it is an essential part of the total machine.

Action of greater psoas muscle in thigh flexion. The attachment of the greater psoas muscle to the femur is shown in Fig. 7-8. If this illustration is visualized as a phase in hip flexion, the femur is shown moving through the sagittal plane, and the fulcrum of the action is on an axis passing through the hip joint in the transverse and frontal planes. If the weight of the leg is 95 N, the muscle must oppose this force. However, the resistance arm is that section of the femur that extends from the axis to the center of gravity of the leg (approximately 36 cm), and the effort arm is only 6 cm. The effort arm is measured along the section of the femur that extends from the axis to the muscle attachment, since the leg is estimated to be horizontal. In Fig. 7-8 the angle of pull of muscle is estimated as 45 degrees. Since the sine of 45 degrees equals 0.707, the muscle force in the vertical direction is equal to

$\uparrow$ E $\times$ EA = $\downarrow$ R $\times$ RA (for equilibrium)
E $\times$ EA = 95 N $\times$ RA
E (6 cm) = 95 N $\times$ 36 cm
$$E = \frac{95 \text{ N} \times 36 \text{ cm}}{6 \text{ cm}}$$
E = 95 N $\times$ 6
E = 576 N of vertical force

To determine the total muscle force acting at a 45-degree angle, divide the vertical force by the sine of the angle. Thus the muscle force always will be greater than that required when the muscle acts at an angle normal to the bone (90 degrees). Thus:

Total muscle force = 576 N $\div$ 0.7
Total muscle force = 823 N

In these calculations 823 N of muscle force required to support a leg weighing 95 N is equivalent to approximately 183 pounds of muscle force supporting a leg weighing less than 22 pounds.

Thus the muscle must exert a force greater than 8 times that of weight of the leg. One might estimate how much force would be required if the legs were held in a tuck position, with the center of gravity of the legs now being approximately 15 cm. If the legs were fully extended, as recommended for maximal difficulty, the resistance arm would be 46 cm. Is it any wonder that many persons cannot elevate their legs to the horizontal position and maintain this position? This analysis is limited to only one muscle to simplify the mathematic processes.

Action of brachioradialis in forearm flexion. Flexion of the forearm resulting from contraction of the brachioradialis is illustrated in Fig. 7-9. The forearm moves through the sagittal plane, and the axis, passing through the elbow joint, lies in the frontal and transverse planes; the fulcrum is on that axis and lies within the joint. The lever includes the radius and the ulna; the effort arm includes that length of the bones which extends from the axis to

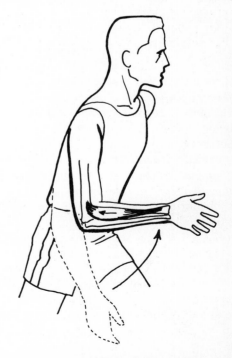

Fig. 7-9. Action of brachioradialis in forearm flexion.

the point of attachment of the muscle, a length of 15 cm. Since the center of gravity of the forearm-plus-hand lies closer to the axis than does the site of the muscle attachment, this is an example of a second-class lever system. This system could be one of great strength, except for the fact that the brachioradialis has such a low angle of pull that there is virtually no movement component to this shunt muscle.

Since the mechanical advantage of the brachio-radialis is poor, this muscle usually acts to stabilize a fast flexion or movement of a large load in which such stabilization is of prime importance. If a weight is suspended at the center of gravity of the segment, the arrangement would remain an E-R-A lever, that is, a second-class lever. If, however, the weight is moved to the hand, the arrangement could become an A-E-R lever, that is, a third-class lever. One would need to calculate the position of the center of gravity of the system (arm plus hand plus weight) to determine the common resistance arm.

One can see readily how a performance may require great muscle effort or very little muscle effort merely by adjusting the placement of external weights on the body and by adjusting the position of the limb in space, which changes the angle of pull of the muscle as well as the effort arm. For efficient movement the forearm and hand should be brought closer to the body, thus decreasing the moment arm for the resistances. A heavier weight can be carried if the forearm is nearly vertical than if the forearm position is that shown in Fig. 7-9.

Action of rectus femoris in leg extension. A major joint action in kicking is leg extension. The action of the rectus femoris in kicking is illustrated in Fig. 7-10. The leg is shown moving through the sagittal plane; the fulcrum is in the knee joint on an axis that lies in the frontal and transverse planes. The rigid bar includes the tibia and fibula and those tarsal and metatarsal bones which are firmly attached to the leg bones from the ankle joint to the point of ball contact. The effort arm is that section of the bones which extends from the axis to the attachment to the tibia, a length of 12.7 cm (5 in),

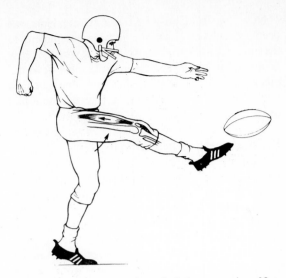

Fig. 7-10. Action of rectus femoris in leg extension. Note position of patella in extension.

and the resistance arm includes those bones which extend from the axis to the center of gravity of the leg-plus-foot, a length of 35 cm.

Since the limb is not horizontal, components of the forces perpendicular to the moment arm described will be as follows: (1) weight of leg times the sine of angle of leg with the vertical and (2) effort times the sine of angle of muscle with the forearm. At the point of contact with the ball, the weight of the ball will produce a resistance moment of force in addition to that created by the weight of the leg. The lever now includes the complete length of the body segment, since the ball acts at the distal end of the segment. In previous calculations in which no external forces existed, the resistance arm was measured only to the center of gravity of the body segment. One might say that the remainder of the lever did not exist. When objects are struck or projected, the entire lever, from an anatomic perspective, must be used in the calculations. This concept will be discussed later in this chapter and also in Chapters 14 and 15. With respect to Fig. 7-10, one must assume this

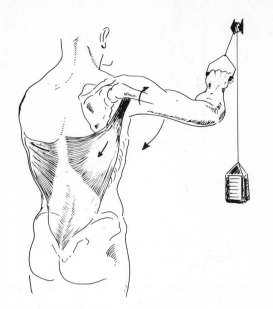

Fig. 7-11. Action of latissimus dorsi in adduction of humerus.

axis that is in the sagittal and transverse planes. The rigid bar of the lever includes the humerus, the radius, the ulna, the carpals, and the metacarpals. The actual resistance arm is the length of the upper arm, since the forearm and hand are the line of application of force passing through the elbow and are parallel to the axis at the shoulder. This moment arm, therefore, is a perpendicular line from the axis at the shoulder to the line of application of force. The effort arm is that portion of the humerus between the axis and the attachment of the muscle.

This analysis has dealt only with adduction of the arm. Since the lattisimus dorsi also causes medial (inward) rotation, there will be a moment of force about an axis passing through the shoulder joint in the lateral-horizontal plane, and the humerus will move in the sagittal plane. A separate analysis of this movement or lack of movement, which is caused by the resistance of other muscles to this action of the latissimus dorsi, could be done.

Muscle-group levers

Effort arm for the action of muscle groups. When more than one muscle contracts to move a segment, the point of application of effort is difficult to determine. In Fig. 7-12 three muscles are depicted, and the effort arm for the action of each is described. If the three muscles contract and pull on the femur at the same time, the amount of force that each exerts, as well as the point of attachment of each, must be known to determine the effort arm for the combined action. The amount of force exerted by each is not known, and to describe the effort arm and its length is therefore impossible. This is true for all situations in which the joint action is caused by the contraction of more than one muscle. The descriptions of single-muscle action have been presented only as a means of developing a concept of body levers. Until information regarding the pulling force of individual muscles is available, the kinesiologist can only estimate the effort arm for muscle-group action.

Action of adductors in lower-limb adduction. The action that occurs in moving a soccer ball to the

situation to be quasi-static and must disregard the force of the leg swing.

Single-muscle levers in frontal plane

Action of latissimus dorsi in adduction of humerus. The humerus shown in Fig. 7-11 is depicted as starting from 90 degrees of abduction and the forearm from 90 degrees of flexion, pointing directly forward. As the latissimus dorsi contracts, the humerus adducts and moves to the side of the trunk through a frontal plane. This shoulder action moves the forearm, although no action occurs in the elbow joint. The forearm moves through a frontal plane also, a concept that some students find difficult to visualize. Such students have found it helpful to perform the action and in doing so to note that, as the distal end of the upper arm moves through a frontal plane, the proximal end of the forearm moves through a frontal plane parallel to that through which the upper arm moves. The distal end of the forearm and the hand move through frontal planes that are parallel to those through which the upper arm moves.

The fulcrum lies within the shoulder joint on an

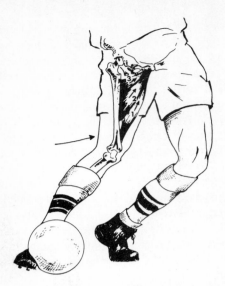

Fig. 7-12. Action of adductors in lower-limb adduction. *1*, Adductor magnus; *2*, adductor longus; *3*, adductor brevis.

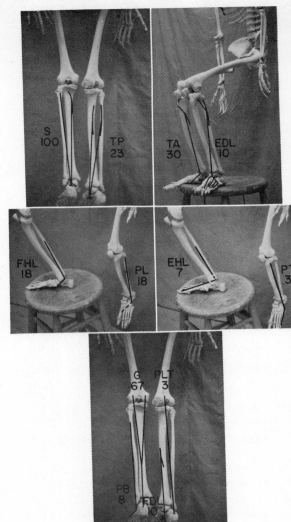

Fig. 7-13. Muscles acting on foot, expressed as percentage of physiologic cross-sectional area (PCSA) of soleus *(S).* All muscles cross ankle, and some also cross knee or metatarsal joints. Relative effectiveness of each muscle may be estimated from PCSA values and attachment sites (direction of force and length of effort moment arms). *(TP*, Tibialis posterior; *TA*, tibialis anterior; *EDL*, extensor digitorum longus; *EHL*, extensor hallucis longus; *PT*, peroneus tertius; *FHL*, flexor hallucis longus; *PL*, peroneus longus; *G*, gastrocnemius; *PLT*, plantaris; *PB*, peroneus brevis; *FDL*, flexor digitorum longus.) (Modified from Mastropaolo, J.: Kinesiology for the public schools, Paramount, Calif, 1975, Academy Printing and Publishing Co.)

left of the body is shown in Fig. 7-12. As the adductors contract, the lower limb moves through the frontal plane on an axis passing through the hip joint in the sagittal and transverse planes. The lever includes the femur, tibia, fibula, tarsals, metatarsals, and that portion of the phalanges which extends to make contact with the ball. The lever bones and length will be the same for the magnus, longus, and brevis muscles. However, the length of the effort arm will differ for the three. If each muscle is considered separately, each effort arm will include that portion of the femur which extends from the axis to the point of attachment of the muscle under consideration. The effort arm for the magnus is longest, and that for the brevis is shortest. In all three situations the resistance arm will include the bones and will be the length just mentioned in describing the total lever.

MUSCLE-BONE LEVER SYSTEMS OF HUMAN BODY

The multitude of muscle-bone lever systems of the human body are presented in Figs. 7-13 to 7-21. In certain cases the vectors are drawn to

Text continued on p. 137.

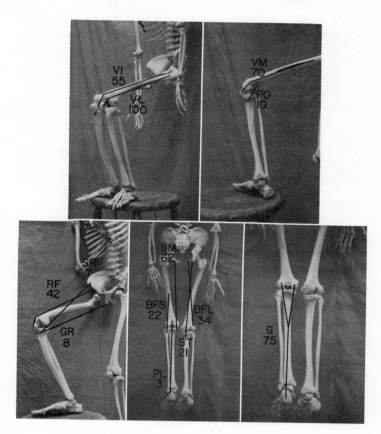

Fig. 7-14. Muscles acting on shank, expressed as percentage of physiologic cross-sectional area (PCSA) of vastus lateralis *(VL)*. Several muscles are biarticular, crossing either hip or ankle, as well as knee. Relative effectiveness of each muscle may be estimated from PCSA values and attachment sites (direction of force and length of effort moment arms). *(VI,* Vastus intermedius; *VM,* vastus medialis; *PO,* popliteus; *SR,* sartorius; *RF,* rectus femoris; *GR,* gracilis; *SM,* semimembranosus; *ST,* semitendinosus; *PL,* plantaris; *BFS,* biceps femoris, short head; *BFL,* biceps femoris, long head; *G,* gastrocnemius.) (Modified from Mastropaolo, J.: Kinesiology for the public schools, Paramount, Calif., 1975, Academy Printing and Publishing Co.)

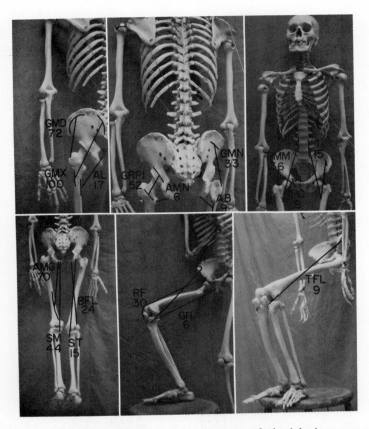

Fig. 7-15. Muscles acting on thigh, expressed as percentage of physiologic cross-sectional area (PCSA) of gluteus maximus *(GMX)*. Several muscles also cross knee and act to move shank. Relative effectiveness of each muscle may be estimated from PCSA and attachment sites (direction of force and length of effort moment arm). *(GMD,* Gluteus medius; *AL,* adductor longus; *GRPI,* group of muscles including piriformis, gemellus superior and inferior, obturator internus and externus, and quadratus femoris; *AMN,* adductor minimus; *AB,* adductor brevis; *GMN,* gluteus minimus; *PMM,* psoas major and minor; *I,* iliacus; *PC,* pectineus; *AMG,* adductor magnus; *SM,* semimembranosus; *ST,* semitendinosis; *BFL,* long head of the biceps femoris; *SR,* sartorius; *RF,* rectus femoris; *GR,* gracilis; *TFL,* tensor fasciae latae.) (Modified from Mastropaolo, J.: Kinesiology for the public schools, Paramount, Calif., 1975, Academy Printing and Publishing Co.)

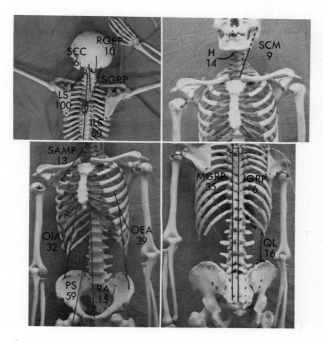

Fig. 7-16. Muscles acting on trunk (spinal column) and head, expressed in percentage of physiologic cross-sectional area (PCSA) of levator scapulae *(LS)*. Relative effectiveness of each muscle may be estimated from PCSA values and attachment sites (direction of force and length of effort moment arm). *(SCC,* Splenius capitis and cervicis; *RGRP,* rectus capitis anterior and lateralis, and longus capitis and colli; *SGRP,* semispinalis capitis, cervicis, and dorsi; *ILS,* iliocostales, longissimi, and spinales; *MGRP,* multifidus, rectus capitis posterior major and minor, and obliquus capitis superior and inferior; *IGRP,* interspinales, intertransversarii, levatores costarum, and rotatores; *QL,* quadratus lumborum; *H,* hyoids; *SCM,* sternocleidomastoideus (dotted line denotes posterior attachment); *SAMP,* scalenus anterior, medius, and posterior [arrows indicate insertion beneath bone]; *OIA,* obliquus internus abdominis; *OEA,* obliquus externus abdominis; *PS,* psoas major and minor; *RA,* rectus abdominis.) (Modified from Mastropaolo, J.: Kinesiology for the public schools, Paramount, Calif., 1975, Academy Printing and Publishing Co.)

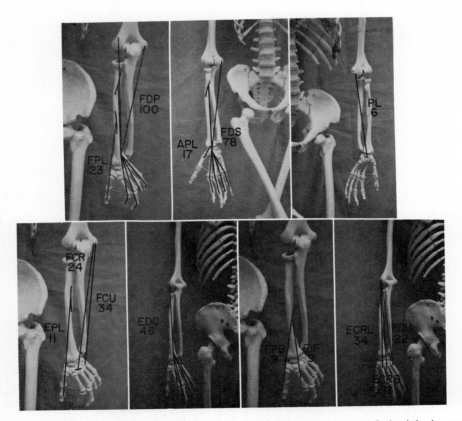

Fig. 7-17. Muscles acting on hand and/or fingers, expressed as percentage of physiologic cross-sectional area (PCSA) of flexor digitorum profundus *(FDP)*. All muscles cross wrists, and many cross elbow and metacarpal and interphalangeal joints and have multiple insertion sites. Relative effectiveness of each muscle may be estimated from PCSA values and attachment sites (direction of force and effort moment arm). *(FPL,* Flexor pollicis longus; *APL,* abductor pollicis longus; *FDS,* flexor digitorum superficialis; *PL,* palmaris longus; *FCU,* flexor carpi ulnaris; *FCR,* flexor carpi radialis; *EPL,* extensor pollicis longus; *EDC,* extensor digitorum communis; *EPB,* extensor pollicis brevis; *EIP,* extensor indicis proprius; *ECRL,* extensor carpi radialis longus; *ECU,* extensor carpi ulnaris; *ECRB,* extensor capri radialis brevis.) (Modified from Mastropaolo, J.: Kinesiology for the public schools, Paramount, Calif., 1975, Academy Printing and Publishing Co.)

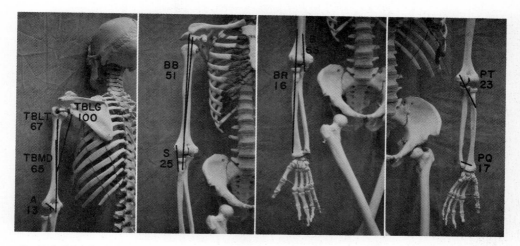

Fig. 7-18. Muscles acting on forearm, expressed as percentage of physiologic cross-sectional area (PCSA) of triceps brachii, long head *(TBLG)*. Except for *TBLG,* a biarticular muscle that crosses both elbow and shoulder joints, and except for pronator quadratus *(PQ),* all muscles cross elbow joint only. Relative effectiveness of each muscle may be estimated from PCSA percentages and attachment sites (direction of force and length of effort arm). These muscles usually move forearm, but they also move humerus when forearm is fixed. (*TBLT,* Triceps brachii, lateral head; *TBMD,* triceps brachii, medial head; *A,* anconeus; *BB,* biceps brachii; *S,* supinator; *BR,* brachioradialis; *B,* brachialis; *PT,* pronator teres; *PQ,* pronator quadratus.) (Modified from Mastropaolo, J.: Kinesiology for the public schools, Paramount, Calif., 1975, Academy Printing and Publishing Co.)

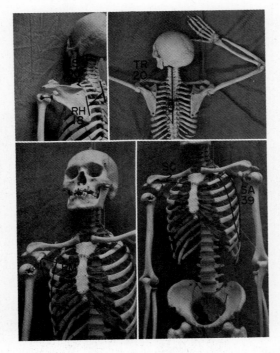

Fig. 7-19. Muscles acting on shoulder girdle, expressed as percentage of physiologic cross-sectional area (PCSA) of levator scapulae *(LS)*. These muscles insert on scapula, clavicle, or sternum. Relative effectiveness of each muscle may be estimated from PCSA values and attachment sites (direction of force and length of effort moment arm). *(RH,* Rhomboideus major and minor; *TR,* trapezius superior, medial, and inferior; *PM,* pectoralis minor; *SC,* subclavius; *SA,* serratus anterior.) (Modified from Mastropaolo, J.: Kinesiology for the public schools, Paramount, Calif., 1975, Academy Printing and Publishing Co.)

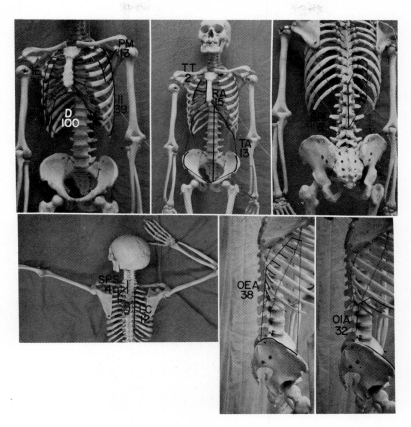

Fig. 7-20. Muscles acting on trunk primarily in thoracic region, expressed as percentage of physiologic cross-sectional area (PCSA) of diaphragm *(D)*. All muscles assist in respiration, having at least one attachment to a rib. Relative effectiveness of each muscle may be estimated from PCSA values and attachment sites (direction of force and length of effort moment arm). (*IE*, Intercostales externi; *II*, intercostales interni; *PM*, pectoralis minor; *TT*, transversus thoracis; *RA*, rectus abdominis; *TA*, transversus abdominis; *SPI*, serratus posterior inferior; *SPS*, serratus posterior superior; *LC*, levatores costarum; *OEA*, obliquus externus abdominis; *OIA*, obliquus internus abdominis.) (Modified from Mastropaolo, J.: Kinesiology for the public schools, Paramount, Calif., 1975, Academy Printing and Publishing Co.)

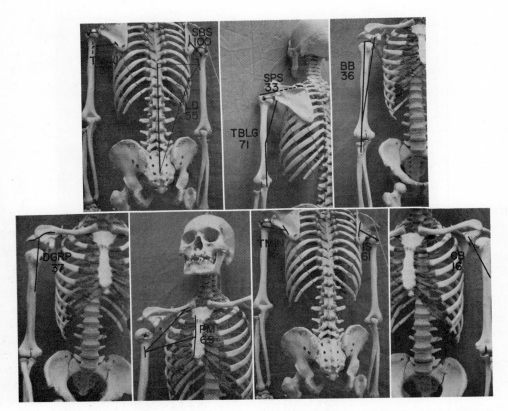

Fig. 7-21. Muscles acting at shoulder to move upper arm, expressed as percentage of physiologic cross-sectional area (PCSA) of subscapularis *(SBS)*. All muscles cross shoulder joints, and latissimus dorsi *(LD)* crosses the vertebrae as well; biceps brachii *(BB)* and long head of the triceps brachii *(TBLG)* also cross elbow. Relative effectiveness of each muscle may be estimated from PCSA values and attachment sites (direction of force and length of effort arm). *(TMAJ,* Teres major; *SPS,* supraspinatus; *DGRP,* deltoid group; *PM,* pectoralis major; *TMIN,* teres minor; *IS,* infraspinatus; *CB,* coracobrachialis.) (Modified from Mastropaolo, J.: Kinesiology for the public schools, Paramount, Calif., 1975, Academy Printing and Publishing Co.)

Table 7-1. Physiologic cross-sectional areas (PCSA) of the largest muscles acting at the major body segments*

Figure	Body segment	Muscle	PCSA (cm₂)
7-13	Foot	Soleus	47.0
7-14	Shank (lower leg)	Vastus lateralis	41.8
7-15	Thigh	Gluteus maximus	58.8
7-16	Trunk (spinal column)	Levator scapulae	35.5
7-17	Hand	Flexor digitorum profundus	10.1
7-17	Fingers	Flexor digitorum profundus	10.1
7-18	Forearm	Triceps brachii, long head	14.1
7-19	Shoulder girdle	Levator scapulae	35.5
7-20	Trunk (respiration)	Diaphragm	35.8
7-21	Upper arm	Subscapularis	19.8

*Modified from Mastropaolo, J.: Kinesiology for the public schools, Paramount, Calif., 1975, Academy Printing and Publishing Co.

illustrate the approximate lines of muscle force as well as the anatomic relationships of the muscles to the joint and bony lever. In other instances the muscle-bone lever system has been separated into two illustrations because of the numbers of muscles acting at that particular joint. Table 7-1 provides further information concerning these muscle-bone lever systems.

Since individuals may increase the cross-sectional area of selected muscle groups because of intense, habitual, and long-term exercise of a particular action, the data presented in Table 7-1 will not coincide with data obtained from these individuals. The table does, however, provide a basis for identifying the most effective—that is, the strongest or fastest—muscle-bone lever systems of a typically average, or normal, human body. The position of the moving body part in space and the plane of movement will determine which of these muscle-bone lever systems are potentially in a position to function. Knowledge of the anatomy of these systems will enable a person to select the most effective movement pattern. Additional anatomic data may be obtained from an anatomy textbook and applied to movement patterns.

Advantages of third-class lever system. As shown in Figs. 7-13 to 7-21, the majority of muscles have their distal attachments near the joints. Therefore the body levers operate primarily as third-class lever systems. Since the muscle effort required in such a system is always greater than the resistance to be overcome, the body would have a mechanical disadvantage when performing activities requiring the lifting of heavy loads. Compensation for this disadvantage is found in the arrangement of the muscle fibers into a featherlike structure. This increases the number of fibers in a given bulk, and since the strength of a muscle depends on the number of contracting fibers, the potential strength is increased. With the increased strength, heavier and longer resistance arms can be moved.

There is an important advantage in possessing third-class levers; this advantage is speed. Given the same amount of shortening of a muscle and the same amount of time to produce this shortening, muscles that have the shortest effort arms will produce the greatest distance of travel of the distal end of the lever (Fig. 7-22).

Referring again to Figs. 7-13 to 7-21, one can see that the muscles with short effort arms usually will have an angle of pull that is mechanically more advantageous than that of muscles with long effort arms. Therefore the design of the human body is one that enables the person to move the

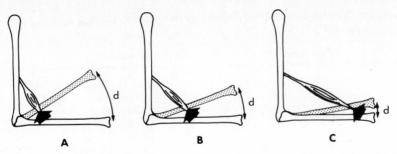

Fig. 7-22. Effect of length of effort arm on movement of distal end of moving segment, given same amount of shortening of muscle.

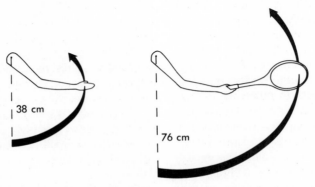

Fig. 7-23. Effect of length of lever on angular displacement, and therefore on linear velocity, of distal end of lever.

limbs rapidly, providing the resistance is not great.

In the sports world, teachers and coaches have capitalized on this human body design by adding to the length of the body lever some external levers of various lengths but primarily of little or negligible weight. The effect of this additional external lever, such as a badminton racquet, is illustrated in Fig. 7-23. The outer end (the hand) of the shorter radius (38 cm), as it moves 90 degrees, will travel through 59.6 cm ([2 × 38 × 3.1416] ÷ 4), whereas the outer end (head of racquet) of the longer radius (76 cm), as it moves 90 degrees, will travel through 119.4 cm ([2 × 76 × 3.1416] ÷ 4).

(NOTE: The division by 4 is made in each case because the illustrated distance is one fourth of a circle.) If the movements are made in the same length of time, the linear velocity of the end of the longer arm will be twice that of the smaller, whereas the angular velocity is the same. Naturally, the angular velocity will not be precisely the same for the two conditions; however, the decrease in angular velocity caused by the added weight of the badminton racquet is minuscule compared to the gain in linear velocity.

Two-joint muscles. Muscles that pass across two joints are called *two-joint muscles*. This arrangement provides another type of human muscular co-ordination in the use of body levers. The action of these muscles on the levers is similar to that of a pulley; the muscles act at each joint over which they pass. For example, the rectus femoris flexes the hip and extends the knee; the gastrocnemius helps flex the knee and extends the foot; the hamstrings flex the knee and extend the hip. In addition, the flexors and extensors of the fingers might be called multijoint muscles, since they pass over the wrist and at least two joints of the fingers.

One outstanding characteristic of these muscles is that they are not long enough to permit a complete range of action simultaneously in the joints involved because of their location on two joints, because the antagonist muscles prevent full range of action on these joints, or because antagonistic action occurs in the two joints (flexion in one and extension in the other). If the rectus femoris contracts, causing flexion at the hip, and at the same time the hamstrings contract to flex the knee, the pull of the rectus is increased at the hip because the muscle does not shorten as much as it would if extension took place at the knee. As an illustration, if there is a downward pull on a rope that passes over an overhead pulley, the tension will be transmitted in a reverse direction to the rope on the other side of the pulley. In the case of the flexors and extensors of the fingers, although the joints move in the same direction, the principle of pulley action is evident. One of the main advantages of using the two-joint muscles is that they maintain tension without complete shortening. This advantage is not enjoyed by one-joint muscles, which lose tension as they shorten.

Two different patterns of action of two-joint muscles have been discussed by Fenn and by Steindler; these patterns are called *concurrent* and *countercurrent*. The simultaneous action of flexion (or extension) at the hip and knee is an example of a concurrent pattern. It has been described as follows: As the muscles contract, they do not lose length and therefore are able to maintain tension. In extension of the hip and knee, the rectus femoris muscle's loss of tension at the knee is balanced by

an increase in tension at the hip. At the same time the hamstrings gain tension at the knee and lose it at the hip.

During certain phases in the kicking pattern the countercurrent two-joint muscle pattern is seen. If the hip is flexed and the knee extended at the same time, there will be loss of tension in the rectus femoris and gain of tension in the hamstrings. Thus, while one muscle shortens rapidly in an action, the antagonist lengthens to the same degree and maintains tension at both ends of the attachment. The result is an effective and coordinated movement.

This discussion does not minimize the importance of one-joint muscles. In a single-joint action they provide the needed force but expend more energy than do the two-joint muscles in the same action. On the other hand, when two joints are involved in the act, the two-joint muscles are more efficient. Elftman found that although, in running, one-joint muscles could do the job, two-joint ones were more efficient; the expenditure of 2.61 hp (1945 watts) by the two-joint muscles could be compared with an expenditure of 3.97 hp (2962 watts) if single-joint ones were used.

ANALYSIS OF LEVER SYSTEMS

Speed of body segments. Little study has been done to indicate the speed with which body segments can be moved. Hill, the English physiologist, has said that in the human body the speed with which each segment moves is related to its length: the longer the segment, the slower its possible speed. This, says Hill, is a safety factor, and he compares these limits to the speeds with which glass rods can be oscillated. A short rod can safely be moved rapidly at a pace that would break a longer one. This relationship of speed to size is seen in the reported number of wingbeats per second of various birds. Hummingbird strokes are as fast as 200/sec; sparrow, 13; pigeon, 8; parrot, 5; stork, 2. The same relationship is shown in the rate of mastication (contractions per minute) of animals, reported by Amar: ox, 70; human, 90 to 100; cat, 1962; guinea pig, 300; white mouse, 350.

Table 7-2. Angular speeds of body segments reported in kinesiology literature

Action	Rad/sec	Degrees/sec
Flexion at wrist	477	3000
Flexion at wrist with tennis racquet in hand	318	2000
Flexion at shoulder during standing long jump	255	1600
Extension at hip, knee, and ankle during standing long jump	236	1480
Transverse rotation at left hip in overhand throw (right hand)	115	720
Wrist flexion with forearm rotation during badminton smash	952	6000

Persons who have observed films of human action know that the wrist action is faster than the action of other joints acting during gross movements. The hand often is not visible as it is moved by action, particularly flexion, at the wrist. Less information exists concerning the rapid movements of the fingers during such rapid movements as are used in playing musical instruments, particularly the flamenco guitar. The speed of various joints given in Table 7-2 represents some of the data reported in kinesiology literature. The fastest movement is that of an internationally ranked woman badminton player.

Linear velocities of distal ends—and therefore of any object projected or struck from the distal end—will be directly related to the length of the lever. One can expect high angular velocities from rotation about the wrist, but linear velocities of the fingers and of balls projected by means of this action will be low. Conversely, low angular velocities from rotation about the shoulder produce high linear velocities of the hand and of balls projected by means of this action. These relationships are shown in Table 7-3, which represents attempts by physical education students to project a ball as rapidly as possible either by using different levers or by modifying the effective radius of a hinged lever (consisting of several joints, as in the arm). The moment arms were measured and the range of motion was predetermined. The ball was released in a horizontal direction, and the distance of projection and height of ball at the time of release were recorded. Since gravity acts to cause the ball to drop to the ground at a known acceleration, the time of flight of the ball could be calculated by using the following formula:

$$t = \sqrt{\frac{2 \text{ height}}{\text{Gravity}}}$$

(This is a rearrangement of $h = \frac{1}{2}gt^2$.)

Linear velocity of the ball was then equal to the horizontal distance of projection divided by the time of flight. One may assume that the linear velocity of the ball is equal to the linear velocity (tangential velocity) of the hand. Thus the determination of the angular velocity of the hand, as well as of the other angular velocities of the other levers that were used, can be obtained by means of the following formula:

$$\omega = \frac{V_t}{r}$$

where r = moment arm, V_t = ball velocity, and ω = angular velocity.

Body segment positioning. A change in the length of the radius is well illustrated by a change in the position of the forearm when the hand is moved by medial rotation of the humerus, a joint action that occurs frequently in throwing and striking skills. To understand these changes better, go through the following movements. First, take a position in which the forearm is fixed in 90 degrees of flexion and the upper arm is abducted 90 degrees and laterally rotated, so that the forearm, pointing directly upward, is vertical. From this starting position rotate the humerus medially so that the forearm is rotated forward and downward in the sagittal plane. The action of the humerus is more difficult to see, but it is also rotating in the same direction and the same plane. The fulcrum, in the shoulder joint, lies on the axis, a line passing through that

Table 7-3. Relationships of moment arm (MA), angular velocity (ω), and linear tangential velocity (V_t)

Axis	MA (meters)	Distance of projection (meters)	V_t(m/sec)	ω (rad/sec)
Hip	0.99	0.66	5.9	6
Shoulder (extended arm)	0.76	0.56	5.3	7
Shoulder (flexed arm)	0.36	0.36	5.0	14
Wrist	0.20	0.20	4.8	24

joint and extending in the same direction as the humerus and roughly along its middle. The radius line must pass through the hand (the point of application of force) to the axis, to which it must be perpendicular. This will be at the elbow. The length of the radius will be approximately equal to the length of the forearm. Next, take a starting position in which the upper arm is in the same position as in the first movement but the elbow is fully extended and the hand is facing upward. Now rotate the humerus medially so that the hand faces forward and then downward; try to eliminate any pronation of the forearm. The radius will now pass through the hand to the axis line, which must be extended through the forearm and hand as well as through the humerus. The length of the radius from the hand to the axis will be 2.5 to 5 cm (1 to 2 in). For the same angular velocity of medial rotation of the humerus, the linear velocity of the hand in the first movement will be some 10 times greater than in the second because of a change in position of parts of the resistance arm; joint action, acting muscles, and bones comprising the resistance arm are identical. The elbow flexion in this movement can vary from 0 to over 90 degrees. The linear velocity of the hand will be least with no flexion; it will increase as the flexion increases, will be greatest at 90 degrees, and beyond 90 degrees will again decrease.

Because medial rotation of the humerus is an outstanding element in the human overarm pattern, because its angular velocity is one of the fastest of the joint actions, and because beginning kinesiology students often fail to recognize it, special ef-

forts should be made to develop the ability to identify this action of the humerus in complex skills. To identify relative positions of upper arms and forearms as medial rotation occurs is also important. This rotation of the humerus on its long axis is usually accompanied by pronation of the forearm.

In studies in which the contributions of various body levers to the total force have been measured, the point chosen for observation has been the release in throws and the point of impact in strikes. All segments between that point and a moving joint are parts of the resistance arm. Thus in a throw the resistance arm for hip rotation would include the pelvis, the spine, the shoulder girdle on the right side (for the right-handed performer), the humerus, the bones of the lower arm, wrist, and hand, and the bones of the fingers up to the center of gravity of the projectile. In spinal rotation the resistance arm would include the same segments except for the pelvis; the shoulder joint would include the segments moved by spinal action except for the spine and shoulder girdle. For all joints acting in the throw the point of application of force is the center of gravity of the projectile; for all strikes it is the point of impact.

The length of the moment arm for any lever and the speed with which it is moving will change during the force-developing phase—for example, in the forward swing in throwing and striking. However, the direct contribution is a result of the length and speed at the time of release. At that instant each acting joint can be considered a separate lever. For example, hip rotation will move the hand, as may spinal rotation and all other joints between the hand and the hip. The linear velocity of each can be determined, and if the measures are accurate, the sum of these linear velocities should equal the velocity of the object projected. This method of evaluating measures of the contributions of each lever will be illustrated as specific skills are analyzed in later chapters.

Anatomic differences. Individuals differ in length of skeletal parts, as is well known. A child's bones are shorter than those of an adult; those of the average woman are shorter than those of the average man. If all persons can move segments at the same angular speeds, those with longer limbs will have greater linear velocities. Some authors have suggested that the distance of the muscular attachment from the joint will differ in individuals. The greater this distance, the longer the effort arm, but the advantages of this length depend on the relationship between the lengths of the effort and re-

sistance arms. If the forearm is 24 cm long and the attachment of the biceps is 2 cm from the fulcrum, the ratio of resistance arm to effort arm is 12:1. If in longer segments the effort arm, although increased in length, remains in the 12:1 ratio, no advantage has been gained. However, an individual in whom the length of the effort arm is proportionately greater than the total length of the arm, and whose muscle strength ratio is also 12:1, will be able to lift heavier weights. Possibly this gain in ability to lift weights because of a proportionately longer effort arm will be accompanied by a decrease in angular velocity. If, when the effort arm is longer, the muscle shortens to the same degree and for the same length of time as when the effort arm is shorter, the distal end of the bone will be moved a shorter distance in the same time, with a resultant decrease in angular velocity. Little information on individual differences in proportionate lengths of effort arms is available, but the pos-

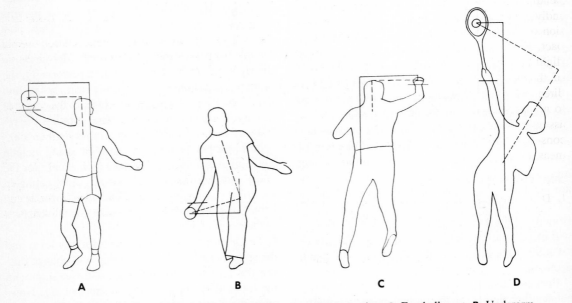

Fig. 7-24. Length of moment arms in various patterns of joint action. **A,** Football pass. **B,** Underarm throw. **C,** Shot put. **D,** Tennis serve. Hip action is shown by unbroken horizontal line from hip axis to center of ball. Spinal action is indicated by broken horizontal or diagonal line from spinal axis to center of ball. Wrist action (not indicated here by a line) is distance from horizontal line through wrist to center of ball.

sibility of such differences suggests the need for investigations that might explain differences in strength and speed of joint actions.

Moment arm measurements for levers common to all patterns. Moment arm lengths for the hip, spine, and wrist are illustrated in Fig. 7-24 with tracings of the body position at the time of release or impact in *(A)* an overarm throw such as a football pass, *(B)* an underarm throw, *(C)* a push such as the shot put, and *(D)* an overarm pattern such as a tennis serve. These tracings also illustrate changes in body levers because of different relative positions of segments.

On each tracing a vertical line has been drawn through the left hip joint to represent the axis of rotation in that joint. In all four cases that rotation will include in the resistance arm the pelvis, spine, right clavicle, humerus, radius and ulna, and bones of the wrist, hand, and fingers; in the tennis serve the racket, as an extension of the hand, is also included. The moment arm lengths will differ, depending to a minor degree on the length of the individual's segments but much more on the position of the segments at the time of release or impact. Horizontal lines perpendicular to the line of flight have been drawn from the axis to the center of the ball. The line of flight is assumed to be directly forward. Although the picture sizes differ to a small degree, for the illustration here all are assumed to be the same: 1 mm on the tracing is considered to be equivalent to 2.5 cm of actual measure.

MINI LABORATORY EXERCISES

1. Draw free body diagrams of the depicted muscle-bone lever systems. Name the classification of the lever system. Determine the muscle force necessary to produce movement. (NOTE: Any amount of force greater than the force necessary to maintain equilibrium will produce movement.)

2. Which situation requires greater force?
3. Draw the moment arms for the following: golf putter, golf driver, racquetball racquet, and tennis racket.
4. Measure the moment arms and rank the contribution of the rotation at the hip with respect to attainment of ball velocities for each sport in Fig. 7-24.
5. Measure the moment arms and rank the contribution of the rotation at the spinal columns with respect to attainment of ball velocities for each sport shown in Fig. 7-24.

REFERENCES

Amar, J.: The human motor, Dubuque, Iowa, 1972, W.C. Brown Co.

Dillman, C.: A kinetic analysis of the recovery leg during sprint running. In Cooper, J.M., editor: Biomechanics symposium, Bloomington, 1970, Indiana University.

Elftman, H.: The work done by muscles in running, Am. J. Physiol. **129:**672, 1940.

Fenn, W.O.: Work against gravity and work due to velocity changes in running, Am. J. Physiol. **93:**433, 1930.

Hill, A.V.: Living machinery, New York, 1927, Harcourt Brace Jovanovich, Inc.

Hill, A.V.: Muscular movement in man, New York, 1927, McGraw-Hill Book Co.

Hill, A.V.: The mechanics of voluntary muscle, Lancet **2:**947, 1951.

Steindler, A.: Kinesiology of the human body under normal and pathological conditions, Springfield, Ill., 1955, Charles C Thomas, Publisher.

ADDITIONAL READINGS

Broer, M.R., and Zernicke, R.F.: Efficiency of human movement, Philadelphia, 1979, W.B. Saunders Co.

Hay, J.G.: The biomechanics of sports techniques, ed. 2, Englewood Cliffs, N.J., 1978, Prentice-Hall, Inc.

Hill, A.V.: Muscular movement in man, New York, 1927, McGraw-Hill Book Co.

Mastropaolo, J.: Kinesiology for the public schools, Paramount, Calif., 1975, Academy Printing & Publishing Co.

Rasch, P.J., Burke, R.K.: Kinesiology and applied anatomy, ed. 6, Philadelphia, 1978, Lea & Febiger.

CHAPTER 8

Innervation of the lever system

Understanding of joint actions and the resulting lever actions is only the foundation for improvement of motor skill. The performer, the teacher, the coach, the therapist, and the industrial engineer must seek means by which the desired actions can be woven into behavior. The action of joints depends on muscular contraction, and muscle action depends on nerve impulses. Joint action is the result; nerve action is the means by which the result is achieved. This concept, still valid today, was expressed by Bard: "The problem of behavior is essentially the problem of explaining how the central nervous system distributes messages to the muscles in such quantities and with such dispersion in time and space as to bring about the sequence of integrated motor events which comprise any normal body movement."* Mountcastle, in this same vein, stated the following:

The motor systems of the brain exist to translate thought, sensation, and emotion into movement. . . .

Movement is the end product of a number of control systems that interact extensively. Their complexity demands that we proceed logically by (1) defining the nature of movement in terms of muscles and joints, (2) presenting an outline of the motor systems so that the relation of the parts to the whole is apparent from the outset, and (3) explaining how "control" is achieved.*

When the details of control of muscles by the nervous system are considered, the general structure of this system should be kept in mind. For convenience in discussion the nervous system is divided into central and peripheral portions. This division does not imply a separation in function, but only in location.

CENTRAL NERVOUS SYSTEM

The central nervous system includes the brain and spinal cord. Both are well protected by the surrounding bones (the skull and the vertebrae).

Brain. The brain, protected by the skull, includes the parts of the nervous system that are the bases of voluntary muscular control, as well as many parts that control reflex behavior. The major portion of the brain consists of the cerebrum, the upper portion (Fig. 8-1). The surface of this portion is composed of gray matter that consists mainly of cell bodies rather than nerve fibers. The activity in these cells is the basis of consciousness and thought. Beneath this surface—the cerebral cortex—are nerve fibers and also other groupings of cell bodies, such as the thalamus and hypothalamus, and mixtures of

*Bard, P.: Medical physiology, ed. 11, St. Louis, 1961, The C.V. Mosby Co.

*Mountcastle, V.B., editor: Medical physiology, vol. 1, ed. 13, St. Louis, 1974, The C.V. Mosby Co., p. 603.

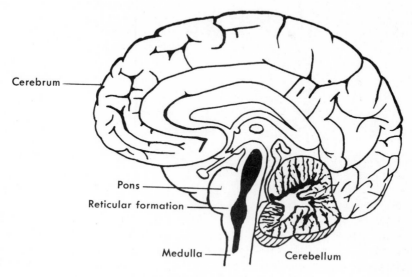

Fig. 8-1. Human brain.

white and gray matter, such as the reticular formation. Connecting these parts of the brain with the cord are the pons and medulla, parts of the *brainstem*.

At the rear of the brain and beneath the cerebrum is the cerebellum, which has an important function in movement. The cortex of this section, like that of the cerebrum, is composed of gray matter, whereas the interior is made up mainly of the white matter of nerve fibers.

Spinal cord. Continuous with the medulla, extending through the spinal canal, and terminating at the upper border of the second lumbar vertebra is that portion of the central nervous system known as the *spinal cord*. Unlike the arrangement of the brain, the gray matter of the cord is in the interior section, in a configuration re-

sembling the letter H (Fig. 8-2). The ends of the H are referred to as the *anterior* and *posterior horns*. Surrounding the gray matter are the white nerve fibers connecting various parts of the brain with cord cells and connecting cells within the cord. The nerve fibers are grouped into tracts, the names of which often indicate the connected areas and also the direction in which nerve impulses are conducted, such as the spinocerebellar and the corticospinal tracts.

Neurons. Nerve fibers and cell bodies are not separate units, since each fiber arises from a cell body. Each cell body with its fibers is known as a *neuron*. Those fibers which conduct impulses away from the cell body are the efferent fibers, known as *axons;* those which conduct impulses toward the cell body are the afferent fibers,

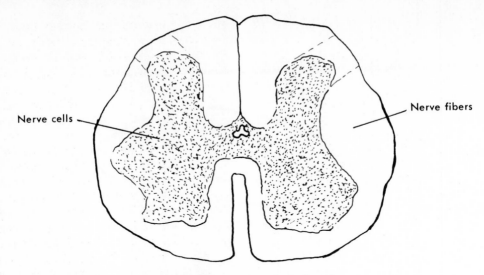

Fig. 8-2. Cross section of spinal cord.

known as *dendrites*. Rarely does a neuron have more than one axon, and this one is usually longer than the dendrites; some axons are as long as 1 m. Often the neuron has several dendrites; near the cell these may be thicker than any axon, but they taper rapidly and branch repeatedly, forming a network of fibers at no great distance from the cell. Impulses do not pass from one neuron to another except at the point where the axon of one cell body is in close contact with the dendrites of another. This contact, known as the *synapse,* is found only within the central nervous system.

PERIPHERAL NERVOUS SYSTEM

The peripheral nervous system includes the cranial and spinal nerves and the peripheral portions of the autonomic nervous system. The latter controls the action of the viscera, glands, heart, blood vessels, and smooth muscles in other parts of the body and is not directly involved in the movement of skeletal parts. The 12 pairs of cranial nerves and 31 pairs of spinal nerves control the action of striated muscle and are thus directly involved in joint actions. The

cranial nerves connect the muscles of the face and head with the central nervous system and also carry impulses to the central nervous system from the receptors of the special senses—the visual, auditory, olfactory, and gustatory senses—and from the more widely spread receptors of pressure, tension, pain, and temperature located in the face and head.

The spinal nerves are most directly involved in movements of the trunk and limbs. The 31 pairs are classified according to the area in which each enters the spinal column: 8 cervical, 12 thoracic, 5 lumbar, 5 sacral, and 1 coccygeal. Each group is numbered from the head downward. In general, the shoulders, arms, and hands are connected with the central nervous system by the fifth, sixth, seventh, and eighth cervical nerves and the first thoracic nerve; the trunk, is connected by all the thoracic, lumbar, and sacral nerves; the hips, thighs, legs, and feet are connected by the second, third, fourth, and fifth lumbar nerves and the first sacral nerve.

Each spinal nerve connects with the spinal cord by an anterior and a posterior root (Fig. 8-3). The posterior roots (afferent nerves) conduct im-

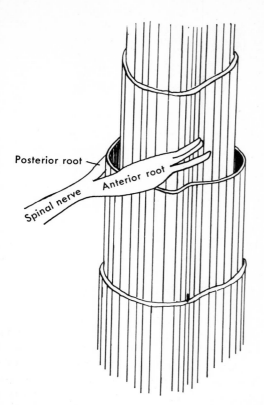

Fig. 8-3. Representation of a spinal nerve and its connections with spinal cord. Anterior root conducts nerve impulses to muscles; posterior root conducts nerve impulses from receptors to central nervous system.

pulses from the sensory receptors of those parts of the body with which the nerves are connected, and the anterior roots (efferent nerves) conduct impulses to the muscles from the central nervous system.

MOTOR UNITS

Each efferent fiber in the spinal nerve arises from a cell body in the anterior horn and is connected with muscle fiber in some part of the body. The majority of skeletal muscles have thousands of muscle fibers, but each is not supplied with a separate nerve fiber. Instead, the axon divides into many collaterals just before

and after entering the muscle; each collateral connects with a single muscle fiber, all of which contract simultaneously when an impulse is sent from the anterior horn cell. The entire neuron and the muscle fibers that it innervates are called a *motor unit*. By this arrangement part of the fibers in one muscle are able to contract while the remaining ones remain at their relaxed length. This arrangement, for partial contraction of a single muscle, is further facilitated by the different degrees of strength in the stimulus needed to excite a neuron. A stimulus that is just strong enough to excite the most sensitive fiber is called a *threshold stimulus*, whereas one that is just strong enough to excite all the fibers is called a *maximal stimulus*. Thus logically a given muscle should be able to develop as many different degrees of strength (because of the contraction of fibers in a unit) as there are motor units represented in that muscle. If 100 motor units were present, 100 different degrees of strength would be possible. Since some muscle fibers are innervated by more than one motor unit, the strength of several motor units contracting simultaneously will not equal the sum of the strength of contraction of the individual units. The number of fibers innervated by a single axon varies. It has been estimated to be 1775 in the medial head of the gastrocnemius, in the tibialis anterior 609, and in the eye muscles from 5 to 8.

Stimulation of motor units. If the muscle fibers in a motor unit are to contract, they must be stimulated by a nerve impulse from the cell body in the anterior horn cell, and this cell, in turn, must be stimulated by impulses that come to it via its short dendrites. The dendrites, in their turn, must receive impulses through the synapses that they make with many nerve fibers, both afferent and efferent. These multiple connections make the motor mechanism of the central nervous system highly complex. A concept of this complexity is shown in the simplified diagrammatic illustration of Fig. 8-4, which indicates that if the intention to move originates in the cerebral cortex, then at the time the nerve impulses from the

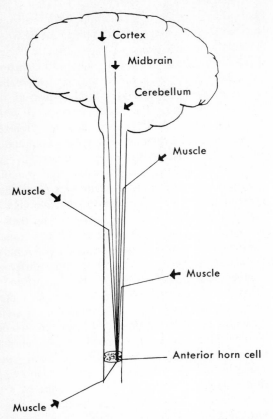

Fig. 8-4. Schematic representation showing possibility for voluntary control of muscle action from cerebral cortex and for involuntary movements caused by impulses from other parts of brain and from other muscles.

cortex reach the anterior horn cell, the impulses from the cerebellum, from nerve cells in the brain below the cortex, and from the afferent fibers arising in other muscles and joints are also likely to be received.

Some comprehension of the complexity of the pathways by which a nerve impulse may reach a motor unit can be gained from consideration of the source of impulses. An impulse originates in the endings of nerve fibers that are specialized to be excited by certain changes in the environment. These endings, known as *receptors,* are each specialized to respond to certain changes

only: those ending in the eye respond primarily to light; those in the ear, to sound; those in the mouth and nose, to chemical changes; and some near the body surface, to pressure. Impulses resulting from these changes may reach the cerebral cortex, and the excitations there have become known as *sight, sound, taste, smell,* and *touch.* The average person is unfamiliar with the many other nerve impulses originating in other types of receptors. Sherrington, to whom we owe much of our knowledge of the nervous system, proposed that receptors be classified as (1) interoceptors, those located in the visceral organs; (2) exteroceptors, those responding to stimuli arising outside the body, such as light, sound, odors, and external pressure; and (3) proprioceptors, those found in muscles, tendons, and joints, which respond to mechanical changes within the body. (The latter are of special interest in the study of movement.)

PROPRIOCEPTORS

Impulses originating in the proprioceptors may travel to the motor unit and be responsible for joint actions that are not consciously directed. They can be the basis for reflex actions, for inherent patterns, for adjustments made during performance, and for learned skills. Several of these receptors have been identified and described, and they are discussed in the following paragraphs.

About 1850 it was found that within muscles there are small groupings of fibers that differ in structure from surrounding fibers in the same muscle. These groupings were later given the name *muscle spindle.* Some persons thought that the muscle spindle might be the specialized receptor in which nerve impulses would be initiated by changes in the degree of contraction in the muscle. In 1894 Sherrington demonstrated that a nerve fiber from the spindle carries impulses to the spinal cord.

A representation (schematic drawing) of a muscle spindle is shown in Fig. 8-5; this drawing has been widely used since it was first presented.

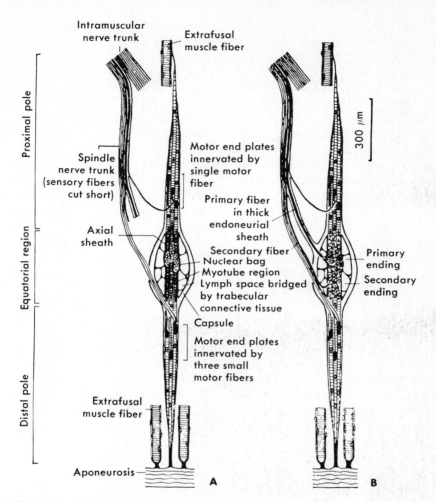

Fig. 8-5. Schematic drawing of structure and innervation of typical spindle organ from mammalian muscle. **A,** Motor innervation only is shown. **B,** Both sensory and motor innervations are shown. (From Barker, D.: Q.J. Micro. Sci. **89:**156, 1948.)

Since that time many investigators have studied the structure and have found details not shown in the drawing. However, it will serve here to give a general idea of the structure and will also serve to increase a realization that there are other receptors, made visible by the microscope, of which the average person is not aware. People have more sense(s) than they realize.

The drawing shows that within a connective tis-

sue sheath, or capsule, there are a number of muscle fibers known as *intrafusal fibers*. Other fibers in the muscle and not within the capsule are known as *extrafusal fibers*. The number of intrafusal fibers shown is not an exact representation. According to Boyd, in a cat's muscle spindle the number varies from 3 to 13, and in humans many more are found. Also not shown in the drawing is the difference in the structure of the fibers. The structure, according to Boyd, differs in several respects, such as length and diameter. The drawing shows in the equatorial region an enlargement known as the *nuclear sac,* or *bag.* It contains a fluid that Boyd says has been referred to as *lymph,* although, as far as he knows, it has not been proved to be lymph. Two types of nerve fibers are connected to the intrafusal ones: one, efferent, carries nerve impulses from the spinal cord to the intrafusal fibers (Fig. 8-5, *A*); the other, afferent, carries impulses from the spindle to the central nervous system (Fig. 8-5, *B*).

The afferent fibers are of two types. They differ in diameter (the larger transmit impulses more rapidly than the smaller) and in type of ending on the intrafusal fiber. The primary, or annulospiral, ending of the larger type rarely branches as it approaches the intrafusal fiber; its ending winds around the fiber in the area of the nuclear sac (Fig. 8-5, *B*). This portion of the fiber does not have contractile ability, as do the outer portions. The secondary, or flower-spray, ending of the smaller afferent fiber also connects with the intrafusal fiber in the region of the nuclear sac, but it is farther from the middle than is the primary ending (Fig. 8-5, *B*). There is only one primary ending on a fiber; there may be as many as five secondary endings, although only one is most commonly found. Whenever the nuclear bag area is stretched, nerve impulses are initiated in primary and secondary endings and transmitted to the spinal cord.

Efferent nerve fibers to the spindle are small in diameter; they connect with the intrafusal fiber, some above the nuclear sac area (Fig. 8-5, *A*), where the muscle fibers have contractile ability. Thus when nerve impulses reach the intrafusal fibers, the latter contract, stretching the nuclear sac area. Since the number of intrafusal fibers as compared to the number of extrafusal fibers in a muscle is small, this contraction appears to make little or no contribution to movement; its function is stimulation of the spindle afferent fibers, which now can be seen as sensory, or at least

afferent, receptors. Some of the efferent fibers do connect at the nuclear sac area, according to Boyd; their function is not clear.

When afferent impulses are initiated in the spindle and transmitted to the spinal cord, they have the possibility of reaching many parts of the body via the complex synaptic connections and nerve pathways in the cord. Some may be carried to the extrafusal fibers in the muscle, in the spindles of which the impulses originated; some may influence the contraction of other muscles acting on the same joint, bringing into action assisting prime movers and synergistic muscle (Chapter 6); some may inhibit the action of antagonist muscles. Such afferent impulses may also activate anterior horn cells in many parts of the spinal cord and thus affect the movement and position of many segments; some may initiate activity in the nerve cells of the brainstem, subcortical brain areas, and cerebellum. They provide the possibilities for complex reflex acts and movement patterns and for the involuntary joint actions that are a part of voluntarily initiated motor acts. These possibilities support the statement that the mind orders an act and leaves the details of execution to lower levels of the nervous system. Without question the muscle spindle plays a major role in movement; by responding to contraction in the active muscles it serves as a coordinator throughout the action.

Golgi tendon receptors are found in the tendons close to their muscular origin and in the connective tissue of the muscle. The end of an afferent nerve fiber is surrounded by layers of tendon fibers enclosed in a connective sheath. Within this encapsulated mass the nerve ending branches; when the tendon or connective tissue is stretched, the pressure on the nerve ending initiates impulses that will be conducted to the central nervous system.

Pacinian corpuscles are widely distributed in the fascia of muscles, especially beneath the tendinous insertion of muscles at the joints. They are also found in the deeper layers of the skin. The nerve ending is surrounded by concentric layers of fibrous tissue, within which the nerve branches. Pressure will be exerted on the nerve endings when muscles contract or are stretched.

Skin receptors, which respond to touch and pressure, are also activated by changes in joints and muscles; they change the amount of pressure on the skin and in the area of the movement.

The nerve fibers connected with these receptors reach the spinal cord by way of the posterior branches of the spinal nerves. They branch as they enter the cord, conducting impulses to anterior horn cells at the same level or to higher or lower levels of the cord. These impulses may result in reflex or subconscious movements. Some impulses may be conducted to the cerebellum and may influence the coordination of movements that are initiated by efferent impulses originating in this section of the brain.

VOLITIONAL CONTRIBUTION TO MOTOR ACTION

Motor acts are often initiated by a decision (activity in the cerebral cortex). That decision does not include conscious, detailed directions of the joint actions that will be needed. Studying motion pictures of one's own performance demonstrates that many joint actions occurred of which one was not aware at the time. The mind orders a "whole," and the details occur without conscious direction. The neuromuscular system selects its own methods of achieving the goal set. As pushups are observed, frequently the body is seen to be lifted by trunk extension before the arms take over the task. According to British neurophysiologist Adrian, "The mind orders a particular movement but leaves its execution to the lower levels of the nervous system."*

A national women's golf champion was asked what she thought about as she prepared to take a shot. She answered, "I see the shot, then feel it, and then I do it." (Further questioning revealed that *seeing* meant visualizing the needed height

and distance.) A basketball coach of national repute was asked how he developed skill in shooting from the free throw line. His reply was identical to that of the golfer. He asked the players to visualize the high point of the shot and to feel it before beginning the movement. A British scientist believes that it is more important to know *what* to do than *how* to do it and suggests that the less a performer knows about the details of the act, the more efficient that act is likely to be.

The lack of cortical control of specific joints and muscles is supported by the investigations of Gellhorn, who reports that stimulation of certain points on the motor cortex results in definite patterns of movement. Among these are such combinations as (1) flexion at the elbow, extension at the wrist, and protraction of the arm, (2) extension at the elbow, flexion at the wrist, and retraction at the shoulder, and (3) flexion at the knee, dorsiflexion at the ankle, and extension at the elbow. Furthermore, Gellhorn found that the same parts of the body could be moved when different cortical points were stimulated: the movement of the lips in speaking and in mastication can be activated from different cortical points, as can flexion of the thumb and closure of the hand, which involve the flexors of the thumb. The concept that movements rather than muscles are represented in the cortex has received increasing emphasis in the two last decades.

The specific movements activated in the cortex are characteristic of the species: they are not unique for each individual. It seems miraculous that even though there are millions of nerve cells in the central nervous system and millions of muscle fibers in the human body, and even though muscles and nerves develop independently in the embryo and during infancy, the connections that develop between muscles and nerves are normally common to all individuals. An explanation for these common connections is given by Sperry, who says that as nerves develop from the central system, each nerve has a predestined terminal contact point and is guided to

---

*Adrian, E.D.: The physical background of perception, London, 1947, Oxford University Press.

this point by a chemical environment. Each nerve fiber as it grows develops numerous ramifications through which it makes contact with numerous cells, but chemical affinity determines which of these ramifications will develop into a specialized synapse capable of transmitting a nerve impulse. Among the supporting experiments that Sperry presents is one in which he transposed the nerves connecting the skin of the left and right hind feet of rats. After the nerves regenerated, a mild shock to the sole of the right foot caused the animal to lift the left. During the experiments some of the animals developed a sore on the stimulated foot, and they then hopped about on three feet but raised the uninjured foot. In another series of experiments the optic nerve of the newt was cut, and the eyeball was rotated 180 degrees. After recovery the animal responded to visual stimuli as if they were seen upside down. The severed nerves had evidently grown attachments to those sections of the eye to which they were normally connected.

Observations such as those of Gellhorn and Sperry provide explanations for the common patterns of human action that are observed to occur without conscious control or awareness.

INVOLUNTARY DETAILS OF MOTOR BEHAVIOR

The involuntary details of common human motor behavior can be attributed to reflex action and inherent motor patterns.

Human motor reflexes

The knee jerk is perhaps the most widely recognized human reflex. A sharp blow on the tendon at the knee initiates a nerve impulse in the afferent nerve, which conducts the impulse to the spinal cord and then to the gray matter of the anterior horn, where the afferent fibers synapse with dendrites of anterior horn cells. The impulse is then conducted via the axon of the motor cells to the muscle fibers of the knee extensors, and as these contract, the leg is rapidly extended. This type of response is also elicited when the pressure on the tendon is a steady pressure rather than a sharp blow. As stated by Bard, "If the pull on the tendon is steadily exerted, the muscle responds with a steady contraction more than sufficient to balance the force of the pull."*

The voluntary concept and the reflex can be visualized in an act such as holding a weight in the hand with the forearm flexed 90 degrees. The intent of the performer is to maintain this angle, with the mind ordering the act in its entirety. The stretch on the elbow flexion signals to the muscle the number of motor units needed. If the weight is increased or decreased, reflex information provides the needed adjustment in strength of contraction.

The stretch, or myotatic, reflex is widely distributed in the body and is especially well developed in antigravity muscles. In the description of the mechanical aspects of standing, the center of gravity of the body is known to be normally in front of the ankle joint. Gravitational force would pull the body forward, causing ankle flexion. The resulting stretch on the ankle extensors initiates the nerve impulses that control the amount of contraction needed to maintain the position that the performer intends. If the forward lean approaches the limits of easy balance, stretch increases and the stimulation to the ankle extensors increases, and the increase in muscle contraction pulls the body back. The intent to stand keeps the ankle joint within a range of flexion that is not consciously controlled.

If the intent is to walk, run, or jump, the degree of ankle flexion is increased, as shown in Figs. 10-4, 11-7, and 12-3 which illustrate joint actions. Ankle flexion is permitted to the extent necessary for the specific act. Then the ankle joint may be held stationary as the foot is raised and later extended at an angular rate that exactly parallels that of the metatarsophalangeal action. Basically these joint actions are the same in the unskilled and the skilled. Some mechanism common to both must be in control.

*Bard, P.: Medical physiology, ed. 11, St. Louis, 1961, The C.V. Mosby Co.

In throwing and striking patterns, it is likely that the rapid backswing, by means of the stretch reflex, produces contraction of muscles needed for the forward swing. Observations of muscle action have shown that the muscles responsible for the forward swing begin their contractions before the limit of the backswing is reached. These contractions not only stop the backswing but also increase the nerve impulses initiated by the stretch and thereby increase the speed of the forward movement.

The myotatic reflex is the simplest of those observed in humans, since often only two neurons are involved. Other, more complex reflex actions that involve action in more than one level of the spinal cord have been observed. These may result in movement of more than one joint and in some cases movement in the contralateral limb. A painful stimulus applied to the foot will result in withdrawal of that limb by flexion of more than one joint (the flexion, or withdrawal, reflex), and this action will initiate impulses that contract extensors in the opposite limb, which are needed to maintain balance (the crossed-extensor reflex). The reflexes that act together to maintain equilibrium are known as the *righting reflexes;* they act in normal standing when the adjustments are barely noticeable and also when there is greater threat to balance. When balance is threatened, many body parts, especially the arms, may be seen moving vigorously and widely. These efforts to bring the body's center of gravity over the feet, needless to say, are not always successful.*

Observers of infant behavior, notably Gesell and McGraw, have reported the age range within which certain reflex acts appear. Their observations suggest that as the infant matures, the reflex action comes under voluntary control and appears as part of a volitional act. The stepping actions that an infant 2 to 3 weeks old will make when held upright with the feet contacting a surface continue to operate reflexly in voluntary walking. The weaving of reflex patterns into voluntary movements may (could well) explain the involuntary details of volitionally initiated movement patterns.

An interesting concept can be drawn from observations reported by Hellebrandt and co-workers. When a weight was lifted by wrist flexion and wrist extension, it was observed that under stress other segments of the body were moved and that head movements resembled those of the tonic neck reflex. These head movements made by infants have been described by Gesell as a turning of the head to the side, accompanied by movements in the upper and lower limbs. On the side toward which the head is turned there are shoulder abduction and elbow extension in the upper limb and knee flexion in the lower limb. On the opposite side there are shoulder abduction and elbow flexion in the upper limb and knee extension in the lower limb. The resulting position is that seen in the fencing lunge (lower limbs) and thrust (upper limb). After observing the appearance of the head movements, Hellebrandt and co-workers found that voluntarily turning the head to the working side increased the work output and turning the head to the opposite side decreased the output. The head position evidently affected the number of nerve impulses sent to the wrist muscles. These findings suggest, as do those of Gellhorn, that the position of segments other than those acting in a given pattern can affect performance.

The neck and labyrinthine reflexes, says Gardner, are among the most important reflex mechanisms in sport and gymnastic skills; for example, divers and tumblers use head movements to facilitate body spin, to flex or extend the limbs and trunk when these movements are desired in a stunt, and to attain correct position at the finish.

Reflexes may facilitate or inhibit volitional movements. For example, the tonic neck reflex inhibits the forward tuck somersault motion be-

---

*For a more detailed discussion of reflex actions see Gowitzke, B.A., and Milner, M.: Understanding the scientific bases of human movement, ed. 2, Baltimore, 1980, The Williams & Wilkins Co.

cause cervical flexion causes the lower limbs to extend. This same reflex facilitates the backward tuck somersault because cervical extension causes the lower limbs to flex. When the head is turned to the side away from the striking arm in racquet sports, the tonic neck reflex causes arm flexion, which causes the person to ''miss the ball.'' The old adage ''Keep the eye on the ball'' is well founded.

Gardner also states that understanding reflex mechanisms is valuable when successful performance requires voluntary inhibition of the associated joint actions, such as pivoting in the golf swing without swaying. She makes this point succinctly by saying, ''One must inhibit 'what comes naturally.' ''

Inherent motor patterns

Although reflex actions are inherent patterns, a division is made here to distinguish those which have a conscious purpose from those which are reactions to stimuli that arise in some part of the nervous system other than the cerebral cortex. Thus withdrawal from intense heat occurs without conscious intent; the withdrawal is often said to occur before one is aware of the pain. A reflex response does not vary; a purposeful inherent pattern, characterized by basic similarities, is not stereotyped. If the human overarm throw is an inherent pattern, the details of performance may differ in individuals and in the same individual at various times, but basic similarities will be present. These responses are not learned: they appear without learning. One writer used the term *action* or *behavior pattern* and defined it as the traditional series of steps by which an objective is achieved. (This definition is closely related to this text's classification of human patterns according to purpose.) The writer also states that an action pattern is as typical of a particular species as is the structure of the animal, and that sometimes species are identified by their action patterns.

Inherent motor patterns in nonhuman vertebrates. According to Lorenz, concerted efforts to identify inherent behavior patterns began about 1930. In-

vestigations in this new field of ethology revealed that motor patterns were common not only to the members of one species but also to those of several species. These interspecies patterns reveal a common ancestry, as do similarities of structure; comparative ethology, as well as comparative anatomy, can provide insight into the origin of a species. Lorenz reports that the behavior of a dog scratching with a hind limb crossed over a forelimb is common to most birds, reptiles, and mammals. The dog scratches by reaching over the forelimb to a point near the head; the bird, in scratching near the head, lowers a wing, which seems unnecessary. Lorenz believes that before the bird can scratch, it must reconstruct the old spatial relationship of the limbs of the four-legged ancestor that it shares with the mammals.

Lorenz has furnished experimental evidence to support observations of innate patterns. By cross-breeding species of ducks he found that genetic factors determine behavior patterns, as well as physical characteristics. The offspring might exhibit movements that were observed in the parents, new combinations of the parents' movements, or even behavior that was exhibited by neither parent.

Evidently the mendelian law operates in determining behavior.

Inherent motor patterns in humans. As human throwing, striking, and locomotion patterns are studied, common elements are evident. Of course, these elements could be learned, but they can be seen in the performance of young children who have had no instruction. We can state with confidence that even children who have an opportunity to observe skilled performers would not be aware of details of action. Fig. 8-6 shows selected tracings taken from a detailed study of the overarm throwing pattern of David, a 33-month-old boy. He had no instruction in throwing; yet the elements of skillful performance are present. In *A* he is seen as forward movement begins. The weight is on the right foot; the left is lifted from the floor; the pelvis is rotated to the right over the supporting foot; the head faces in the direction of the throw. In *B* the left foot has been placed forward to facilitate rota-

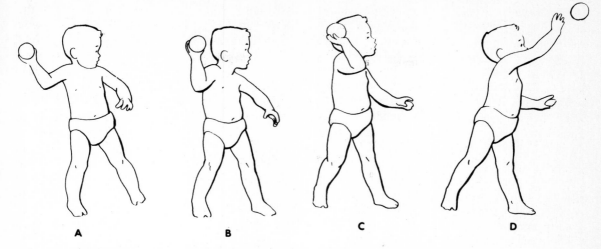

Fig. 8-6. Tracings based on film showing overarm pattern of boy 33 months of age who had had no instruction. Joint actions and their sequence resemble those of highly skilled performers and suggest that basic pattern is inherent.

tion of the pelvis over that limb; the position of the throwing arm has changed little. In the 0.23 second between *B* and *C,* lateral rotation in the left hip has turned the torso in the direction of the throw, and rotation of the humerus has carried the elbow ahead of the ball. This is an interesting aspect of timing—forward rotation of one segment and simultaneous backward rotation of another. It is interesting to speculate what the actions would be if they were attempted by conscious direction. Two elements that would be seen in a more skillful performer are lacking: (1) no vertebral action is in evidence—the torso acts as a unit—and (2) the humerus has not held its position in the transverse plane but has been adducted. The position at release is shown in *D,* 0.03 second after the action shown in *C.* Rotation of the torso has continued, the humerus has rotated medially, the elbow has extended slightly, and the hand has undoubtedly flexed. The observer can only marvel at the coordinations that result from the intent to throw. Underarm and sidearm patterns were also demonstrated by this boy and other boys of preschool age.

Locomotion patterns—walking, running, jumping, and leaping—can be seen in the performances of the young child. As everyone knows, the complicated coordinations of walking and running develop without instruction. Detailed observation shows that the young child's nervous system controls movements within the limits that ensure balance. As running movements first appear, at no time are both feet off the ground. The forward foot is on the ground before the rear foot leaves. With experience the flight phase develops, and as skill is improved, the proportion of time of the flight phase increases. As a two-footed takeoff for a jump is attempted, the nervous system of the young child refuses to allow the center of gravity to move forward unless one foot is moved ahead to receive the weight. This tendency can be seen at all ages perhaps because of lack of experience in attempting a two-footed takeoff. Projecting the body from one foot seems to be the natural, innate pattern.

Another tendency to guard balance has been observed in the use of the arms in the standing broad jump. Effective use would be a forward swing in the sagittal plane on takeoff and a backward swing during flight, followed by a forward swing on landing. Film studies at the University of Wisconsin have shown that elementary-school children and college women whose jumps are shorter than those of their peers do not swing the arms in the sagittal plane. Rather, the arms are held at horizontal abduction throughout the jump. This resembles the action patterns of birds, whose wings are stretched to the side as they take off for flight and also during landing as the legs reach forward. This brings to mind Lorenz's comment on comparative ethology. Unlearned joint action can also be observed in young children. A child under 3 years of age was observed as he jumped from a height equal to his own. The hips had been fully extended on takeoff; yet during flight the hips flexed to bring the feet forward for landing. This was not a learned movement; it was the first experience in that situation. What but inherent patterning could be the basis for the action?

Lorenz has stated that undoubtedly animals in general inherit behavioral traits. To suggest that human behavior follows a different pattern would be illogical. It differs only because of the greater human capacity to modify details of motor inheritance.

LEARNING MOTOR PATTERNS

If motor patterns are innate, one may logically question the need for learning. Apparent are at least two reasons for learning experiences. One is that even innate patterns improve with practice, and the possibility is that if not practiced during the time at which they appear naturally, they will never be as skillful. Riesen reports that newly hatched chickens kept in darkness for 14 days after hatching failed to peck at spots on the ground when brought into the light; he concludes that prolonged lack of practice can interfere with the development of instinctive reflex behavior. He also reports that vision in chimpanzees will not be normal if the eyes are not exposed to light for an extended period after birth. Hess has shown that the instinctive following of a moving object, characteristic of the

young of many animals and known as *imprinting,* is most strongly developed in mallard ducks if the experience occurs within 13 to 16 hours after hatching.

Since children at an early age—certainly before 6 years—have the basic patterns of throwing, striking, and locomotion, it is possible that if these patterns are not experienced at the time the nervous system is ready for them to be used, they will never reach their full potential. Ranson suggests this possibility when he says that the neurons of the nervous system of an adult human are arranged in a system, the larger outlines of which follow a hereditary pattern but many of the details of which are shaped by the experiences of the individual.

The second reason for learning is that basic human patterns should and can be modified for specific situations. If the individual is aware of success or failure after performance, the pattern can often be modified without any conscious direction of joint action. This can be illustrated by the experience with the previously mentioned 33-month-old boy. The boy had a running pattern, and an attempt was made to modify the run into a leap. A verbal description of how to do a leap was not attempted; instead a rolled mat was placed in the runway, and the boy was asked to clear it as he ran. In the first attempt he took off from a running step and landed with both feet *on* the mat. No comments were made, and he attempted a second trial. This time he took off from the mat; he had moved the takeoff too far forward. The third trial was successful; he cleared the mat and landed on both feet (Fig. 8-7). He was then asked to continue running after clearing the mat. He then achieved a one-footed landing, which was not balanced but which improved with successive trials. He had in mind a definite purpose as these adjustments were made; that intent was sufficient to modify joint action when he was aware of his failures. His mind had ordered a ''whole'' but had left the details of execution to those parts of the central nervous system below the level of consciousness.

In addition, this boy was led from a modification of the walking step into a standing broad jump.

First trial   **Second trial**   Takeoff   **Third trial**   Landing

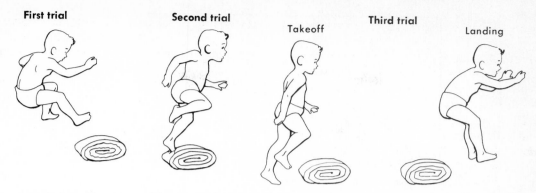

Fig. 8-7. Motor adjustments made by boy 33 months of age as he attempted to clear obstacle by leap. He was given no instructions.

When he was asked to execute a two-footed take-off, one foot came forward to catch his weight. In an attempt to devise a situation that did not resemble so closely that of walking, he was placed on a platform 8 inches above the floor and asked to jump off. He was able to jump without difficulty, although he had a tendency to lead with one foot. The height was increased to 15, to 20, and to 30 inches. The joint action of the lower limbs as he jumped from these heights took on the pattern of the standing broad jump. After this experience he was able to execute a standing broad jump. Evidently the mind had developed the ability to order a given "whole." If the boy had been asked to jump toward an object held over his head, he could also have performed a standing jump for height. A purposeful intent brings into action the necessary joint movements. The learner can modify the innate patterns if the situation calls for the needed adjustments. The function of the teacher is to set up a situation that calls for the needed response.

Inexperienced jumpers can learn to develop the arm swing more rapidly if verbal suggestions are given. Young children of school age who fall backward on landing can swing their arms forward after verbal direction. After the suggestion to reach forward with the arms is given, this goal often results in a forward loss of balance on landing. Verbal suggestion adds a new goal—that of con-centrating on a moving segment while one is executing a basic pattern. This is possible because the mind can be aware of movement.

PERCEPTION OF MOVEMENT AND POSITION

Everyone can describe with substantial accuracy the position of various parts of his or her own body, even with closed eyes. The skilled basketball player knows as soon as the ball is released whether the free throw movements felt right. As stated previously a skilled performer feels the action before executing it. A number of motor-learning studies have shown that a skill can be improved with mental practice, that is, by recalling the feel of the action and substituting successive recalls for physical practice. These recognitions of position and feel are examples of memory of previous motor experience and of recalling activity in the cerebral cortex that accompanied motor acts and cerebral activity initiated by proprioceptors.

Many kinds of memories are developed from cerebral activity—memories of sounds, sights, smells, touch sensations, and tastes. Each type of memory results from activity that was stimulated by a nerve impulse from a corresponding type of receptor. Memories of sound develop from impulses initiated in audioreceptors, and visual memories, from those initiated in vision receptors. Yet, as far as is known, the nerve impulse initiated

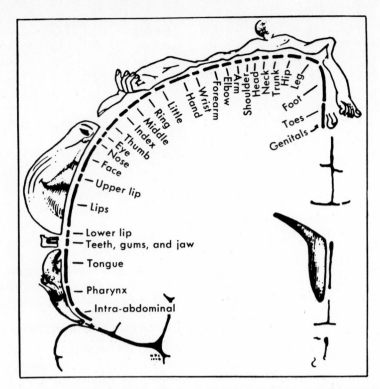

Fig. 8-8. Topographic representation of somatic sensibility in postcentral human gyrus. (From Penfield, W., and Rasmussen, T.: The cerebral cortex in man; a clinical study of localization of function, New York, 1950, The Macmillan Co.)

in one type of receptor does not differ from that initiated in any other type as the impulse travels nerve pathways. The difference in recognition in the cerebral cortex results from the location in which the activity occurs. Cerebral activity initiated by visual receptors is in the lower rear of the cortex. Impulses from proprioceptors arrive in the cortex in a fairly large area that extends from the upper middle surface downward (Fig. 8-8).

The entire body is represented in Fig. 8-8, but the size of representation does not correspond to the size of body parts. The area that receives stimuli from the thumb is as large as that representing the trunk. The cortical representation parallels the density of sensory innervation from the part. When movement occurs, impulses are sent to that part of the cortex which represents the moving seg-

ments. The resulting cortical activity becomes associated with a specific movement, is recognized as accompanying the movement, and is the basis for memory of the act.

It is not known that impulses initiated in all types of proprioceptors reach the areas of the cortex shown in Fig. 8-8. When Sherrington demonstrated in 1894 that a nerve fiber from the muscle spindle conducted impulses to the spinal cord, it was thought that these impulses would reach the brain and be the basis for the cerebral activity that resulted in perception of movement and motor memory. Recent investigations agree that impulses from the spindle do go to the spinal cord but question whether they stimulate activity in the cortical area shown in Fig. 8-8. It is thought that on reaching the spinal cord these impulses may be directed to many muscles involved in the act, including the muscle in which they originated. In other words, these impulses coordinate the movement rather than develop memory or awareness.

Memory and awareness develop from impulses that originate in the proprioceptors found in tissue surrounding joints—ligaments, joint capsules, and adjacent connective tissue. As impulses from these receptors enter the spinal cord, they travel on fibers that extend up the posterior portion of the cord and terminate in the medulla, where they synapse with dendrites of cell bodies located in the medulla. The fibers of this second neuron cross to the opposite side of the brain as they ascend, thus conducting impulses originating in the right side of the body to the left side of the brain and vice versa. These fibers terminate in the thalamus and synapse there with a third neuron, which conducts the impulses to the brain areas shown in Fig. 8-8.

NEURAL ADAPTATION

Electromyography has provided important information concerning tension-load and tension-velocity relationships, fatigue, strength development, learning, and responses to training. For example, there is a positive linear relationship between muscle tension and load, as well as between tension and velocity of performance. Thus various motor units and muscle fibers may be in a state of tension depending on the speed and strength necessary to perform the movement.

Tension to produce a movement with the right arm will show irradiation to the contralateral arm. Contraction of one muscle to lift a very heavy object will require tension in many other muscles designed to stabilize body parts. Tension in a beginner will differ from that in a skilled performer. As strength increases, as learning occurs, and as proficiency develops, the amount of tension and number of muscles producing tension will change, that is, will be reduced. Since these changes are not accounted for solely by physiologic changes in the muscles, the concept of neural adaptation has been proposed. The nervous system adapts the muscular contraction patterns until the most effi-

cient one is found. Patterns of muscle tension in the prefatigued and fatigued state indicate that there are a variety of ways in which persons utilize their muscles during activities requiring endurance. The relationship of each pattern to the endurance time of performance has not been determined. Since this area of research is relatively new, one can only speculate that the training of the nervous system may be the most important discriminator of the highly skilled performer of movement.

MINI LABORATORY EXERCISES

1. List eight different types of movement patterns.
   a. Identify reflexes that might operate during any phase of each of these patterns. Does the reflex facilitate or inhibit the performance?
   b. List common errors in performance of these patterns. Do the errors occur because of existing reflexes?
2. a. Measure reaction time of proximal and distal body segments.
   b. Compare reaction times of right and left limbs.
3. Measure movement time in various planes of movement for upper and lower extremities.
   a. Rank the movement times for movements of a given limb in the various planes.
   b. Obtain physical activity profiles from the performers and speculate reasons for the rankings.
   c. Interpret the data also from anatomic facts.

REFERENCES

Boyd, I.A., et al.: The role of the gamma system in movement and posture, New York, 1964, Association for the Aid of Crippled Children.

Gardner, E.B.: Proprioceptive reflexes and their participation in motor skills, Quest **12:**1, 1969.

Gellhorn, E.: Physiological foundations of neurology and psychiatry, Minneapolis, 1953, University of Minnesota Press.

Gesell, A.: The embryology of behavior, New York, 1940, Harper & Row, Publishers.

Hellebrandt, F.A., Rarick, G.L., Glassow, R., and Carns, M.L.: Physiological analysis of basic motor skills, Am. J. Phys. Med. **40:**14, 1961.

Hess, E.: Imprinting in animals, Sci. Am. **198:**81, March, 1958.

Lorenz, K.Z.: The comparative method in studying innate behaviour patterns. In Danielli, J.F., and Brown, R., editors: Symposia of the Society for Experimental Biology, No. 4: Physiological mechanisms in animal behaviour, Cambridge, England, 1950, Cambridge University Press.

Lorenz, K.Z.: The evolution of behavior, Sci. Am. **199:**67, Dec., 1958.

McGraw, M.: The neuromuscular maturation of the human infant, New York, 1943, Columbia University Press.

Ranson, S., and Clark, S.L.: Anatomy of the nervous system, ed. 10, Philadelphia, 1959, W.B. Saunders Co.

Riesen, A.: Arrested vision, Sci. Am. **183:**16, July, 1950.

Sherrington, C.: The brain and its mechanism, Cambridge, England, 1933, Cambridge University Press.

Sherrington, C.: Man on his nature, ed. 2, Garden City, N.Y., 1953, Doubleday & Co., Inc.

Sherrington, C.: The integrative action of the nervous system, New Haven, Conn., 1961, Yale University Press.

Sperry, R.W.: Action current study in movement coordination, J. Gen. Physiol. **20:**295, 1939.

Sperry, R.W.: The eye and the brain, Sci. Am. **194:**48, May, 1956.

Sperry, R.W.: The growth of nerve circuits, Sci. Am. **201:**68, Nov., 1959.

ADDITIONAL READINGS

Gowitzke, B.A., and Milner, M.: Understanding the scientific bases of human movement, ed. 2, Baltimore, 1980, The Williams & Wilkins Co.

Hellebrandt, F.A.: The physiology of motor learning, Cereb. Palsy Rev. **10:**9, 1958.

Moore, J.C.: Neuroanatomy simplified, Dubuque, Iowa, 1969, Kendall/Hunt Publishing Co.

O'Connell, A.L., and Gardner, B.: Understanding the scientific bases of human movement, Baltimore, 1972, The Williams & Wilkins Co.

Sale, D.: Chronic plasticity in reflex pathways: effects of training, and disuse, paper presented at the Symposium on Spinal Regulation of Muscle, American College of Sports Medicine, Las Vegas, 1980.

Analyzing and improving performance

CHAPTER 9

Qualitative and quantitative assessment

Information in this chapter includes ideas and discussions on several topics related to analyzing and improving performance, from both a qualitative and a quantitative point of view. The concepts are introduced by reviewing some of the movement-related occurrences that take place before and just after birth and the ways they influence later movement patterns. A section is presented on rhythmic movement patterns and their effect on motion. Certain principles and beliefs related to improvement of performance are included as suggestions of general methods and procedures that might be instituted. An observational course of action is offered in which only the naked eye is available, and a sample analysis plan of execution is contained in the presentation. Some basic cinematographic elements are proposed as a form for use in analysis, and a general plan for studying motor acts is included. Finally, laboratory exercises are presented in which the rectangular coordinate system is used to analyze a movement in quantitative terms.

EMBRYOLOGIC BASIS FOR UNDERSTANDING HUMAN MOVEMENT

A review of some movement-related occurrences during the first few months of human life or even before may help the student to better under-

stand the ideas developed later in this chapter. It may also help to explain why individuals move and act differently and may show the reader that "nature" does not have a set of molds into which every human being is poured. Rather, the way an individual reacts to the environment from the very beginning helps determine what he or she will be. There is no clear set of blueprints that may be taken and studied in the belief that all people develop accordingly.

Although information presented here may or may not be related directly to the understanding of adult movement, a discussion of this topic must have a beginning. It was decided that it would be convenient to present the movement development of the fetus or neonate as the proper foundation for the understanding of adult human movement.

The prenatal and natal influences serve to temper ultimate human movement patterns, but just because a human fetus lives in a watery environment and at one stage in its development resembles a fish is no reason to say that children will automatically breathe under water. Rather, they will not breathe under water because they are not designed to live in water. They climb trees to help develop their arms and total body and because they enjoy such movement.

Even though the exact evolution of human structure is not known, that the structure of a part will affect its function is known. Conversely, the function a part performs will ultimately affect its structure. These points should be kept in mind as the information in Part Three is presented.

A discussion of the behavior of the human being must begin with the time of fertilization. It is true in a sense that "all life comes from previous life." It has been stated that reproductive cells trace themselves back through previous generations. In addition, a movement made by the organism involves not only the skeletal, muscular, and nervous systems but also some of the sense organs.

Many experiments have been conducted to determine whether the unborn child will respond to external stimuli such as loud noises, electrical stimuli, or stroking. There is a great deal of evidence to support the idea that 4 or 5 weeks before birth the human fetus can respond with sudden movements to a loud sound or other stimuli originating outside the mother's body.

Some of the organic senses (hearing, at least) are activated before birth, and some (taste, smell, and vision), not to any great extent until after birth. Proprioceptors (muscle, or kinesthetic, sense) appear to be operative long before birth. An individual, even an unborn child, responds with movement to its environment. Whatever the environment in which a human being finds himself or herself, the first response may be to the location itself. Then, as movement takes place, the response is related more to the manner in which movement takes place. Thus the response is first "on the environment" and then "to the environment."

As we look at the movement development of human beings more closely, we need to understand the mechanisms that help in this evolvement. The righting responses, postural tonus, general body reaction to gravity, and visual and tonic neck reflexes are considered to result from the stimulation of receptors (nonauditory labyrinthine and associated) (Chapter 8). However, it is believed by several investigators that it is the labyrinthine senses and some others as they relate to postural adjustments that are important in adult locomotor activities such as walking. An explanation of how these movements are accomplished involves the point that after a response is made, it may then become the stimulus for the next response. These "feedback" systems (mentioned by Weiner), in which the incoming nerve impulses relate motor reactions, are similar to electronic feedback systems (called servomechanisms) used in industry.

Even the part self-stimulation plays in the development of a very young human being cannot be overlooked. The stimulation that results from nonpurposeful, uninhibited neuromuscular activity modulates future human development. In a sense, it is an organismic response to the environment. This autogenetic occurrence often helps account for the differences in human movement patterns. Young children's undirected play is a creative sculptor device—they are molding their own image.

Finally, environment has great impact on the child. Perhaps the mere location in the uterus influences behavior. It is known that because of differences in such body dimensions as height, weight, and length of legs, each individual perceives environment differently. For example, children who have a slow growth pattern may exhibit a reluctance to play games with a faster-growing group, especially if they are made to feel inferior. Conversely, rapid growers tend to be in greatest demand for membership on teams and are looked up to at the time. Later, they may be hard pressed to adjust to the fact they are not able to excel as before because slower growers have caught up with them. However, a fast grower has an advantage, especially early in life, both physically and psychologically.

It might be stated that the child's physical maturity controls certain limits and to a great extent helps determine physical and social environment. Determining factors include not only height and weight but the relative proportion of limbs and other parts of the body. This information needs to be kept in mind when one is studying movement.

ROLE OF RHYTHMIC MOVEMENT PATTERNS

The rhythms of human beings in action are characterized by signs, motions, and sounds made by their bodies or parts thereof to express themselves in some manner. The word *rhythm* comes from the Latin word *rhythmus* and the Greek word *rhythmos*. It is related to the Greek word *rhein,* which means to flow. It also has a musical connotation because of the elements of accent, meter, time, and tempo. Thus the sounds and motions of a human being who is moving often have an orderly sequence of closely related elements called rhythm.

The universe has an order and a rhythm about it as the sun, planets, and moon move in relation to each other. The living creatures on the earth respond to internal and external signals that, in turn, elicit rhythmic reactions. The mating season among animals and fowl brings about many outward manifestations of unusual responses. For example, geese hiss in a different manner during this period. Male birds strut and puff up, fish dance, songbirds sing differently, and bulls bellow in a different manner.

The organs and systems of the human body are capable of emitting signs that indicate to the skilled listener that certain conditions are present. As more-sophisticated instruments are developed, a greater understanding of these rhythmic communications will become known. It now is possible to detect the onset of fatigue, the effect of stress, and the lack of concentration, as well as which muscles are supplying the most effort in a given action.

The examination of a sample of blood through

the use of an electron microscope may reveal to the medical laboratory technician the state of health or disease of a given individual. The beat of a person's heart, especially as seen in an ECG record, gives the exercise physiologist valuable information about a person's heart and body functions, especially if subjected to a stress test.

A device called light tracing, whereby tiny lights are placed on certain parts of the body, reveals to a kinesiologist the path of the rhythmic action of a performer (Fig. 9-1). One record may be compared with another.

The computer's role in the assessment of the rhythm of an action is almost unlimited. The records plotted by a computer can reveal much about the temporal aspects and the path of the various body parts in an action situation.

Rhythmic movement can even be detected in the changing angles of the joints as action takes place. The electrogoniometer translates the action into an understandable record. A rhythmic pattern can be seen in the beat, meter, and accent of an action. The same may be said of a force platform record. The accents, the rise and fall of the body's weight, and the direction of the body as the force of the foot, hand, or other part strikes the force plate disclose the rhythmic aspects.

The rhythm of physical skills used in sports can be recorded in musical notation. Usually the sounds made by the feet, hands, and instruments such as a bat as they strike a surface are recorded in a tape recorder, and then the patterns are transcribed into musical symbols.

We have transcribed some specific sports actions into musical notation, and they are presented on pp. 166 and 167.

Following is a summary of observations based on studying and analyzing the results of the rhythmic patterns of sports movements:

1. Every performer has a certain individual composite rhythm.
2. Each segment of each performer's body has a rhythm all its own.
3. The complete rhythm of movement is difficult to record.

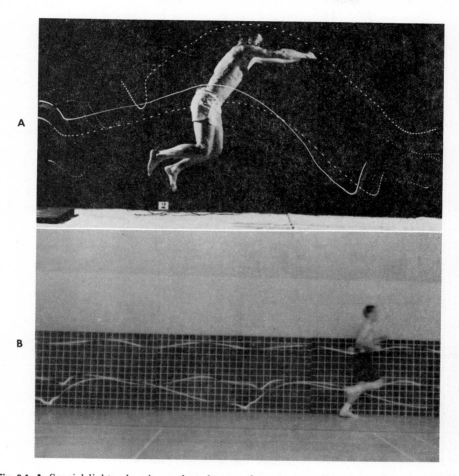

Fig. 9-1. A, Special lights placed on selected parts of runner, revealing rhythmic motion. **B,** Light-tracing photograph depicting path of action of hip, knee, and ankle. (**A** courtesy Motor Learning Research Laboratory, University of Wisconsin; **B** courtesy Indiana University Biomechanics Laboratory.)

Punching bag

(Regular rhythm — very fast)

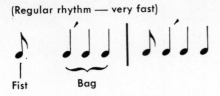

Fist   Bag

Finish

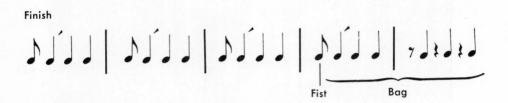

Fist   Bag

Tumbling — back handspring and backflip

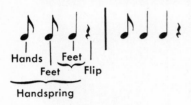

Hands   Feet
    Feet   Flip
Handspring

Discus — two performers varied

Uneven

Step Toe-   Feet
      tap

Even

Basketball

Setup   (♪) Swish of ball in basket

Foot   Foot   Takeoff Landing
    Ball

These musical symbols indicate pertinent action only; the completion of the performance is not included.

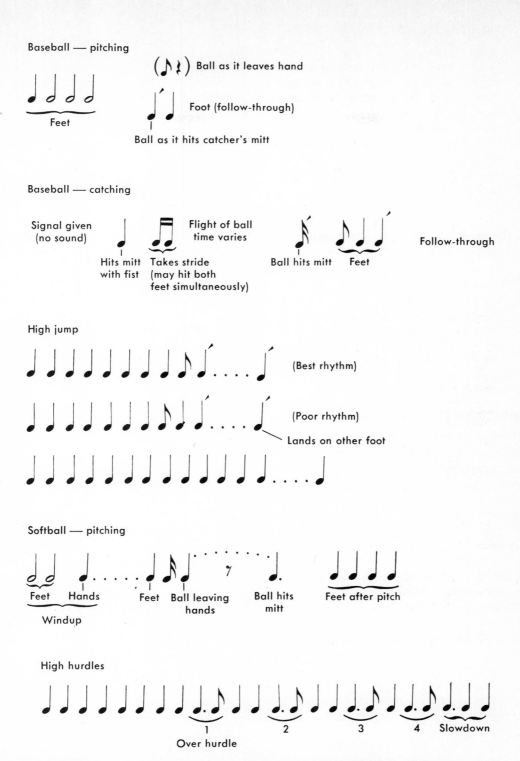

These musical symbols indicate pertinent action only; the completion of the performance is not included.

4. In some sports, such as boxing or baseball, the opponent tries to "feel" one's rhythm.

5. The tempo of a performer's rhythm is not necessarily smooth and even. It is often uneven but consistent in pattern.

6. Usually the tempo (speed) of movement is one of the biggest single factors in distinguishing the good from the poor performer.

7. Most performers do not know what their rhythm is and only subconsciously recognize it.

8. There seems to be a rhythmic pattern that is best for an individual to use; this pattern may also be best in general for all good performers.

9. As people discover better and more effective ways to accomplish a task (perform a skill), they may develop different rhythmic patterns from the ones now used by top performers. (Additional information on this subject may be found in the article by Cooper and Andrews in *Quest*.)

IMPROVEMENT OF PERFORMANCE

Often the kinesiologist is consulted by the physical educator and others interested in improving the performance of individuals in sports settings or in various movement situations. Anyone teaching motor skills is also confronted with the improvement aspect. The following eight suggestions, offered from a kinesiologic (biomechanical) viewpoint, may also involve the aid of other experts in various subdisciplines. A few of the suggestions have been developed in detail elsewhere, some will only be mentioned because of space and other problems, and others will be explained rather fully.

1. Cajoling, demonstrating, explaining the reason for a movement, using social pressure by peers of both sexes, and encouraging the verbalizing of concepts and ideas have helped average performers to become skilled performers. For more information, consult a motor learning expert.

2. Using observational procedures (presented later) and making on-the-spot corrections may bring about improvement. Especially will this be true if the observations are recorded in accordance with a carefully prepared checklist (as reported later).

3. Making precise mechanical analyses of an action and making use of the findings may help a performer to improve. (More information on this subject is available elsewhere.)

4. Determining components and actions of a movement and field testing them under gamelike conditions may be done for any movement. For example, pole vaulting might be broken down into the following:

   a. The run-up, which is usually 24 m (80 ft) to 30 m (100 ft) could be increased to 36 m (120 ft) to gain horizontal velocity. It is known that sprinters can increase their velocity or accelerate up to 18 m (60 yd).

   b. The pole carry should be such that the pole is carried across the body for part or most of the run-up. The recessive weight of the pole is reduced by such a procedure.

   c. The speed of the run might be increased to generate greater horizontal velocity.

   d. The spacing distance of the hands on the pole might be reduced or increased to facilitate greater arm pull-up.

   e. After takeoff, maintaining a body position that is close to the pole might be used to reduce the body's resistance arm.

   f. Action over the bar should be such that the center of gravity of the body is a doughnut shape. The center of gravity would then be under the bar as the body goes over it.

   Similar procedures could be used to determine whether the actions of any movement are sound or whether they need to be altered and refinements made.

5. Other uses of motion might be studied. As a case in point, midget-car drivers approach a

curve with the car under control and then accelerate on the curve. Runners should do the same. Football coaches should look to basketball for discovery of deceptive moves and the development of finesse. The physical therapy field is rich with ideas and information that can be used by persons interested in movement. The United States Navy and Army researchers study humans and animals in many environments and publish their findings; some of these ideas are very useful. Other countries in the world are working on improvement of motor performance, and their findings should be carefully scrutinized for usable ideas.

6. Limitations can often turn into assets:

   a. Each individual has a maximal rhythm of the hands and feet that is effective; yet often by diligent effort a slow rhythm of movement can be increased. Using other body parts such as a hip can aid in the process.

   b. In most movements, especially in sports, greater flexibility of the joints is an asset. Most sports performers lack sufficient flexiblity.

   c. Lack of height is a limitation in some activities and an asset in others. In a sense, to be able to jump high increases height in action. Height is decreased in gymnastic activities by curling the body into a tight ball, such as is done in tumbling. Lowering the center of gravity in a stance, coupled with a wide base of support, keeps the body height low.

   d. Being heavy is an asset or a libability, depending on the circumstances. Having great weight helps in contact but hinders mobility. Reduction in weight increases mobility. Lightweight individuals in contact sports must move first and place their center of gravity under the opponent's to counteract the weight advantage.

   e. Modification of the implements used may improve performance. Increasing the moment arm, changing the center of gravity of the implement, or changing the resistance arm may improve performance.

   f. In actions calling for rapid backward movement, displacement of the center of gravity in the new direction and even running forward in the backward or new direction may help the performance. The reason is that human beings run faster forward than backward because of structural and muscular design.

   g. Movement that is always the same is not only tedious but in sports situations is so stereotyped that often a less gifted performer can equal a more gifted one by anticipating the action.

   h. Once a performer starts a movement, it is difficult to stop; thus an opponent can take advantage of this fact. On the other hand, the performer must time the movement so as to avoid, if possible, trying to stop the action.

   i. A movement to stop an opponent should be started before the opponent's movement. On the other hand, in many actions the offensive performer has the advantage, since offensive movements frequently use a short range of movement and often cannot be precisely anticipated.

   j. Certain requirements of a sport, such as strength and endurance, are usually of such short duration that they are not developed sufficiently under playing conditions. Artificial means, such as weight training and endurance practice, are then necessary.

   k. In almost all kinds of action where flexion or extension of the limbs takes place, the limbs are first moved in the opposite direction. This maneuver aids in performance but gives a clue away to the opponent.

   l. Human beings are one-eyed, one-handed, and one-footed in a movement as the action reaches a climax. This improves the ability to concentrate on a given target. It might aid an opponent, however, to know which side is the dominant one.

7. A review of some basic laws and principles as the performance of an individual is observed may aid in discovering flaws. For example, observing the way inertia of the body is overcome, interaction is accomplished, and gravity is utilized provides information that can be used for improvement.

NAKED-EYE OBSERVATIONAL PROCEDURES

Through years of trial and error the trained teacher or observer of movement learns to recognize many (but not all) skilled and unskilled movement habits. Some habits are sensed; some are recognized. However, only the most competent and keenest of analysts is able to recognize what a performer does or should do to correct faulty movement. Such analysts also are able to encourage certain movement tendencies for optimal performance. It is almost impossible, without cinematographic records, to accurately view with the naked eye the distal ends of the limbs in a fast action. Both the starting position and the terminal position are seen, but the propulsive phase is almost a blur. Yet, after an observer has had years of practice, some educated guesses are reasonably accurate and certainly are enhanced by kinesiologic knowledge.

To be consistent and reliable both in observing performers who are learning motor skills and in evaluating movement for practical or research purposes (either in action movement in a game or work situation or in action viewed from film), one must adopt a definite observational plan.

Principles. Certain principles should also be kept in mind before an observational checklist is developed. Some of these principles are as follows:

1. It is difficult to identify fast action without first observing the origin of the movement. One must look at the large parts before observing the small parts of the body.

2. An observer can usually see only one part of the body in action at a time. One should then plan to observe the action of one part at a time—for example, the head or arms—before analyzing a motion. Several viewings of a performance are thus required.

3. The observer who is too close may be unable to see the action, or it may be impossible to distinguish one part of the movement from another because of the speed of movement. Looking through (not at) the performer to include the entire background helps in gaining proper orientation. One might even look out of the corner of one's eyes part of the time to observe unusual actions.

4. The action should be viewed many times. The observer's analysis should not be made on the basis of only one or two observations because beginners and other unskilled performers rarely repeat one and only one error.

5. The powers of human concentration are such that an observer usually sees only what is expected. The observer must learn to look for unusual clues to eliminate biases and to make an effective study of the movement.

6. Some actions are too fast for the naked eye to observe them accurately under any circumstances. However, after an action is seen in a slow-motion film, it may sometimes be identified by the naked eye.

7. One action is related to a previous action. Consequently, the total motion may be traced from the follow-through back to its inception to discover how the action was performed.

8. It might help to observe the action from many vantage points—at a distance, close up, from above, from the rear, from the front, and even lying flat on the ground. Each position may reveal different things.

9. The observer should have a kinesiologic model of the skilled manner of performing the action and should attempt to compare the performance with this model.

Sample procedure for analyzing a movement without using sophisticated tools. There are many approaches to making a careful study of a specific performer in action when no sophisticated equipment is available. Sequential steps to be used in making such an analysis are suggested as follows:

1. View the movement several times with the naked eye. If film or videotape is available, project it on a screen so that the action is observed at least 7 to 10 times.

2. Record what seems to occur, using a checklist such as the one mentioned later. Unless a checklist is used, beginning analysts overlook many actions that are important to the total movement. It is probably best to begin by observing the large parts of the body and then proceed to the smaller parts, usually from the proximal to the distal ends.

3. Field-test what has been recorded on the checklist in several game or work situations, again observing the action and comparing it with what was recorded. If possible, the action should be filmed, regardless of the type of camera available (16 mm, super 8 mm, videotape, etc.).

4. Make estimates (or if film data are available, make some measurements), determining or estimating such factors as distance, duration, velocity, and angles.

5. Establish some principles of performance that are related to the action under scrutiny; for example: How does the performer overcome the inertia of the body? Does the performer make use of centrifugal force?

6. Present the principles, observations, and findings (even if not precise ones) to performers, coaches, teachers of motor skills, and researchers interested in the movements. Secure their reactions to the concepts proposed.

7. Restudy the information and revise if necessary.

Checklist. A typical checklist that has been devised for carrying out the steps presented above is presented here. This list does not necessarily include all the important items that would apply to every action being analyzed. However, it is believed to be a fairly comprehensive list of the actions that many performers may make in the execution of a skill. When necessary, other items may be added or deleted to make the checklist more appropriate. Therefore alteration, addition, or elimination of some items may have to be made when the action of a given skilled movement is recorded. Some of the comments contained in the checklist are put into question form for clarity. The basic outline for the questions is derived from the theoretical model presented in Chapter 2.

1. Locate as accurately as possible the center of the body while it is in action. A statement often used—"Look at the hub of the wheel before observing the rim"—is apropos here. The center of the mass (center of gravity) of the individual(s) under study is the most slowly moving part (with the exception of the base of support) and the easiest to locate. It should be the orientation point for the observation of subsequent parts.

2. What is the height of the center of gravity from the base of support? Is it low or high during the movement? Does it change during the crucial part, such as at the moment of impact of the bat against the ball? Usually the center of gravity is high for quick, speedy action in a linear direction. It is low when great force is exerted or when stability is needed. The imaginary point of the center of mass should move in a parallel plane or steadily upward as the velocity increases.

3. If hip (pelvic) movement is essential, what are the extent and direction of movement during the action? In many sports the failure to use the pelvis (hip region) properly is the difference between a skilled and an unskilled performance. When top performers are studied carefully, the hip region's leading of the rest of the body in action is very pronounced in the discus throw, the golf

swing, the bat swing, and similar movements.

4. Where is the body weight at both the start and the finish of the action? Often the weight should be moved so that it is centered over the leading, or front, foot as the action comes to a climax. Unskilled performers in golf, for example, often have their body weight centered over the rear foot as they contact the ball with the club head. In a throwing action designed for the purpose of gaining great ball velocity or distance, the body weight of the performer must be moving forward as the action is completed if the performance is to be effective. In some sports movements the body weight may move so that it is centered over the front foot as the action is being completed.

5. What happens to the head during the action? The position of the head initially, as well as during and at the end of a movement, may be revealing. Usually the head should remain as stationary as possible during the action. A rapid change in its position may cause an undesirable change in the direction in which the body or its parts are moving. For example, the swing of the arms in batting may be altered upward if the head is raised, thereby affecting the resultant force on the ball. On the other hand, in twisting and tumbling actions the head initiates the action and determines the direction the body will take.

6. How do the shoulders move during the action? In many movements the shoulders and head move almost as one unit. In most throwing and striking actions the shoulder is "turned" to promote effective performance. Yet in some movements there is often a problem with a shoulder "dip." For example, the arc of the swing of a golfer may be altered during the course of the striking action, often causing an ineffective performance.

7. How wide is the base of support? In many movements a narrow foot stance means that an unstable position has been assumed by the performer, and the total movement may be affected adversely. However, a very quick step may be taken from a narrow base. A wide stance signifies stability, but an extremely wide base restricts quick movements.

8. In what direction do the feet move before, during, and after the action? The direction in which the feet move is usually the direction in which the action will take place.

9. How often will sway, dip, and unusual twists of the body occur during the action? A sway, dip, or twist of the body usually means that forces other than those moving in the desired direction are at work and most likely will diminish the total force. On the other hand, hip twist may cause the arm to attain a wide range of motion. One must differentiate between movements that position the body for the desired direction of force and movements that prevent the application of force in the desired direction.

10. What are the extent, direction, and pattern of the follow-through of the body, arm, hand, leg, or other body parts? The follow-through of the parts of the body after the main action has taken place gives an indication of the direction in which the body moved in force and also may—in the case of the leg, for example—indicate just how much force was expended.

11. In what direction (including path) do the arms and legs move during the action? Sometimes in a striking motion a performer moves one arm away from the desired direction and thus interferes with the effectiveness of the total action. Pulling the inside arm against the body in a golf stroke reduces the force that the arm is able to contribute to the swing.

12. What are the total range, the patterns, and the path of movement through which the

body and appendages move during the action? Sometimes the range of movement is too wide to be effective in some sports. In others the lack of enough range of motion hinders the performer. More force may be generated by a wide range of movement, but accuracy may be sacrificed, because the wider the range of motion, the more an error is accentuated.

13. How does the hand or sports implement act during the moment of impact in sports involving striking? Is the hand or club moving so that the full portion of the hand or club contacts the object? If not, some force is probably lost.

14. What is the action of the wrist, hand, and fingers at the moment an object is contacted or released? Usually a trained eye may come close to detecting the uncocking of the wrist and the inward turn of the hand, which are components of skilled throwing or striking performance. The index and middle fingers supply the final force in throwing, especially when great speed is desired.

15. What is the angle at which the object leaves the hand or sports implement in a striking or throwing activity? Theoretically the maximal angle for distance is usually 45 degrees. Lesser or greater angles usually occur because of movement situations.

16. Does the hand or sports implement cut across the object to be struck as the striking action takes place? Usually the follow-through of the body, and especially of the appendages and implement, indicates the manner in which the object was struck.

17. During a striking or throwing motion, are the eyes of the performer fixed on the object to be struck or on the target? A slight movement of the eyes toward the anticipated flight of the object, or the shifting of the eyes to some distracting influence as the action takes place, may move the head and

change the arc of the swing of the arm or implement and thus may interfere with accuracy or force, moving the body away from the desired direction.

• • •

The above checklist questions are specific in nature. The following questions are concerned with general observations of the performer after details of the movement have been ascertained.

• • •

18. What is the total visual image of the performer as pictured by the observer? Is the action smooth, continuous, and rhythmic? Is there any unnecessary hesitation during the action? Usually smooth action means effective movement, but this is not always true. A performer may appear to be awkward in the action until a thorough study reveals that each phase complements the next. Thus the movement is effective because there is a continuously accelerating motion during the crucial portion of the action.

19. How effective is the total body movement? The analyst (observer) should be aware that the observed starting position is sometimes alternated as the action begins. This last-minute change may affect performance and interfere with correct analysis if it is not taken into account. A starting stance is often changed just as the action begins to make the movement less effective or even more effective. In evaluating the movements of a performer, special attention should be given to those actions performed at the time and in the position that are the most crucial to the total performance. For example, a baseball batter may have a peculiar, awkward stance at the plate, but just as the action of batting begins, the batter moves to a mechanically good position in preparation for striking the ball.

BASIC ELEMENTS OF CINEMATOGRAPHIC ANALYSIS

Photography and cinematography (motion pictures) are widely used to record objective evidence in physical education and athletics. The practice of taking moving pictures of football games is very prevalent in both colleges and high schools. The same is true of basketball games in some areas of the country. The use of game films has added greatly to the ability of the coach to subjectively analyze the performances of his players. Although this qualitative approach has proved useful in gross evaluation, it has added little to the more exacting requirements of cinematographic analysis. Quantitative analyses are desired to provide more precise and accurate information about the performance of the various skills.

Film analysis procedures

There are three basic methods available for obtaining quantitative data from film. The oldest and most time-consuming procedure involves projecting the image onto a flat surface such as a wall. Segmental endpoints are then drawn onto graph paper attached to the surface. Care must be taken to ensure that the projection is at right angles to the drawing or wall surface; otherwise, there will be distortion of the image. One way to check this is to measure the dimensions of the four sprocket holes at the edge of the frame. If the projector is properly aligned, they should all be the same size. It is also necessary to mark stationary background references (two or more) on the paper to ensure that each frame is projected onto the same place on the drawing surface. Although this method does have a number of disadvantages, it provides a large image size and therefore considerably reduces measurement error. Any stop-action, single-frame-advance movie projector may be used for this type of analysis.

The second and most widely used technique involves the use of a 16 mm Recordak Film Analyzer. The image is projected onto a ground-glass screen providing a magnification of 20 to 40 times the frame size. As with the first method, precau-

tions must be taken to ensure that the frame orientation remains the same as the film is advanced (reference points). The Recordak does not have a frame counter, and therefore care must be taken to properly mark and record the frames analyzed. This method is not recommended for highly refined film analysis; however, it is acceptable as an excellent teaching aid and in the performance of small projects. Most libraries have film readers for 35 mm film that are adaptable to 16 mm film analysis by changing the film reels.

The third method is the use of a digitizing tablet. The film is projected on a tablet, and a pen, cursor, or other device is used to work the position of a joint or other points of interest on the tablet. A digitizer automatically displays the x- and y-coordinates of the point (Fig. 9-2). The investigator may copy the coordinates and calculate distances and angles, or the digitizer may be connected to a microprocessor or computer and calculations performed by the device.

Ways of graphically depicting tracings from film

The contourogram, or traced outline of a performer, provides a clear overview of the performance because it resembles the view seen by the observer. Line segments provide the analyst with information concerning the body segments. Angles and inclinations with the vertical can be identified. Line segments are obtainable by drawing straight lines between joints. The x- and y-coordinate system is shown in Fig. 9-2. The segmental endpoints are plotted. From this information the path of the center of gravity, the velocities, and the accelerations can be calculated as more images of the performer are shown.

Film measurements

Angles, distances, and time data can be obtained from the film, and velocities and accelerations can be calculated from these data.

Angles. Any angles to be measured can be obtained through the use of a protractor if a Recordak or projector is being used. It is not necessary to adjust angular measurements to compen-

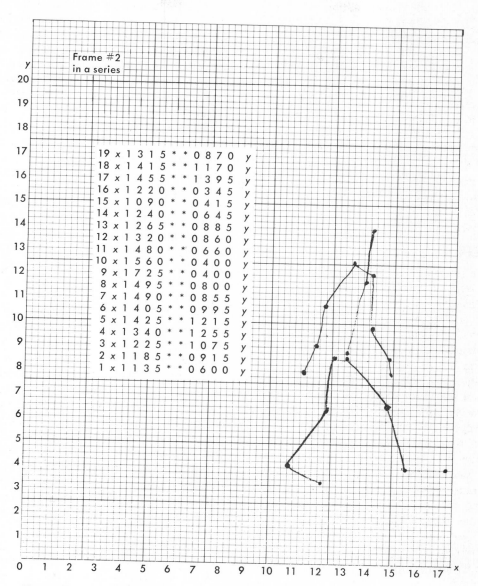

Fig. 9-2. The *x*- and *y*-coordinate system used to analyze movement of soccer player.

sate for the reduced size of the projected image. However, the angles must be in the plane of the projection. It should be noted that by measuring angles at specific times, it is possible to determine the angular velocity of the body as well as its angular acceleration. This knowledge may lead to a better understanding of the relative contribution to movement made by each segment of the body.

Distance. Accurate determination of vertical and horizontal displacement of the human body almost always depends on the accurate determination of the center of gravity of the body or one of its segments in a succession of positions. Computation of segmental and total body centers of gravity must be performed before determination of displacement measurements can be made accurately. It is important to realize that, in determining any distances from the film, they must be converted to life size, since the projection will be considerably smaller than true size. Consequently all measurements taken from the picture must be adjusted by using an object of known length in the picture. By comparing the actual size and the projected size, one can determine a multiplier that can be applied to distances measured on film.

EXAMPLE 1: Assume that a 1-m measuring stick measures 10 cm (0.1 m) on the screen. It should be evident that 1 cm on the screen is equal to 10 cm in life. The actual computation of the multiplier is as follows:

$$X \text{ cm on screen} = Y \text{ cm in life}$$

$$1 \text{ cm on screen} = \frac{Y \text{ cm in life}}{X}$$

or

$$\text{Multiplier} = \frac{\text{Life size}}{\text{Projected size}} = \frac{100 \text{ cm}}{10 \text{ cm}} = 10$$

EXAMPLE 2: To compare English measurements, assume that a yardstick measures 3.6 inches on the screen. It should be evident that 1 inch on the screen is equal to 10 inches in life. The actual computation of the multiplier is as follows:

$$X \text{ inches on screen} = Y \text{ inches in life}$$

$$1 \text{ inch on screen} = \frac{Y \text{ inches in life}}{X}$$

or

$$\text{Multiplier} = \frac{\text{Life size}}{\text{Projected size}} = \frac{36 \text{ inches}}{3.60 \text{ inches}} = 10$$

Thus a measurement taken from the film in centimeters or inches must be multiplied by 10 to convert the distance to life-size units of centimeters or inches. (If life-size units in feet are desired, the multiplier is equal to 0.83 to convert screen measurements to feet.)

If a grid screen is provided in the film background, then displacement values can also be obtained by simply counting the number of grid lines crossed between frames. For example, assuming that you are using grid lines equal to 10 cm in life, and a body segment under study has moved through 16 grid lines, then the displacement would be equal to 10 × 16, or 160 cm (1.6 m). To use English measurements, assume that you are using grid lines equal to 4 inches in life, and a body segment under study has moved through 16 grid lines, then the displacement would be equal to 4 × 16, or 64 inches (5.3 feet). The use of a grid screen will help to reduce the possibility of perspective error.

Time. Since the camera is operating at a known speed, the time elapsed per frame can easily be determined. If it is moving at 128 frames/sec, the time per frame would be 1/128 second. If the camera speed is other than 128 frames/sec, then the time per frame is merely 1 divided by the number of frames per second.

Velocity. The velocity of an object or body part can be computed from the distance traveled and the time elapsed during the movement. Displacement can be secured by measuring the distance covered on the film and applying the multiplier or by counting the grid lines and multiplying by 10 cm or 4 inches. The time is obtained by counting the number of frames during that phase of the movement and multiplying by the computed time per frame. The following formula should then be used:

$$\text{Velocity (average)} = \frac{\text{Distance}}{\text{Time}}$$

EXAMPLE 1:

$$\text{Distance} = 16 \text{ grid lines} \times 10 \text{ cm} = \frac{160 \text{ cm}}{10} = 1.6 \text{ m}$$

$$\text{Time} = \frac{1}{128 \text{ frames/sec}} \times 14 \text{ frames} = 0.109 \text{ second}$$

$$\text{Velocity} = \frac{1.6 \text{ m}}{0.109 \text{ second}} = 14.8 \text{ m/sec}$$

EXAMPLE 2:

$$\text{Distance} = 16 \text{ grid lines} \times 4 \text{ inches} = \frac{64 \text{ inches}}{12} = 5.3 \text{ feet}$$

$$\text{Time} = \frac{1}{128 \text{ frames/sec}} \times 14 \text{ frames} = 0.109 \text{ second}$$

$$\text{Velocity} = \frac{5.3 \text{ feet}}{0.109 \text{ second}} = 48.62 \text{ ft/sec}$$

Acceleration. Acceleration can be calculated by determining the rate of change in velocity as computed from the film. The data obtained, however, are not without error and in many cases are unreliable unless the original displacements have been smoothed mathematically before velocity and acceleration are calculated.

GENERAL PLAN FOR STUDYING ACTION

Three body systems, namely, the nervous, skeletal, and muscular systems, are the primary components of the human motor mechanism. They are discussed in other chapters. To summarize with extreme brevity, we can state that movement initiated within the body requires first that nerve impulses reach muscle fibers. In the fibers the impulses start a chemical reaction that results in contraction of the fibers. As the muscle shortens during contraction, it tends to pull its bony attachments toward each other. The moving bones act as levers, transmitting energy from the muscle to a body part or an external object.

Students of motor skill analyze movement in reverse order; they begin with the final phase—the actions of the levers and the joints, which determine the degree of skill. If the levers are not producing the desired amount of force in the desired direction, they know that lever and joint action should be changed.

However, changes must be made through the nerve-muscle chain. Little is known about that chain except in a general way. Sometimes nerve action can be started in a simple way: a decision may be made to move or not to move a joint that is part of a complex pattern. What occurs between decision and muscle contraction is not known in detail; when such knowledge is available, the teaching of motor skill should be more effective. Meanwhile, efforts should be made to apply present knowledge.

It is logical to begin the study of motor skill with a consideration of human levers and their efficient use. This is not a simple task. First, it is complicated by the number of directions in which each lever can be moved. Every segment can be moved in at least two directions from its anatomic position. If flexion, medial rotation, or adduction is a possible action for a segment, the opposing action—extension, lateral rotation, or abduction—is possible also. In addition, a segment can be moved in two directions simultaneously; for example, the humerus can adduct and rotate at the same time.

Second, in most skills more than one lever is moving at the same time; as many as five or six levers may be involved. This feature, combined with the number of directions in which a segment can move, provides thousands of possible combinations. Suppose that only two levers are moving at the same time. Lever A can move in a, b, c, d, e, and f directions and lever B in a, b, c, and d directions. Theoretically each A action could be combined with each B action—AaBa, AaBb, AaBc, and AaBd. Also, Ab, Ac, Ad, Ae, and Af might act with each B action. The thousands of possibilities are evident.

If the study of human movement warrants the title *kinesiology,* pertinent information, like that in every science, should be systematically organized. One kinesiologic grouping is widely used—the grouping of joint action: flexion, extension, rotation, abduction, and adduction. The definition of each term in this classification should be such that it could be applied to movements of any body segment. Application of this classification based on description is limited to the action of a single joint. Since the great majority of motor acts are complex, involving several segments and joint actions, there should be some type of grouping that could be applied to the many possible combinations.

An outstanding student of human movement has said, "Voluntary movement is goal-oriented."* This statement suggests that voluntary actions could be classified on the basis of purpose. Such grouping was recommended by one of us (R.B.G.) in 1932, by Wells and Luttgens, and by Broer and Zernicke in *Efficiency of Human Movement*. Although originally the grouping was based on voluntary acts, it is now evident that it applies to inherent movement patterns also.

Major divisions in the recommended classification include moving external objects, moving and balancing the body itself, and stopping moving objects. These types of activities have for centuries been essential for human survival, and human beings, like all living organisms, developed structure and motor behavior to cope with the environment. Motor patterns, unique combinations of nerve-muscle-bone actions, were developed to accomplish certain purposes. Today these patterns are the foundation of human motor skills. They need not be learned; coordinations related to purpose are inherent. Children as young as 3 years of age, when in situations not encountered previously, respond with effective movements. Basically these movements are those which would be used by skilled performers; the child needs no instruction to bring forth the fundamental pattern.

However, a purpose is not always accomplished with the same movement pattern. An external object can be moved with a throw, strike, pull, or push. A throw can be made with an overarm, an underarm, or a sidearm pattern; a strike may also be made with these patterns. The human body moves itself by a run, walk, or jump. Similar patterns can be identified by even the casual observer

*Gardner, E.B.: Proprioceptive reflexes and their participation in motor skills, Quest **12**:1, 1969.

in a general way, but for identification of details other methods of observation are needed.

Film sequences of skills have shown that there are similarities in an underarm throw, an underarm volleyball serve, and a badminton serve. In addition, an overarm throw, a badminton clear, and a tennis serve are basically the same, as are a sidearm basketball throw, a tennis drive, and a baseball batting action. The similarities in the pattern of the lower limbs in a one-footed takeoff in the basketball lay-up, the volleyball spike, and the hurdle for the running dive are known.

Another means of identifying similarities has employed detailed analysis of film. From photographs such as those shown in Fig. 9-3, each acting joint can be identified. The number of degrees that each segment moves from frame to frame can be measured, and since the clock in the picture gives the time per frame, the angular velocity can be determined. If the change in degrees is plotted against the time, the graph of all joints presents a picture of what is occurring during the total performance. Here can be seen the sequence and range of joint actions in relationship to each other. The joints acting in the final phase, such as the release in a throw, the impact in a strike, and the takeoff in a jump, can be identified.

In this final phase the length of the moment arm of each acting joint can be measured from the view best suited to provide the length (side, front or back, or overhead). When the length of the moment arm and the angular velocity of the joint are known, the linear velocity of each moment arm can be calculated. The contribution made by each acting joint to the final application of force can then be determined.

The use of triplane photography (Fig. 9-3) has been helpful in the development of research technique. The earliest film studies were based on views taken with one camera, usually from one side. Only joint actions that occurred in the picture plane could be measured directly. As research progressed, cameras were added to obtain overhead and rear (or front) views. The overhead camera is likely to present the most difficulty in the filming

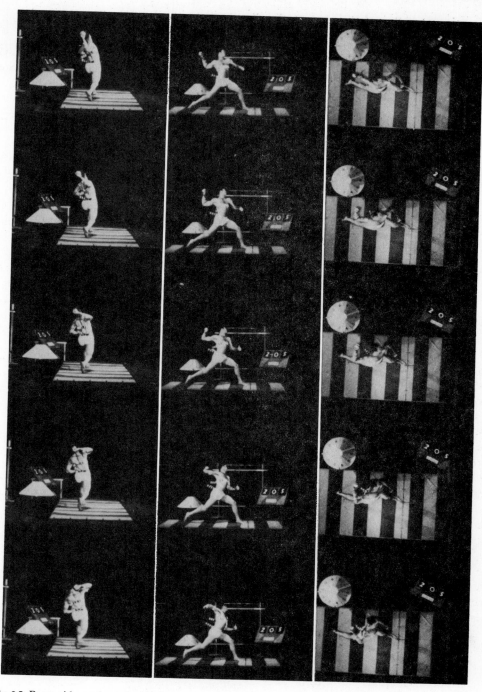

Fig. 9-3. Rear, side, and overhead views taken to study overarm throw. Number 205 identifies subject and trial in series; note presence of cone-shaped timing device, as well as uprights and crossbars that establish vertical and horizontal lines to aid in measurement. (Courtesy Kinesiology Research Laboratories, University of Wisconsin, and A.E. Atwater, University of Arizona.)

Continued.

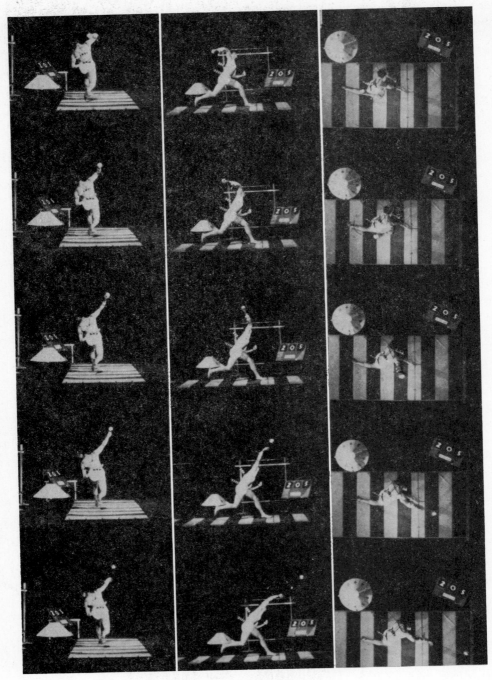

Fig. 9-3, cont'd. For legend see p. 179.

situation. The distance between that camera and the subject must be great enough (1) to include the field to be photographed and (2) so that the photographed size of an object at the side of the field will not differ significantly from its size when it is photographed in the middle of the field.

The newest development is a phase-lock camera system in which one camera is the master and one or more are "slaves" to it. In other words, all cameras are synchronized so that the film frames are identical as to action but the action is viewed from a different angle (Dawson and Al-Haroun).

Devices such as the cone-shaped clock in Fig. 9-3 are now used. When film studies were based on one-plane views, a flat-faced clock could be used; with biplane photography, the clock could be placed at an angle and be seen in both views. When three cameras were used, the cone-shaped clock, which can be read in all three views, were suggested. Roberts has recently added an electrical device to the cone that permits recording of time intervals and eliminates the necessity of reading the clock. The velocity of thrown balls and the forces made by the feet in a throw can be determined by the use of a laser beam and force platforms. The accuracy of recording is improved with these devices.

Tracings from a film study are shown in Fig. 9-4. A primary purpose of the investigator was to observe the path of the ball before release when the subject used the overarm throwing pattern. The tracings are from the side and overhead views and illustrate the value of biplane photography. The circles are tracings of the ball in successive frames and represent the same points of time in the two views. (Note the lettering and numbering.) The time relationship is more easily identified by the blackened circles. With reference to the performer, the circles indicate the ball as it progresses from the back toward the front. Only the side view shows the downward and upward progress (vertical plane), and only the overhead view shows the movement from right to left and then to right again (horizontal plane). This investigator chose to trace the performer when the ball had been released. A

similar tracing could be made to accompany any ball position.

This type of detailed observation and measurement shows similarities and differences in movement patterns. Equally important is the understanding of the mechanics of body action that it provides. With such understanding, students of movement are freed from imitation of the expert. If a joint action is recommended in a pattern, they should ask, "What will it contribute?" They should not be satisfied with developing a pattern because they are told that it is "good form," the pattern of some well-known skilled performer. If reference is made to the pattern of an expert, the mechanical advantages of the expert's joint actions should be understood. Students should not strive to develop a description of expert performance; they should strive to develop an understanding of a pattern that is mechanically and physiologically efficient.

Insight into the mechanics of a skill can be gained from studying film of poor performers and comparing it with film of good performers. For example, the graph of the moving segments of a highly skilled girl as she executes the standing broad jump shows that in the final phase most of the power is derived from the movements of the thigh and the foot. Since the thigh is moved by extension at the knee joint, study of the graph suggests that knee extension is a major factor in attaining power in the standing broad jump. This concept is given support by a comparison of knee action in observations made by Felton. Five college women whose jumps averaged 85 inches were extending the knee at takeoff at an average velocity of 729 degrees per second, whereas five women whose jumps averaged 48 inches extended the knee at an average velocity of 183 degrees per second.

Knee action has been shown to be an important factor in producing power in another form of locomotion—the run. Knee action of a skilled performer was compared with that of an unskilled runner. Measurements from film showed the range of knee extension to be 32 degrees in the skilled

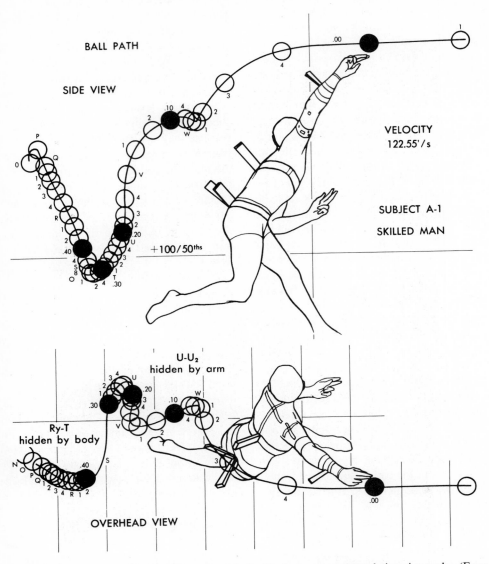

Fig. 9-4. Tracings from film to show path of ball. Circles represent equal time intervals. (From Atwater, A.E.: Movement characteristics of the overarm throw, dissertation, University of Wisconsin, 1970.)

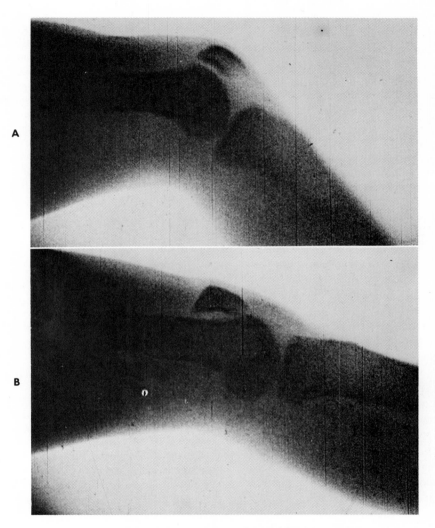

Fig. 9-5. X-ray motion pictures of knee in kicking action.

and 6 degrees in the unskilled; the velocity of knee extension was 711 degrees per second in the skilled and 80 degrees in the unskilled.

The similarity in the mechanics of jumping and running, as described in the preceding paragraphs, and of other activities that will be discussed later in the text, suggests that these skills are modifications of the same basic pattern. Running and jumping have a common purpose—to move the body. For any given purpose, the human mechanism is likely to have inherent patterns that to some degree will achieve the desired end. By recognizing these patterns in attempts to improve skill, the student can utilize the nerve-muscle chains that move the body levers. Each situation will require its own modifications of the basic pattern. The modifications should be made to improve the mechanics.

Videotape is used extensively in the teaching of motor skills. When camera speeds are increased in the future, it will be used in quantitive analyses. Split-screen effects help in the understanding of the dimensional aspects of movements. The use of web graphics has been mentioned as a possible means of appraising movement. Its possibilities are intriguing.

The use of notation systems gives a different approach to the teaching and analyzing of a movement. Many other types of movement analysis procedures and equipment will appear on the horizon in the future, giving the kinesiologist greater insight into the understanding of movement.

X-ray motion picture data were used until the radiation problem was given prominence. Still pictures from such film data are seen in Fig. 9-5.

Other tools in addition to cameras are used in kinesiologic (biomechanical) research. Many are listed in Chapter 3, and one of them, the force platform, is now used extensively with film data. For example, the curve of the forces made by the feet, including the length of time the forces are applied, gives valuable information to the analyst. The impulse (F × T) of one high jumper as compared to another may indicate the reason that one is better than another. The top jumpers always have a greater net impulse. Information gained from other tools, often with the aid of a computer, may be just as revealing.

LABORATORY EXERCISES: DETERMINING MOVEMENT*
Position and displacement

The first problem in describing the motion of an object or body is to define its position by establishing a reference system whereby change of position (displacement) can be defined. The *rectangular coordinate system* is such a reference system. This Cartesian system consists of a set of axes that measure units of displacement in two directions in one plane. Looking at the following drawing, you can see that the position of the ball at various times can be *pictured* on the coordinate system. Its position can be *described* by use of coordinates. Coordinates are numbers that describe a position or locate a point on a coordinate system.

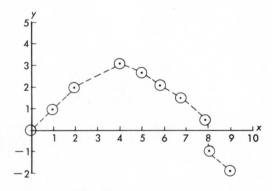

Two numbers (coordinates) are needed to define a position in a given plane. One number refers to position relative to the *x*-axis, or horizontal axis, and the other number describes position relative to the *y*-axis, or vertical axis. Either number may be positive or negative because it simply defines position *relative to* a given zero point, where both axes are zero. In the drawing above, the ball is at the zero point on both axes in its first position. The coordinates at this point will then be (0,0). Coordinates are written so that the *x*-coordinate, or number, is first, followed by a comma and the *y*-coordinate. Usually the coordinates of a single point are called

---

*Developed by Betty Haven, Mary Dawson, and others at Indiana University, Bloomington, Indiana.

a set of coordinates and are enclosed in parentheses. In the second position the center of the ball is at the point (1,1), whereas in the last position the point can be described as (9,−2).

■ *Locate the following points on the coordinate system provided in the following drawing: (0,4), (1.3,5), (1.5,2), (2,0), (2.5,−2), (3,−2), (3.5,−2.5), and (4,−3).*

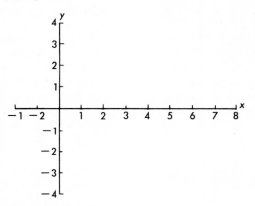

Distance between two points

The distance between two points in a plane can be found by calculation. Consider three different situations:

1. When you wish to find the distance between two points that have the same *y*-coordinate (that is, both points lie on a line parallel to the *x*-axis), you simply find the difference between the two *x*-coordinates.

■ *What is the distance between the point (5,2) and the point (3,2) in the following drawing?*

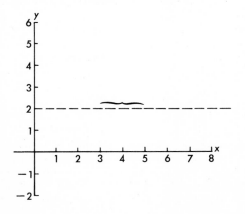

2. When you wish to find the distance between two points that have the same *x*-coordinate, you simply find the difference between the *y*-coordinates.

■ *What is the distance between points (3,2) and (3,−4) in the following drawing?*

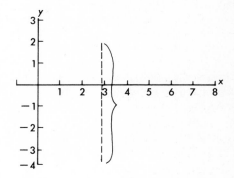

3. When you wish to find the distance between two points that are not on the same horizontal or vertical line, the distance must be calculated in a different manner. We are given two points: P_1 with coordinates (x_1, y_1), and P_2 with coordinates (x_2, y_2). These are two distinct points not on the same vertical or horizontal line, as shown in the following drawing.

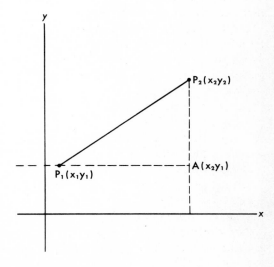

If a line is drawn through P_1, parallel to the x-axis, and another line is drawn through P_2, parallel to the y-axis, these lines will meet at point A, with the coordinates (x_2, y_1), and form the right triangle $\triangle P_1P_2A$. Then P_1P_2 is the length of the hypotenuse of the right triangle, whose sides $\overline{P_1A}$ and $\overline{AP_2}$ are of the lengths $x_2 - x_1$ and $y_2 - y_1$, respectively.

Pythagoras' theorem states that the square of the hypotenuse of a right triangle is equal to the sum of the squared sides, or in this case:

$$\overline{P_1P_2}^2 = \overline{P_1A}^2 + \overline{P_2A}^2$$

Since P_1 and A are both points on the same line, and since both P_2 and A are on the same line, their lengths can be determined as above. Then:

$$\overline{P_1P_2} = \sqrt{(x_2 - x_1)^2 + (y_2 - y_1)^2}$$

- *Calculate the distance between points $(-3,2)$ and $(5,8)$.*

Now let us apply these procedures to finding the length of some segment of the body if we are given the coordinates of the proximal and distal ends of the segment.

- *In the following drawing, first find the length of the right thigh in scale units. Second, find the length of the left leg (hip to ankle) in scale units. If one unit equals 10 cm, how long is the runner's left leg? If one unit on the scale is equal to 4 inches, how long is the left leg?*

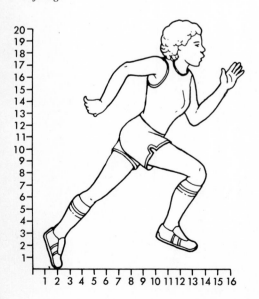

If the runner in the drawing then continues to run, her right hip will move—her hip will be displaced along both the vertical axis and the horizontal axis. If we consider only the horizontal movement of the right hip and are able to find the coordinates of that hip at several points in time, we can plot a displacement curve that describes the horizontal displacement of the right hip with respect to time. NOTE: Horizontal displacement (the x-coordinate) does *not* have to be plotted on the horizontal axis. Ordinarily the displacement-time plot is constructed so that time is on the x-axis, or horizontal axis, and displacement (in any direction) is on the y-axis.

- *Given the following information, plot a horizontal displacement line for the runner's right hip with respect to time.*

Time	Horizontal displacement (x-coordinate of right hip)
0.00	3
0.01	3.5
0.02	3.8
0.03	4.5
0.04	5.0
0.05	5.1
0.06	5.8

With more drawings of the action, velocity and acceleration can be calculated.

REFERENCES

Al-Haroun, M.R.: Three-dimensional cinematographic analysis of selected full twisting movements in gymnastics, unpublished dissertation, Indiana University, 1980.

Broer, M.R., and Zernicke, R.F.: Efficiency of human movement, Philadelphia, 1979, W.B. Saunders Co.

Cooper, J.M., and Andrews, E.W.: Rhythm as a linguistic art: signs, symbols, sounds, and motion, Quest **23**:61, Winter, 1975.

Dawson, M.L.: Dynamics of the approach run of the flop-style high jump technique, unpublished dissertation, Indiana University, 1979.

Felton, E.: A kinesiological comparison of good and poor performers in the standing broad jump, thesis, University of Wisconsin, 1960.

Roberts, E.M.: Cinematography in biomechanical investigation. In Cooper, J.M., editor: Proceedings of the Committee on Institutional Cooperation, Symposium on Biomechanics, Chicago, 1971, The Athletic Institute.

Weiner, N.: Cybernetics, Garden City, N.Y., 1953, Doubleday & Co., Inc.

Wells, K.F., and Luttgens, K.: Kinesiology, ed. 6, Philadelphia, 1976, W.B. Saunders Co.

ADDITIONAL READINGS

Ariel, G.: Computerized biomechanical analysis of human performance. In Mechanics and sport, Applied Mechanics Division, vol. 4, New York, 1973, American Society of Mechanical Engineers.

Bates, B.T.: The development of a computer program with application to film analysis: the mechanics of female runners, doctoral dissertation, Indiana University, 1973.

Hay, J.G.: The biomechanics of sports techniques, ed. 2, Englewood Cliffs, N.J., 1978, Prentice-Hall, Inc.

Ramey, M.R.: A simulation of the running long jump. In Mechanics and sport, Applied Mechanics Division, vol. 4, New York, 1973, American Society of Mechanical Engineers.

Walton, J.S.: Close-range cine-photogrammetry: another approach to motion analysis. In Terauds, J., editor: Science in biomechanics cinematography, Del Mar, Calif., 1979, Academic Publishers.

CHAPTER 10

Walking

LOCOMOTOR PATTERNS ON LAND

The essential feature in all gross body locomotion on land is the movement of the entire body from the point of contact between a body segment and the supporting surface. Achieving this movement requires that some part of the body such as the feet must apply force to a surface and that the surface must resist, not give way to, the force. The resisting force pushes back, and this reaction moves the body in accordance with Newton's third law of motion, which states that whenever one body exerts a force on another, the second always exerts on the first a force that is equal in magnitude but oppositely directed.

Walking, running, and jumping are modifications of stepping, which begins as a human reflex pattern. This pattern can be, and often is, elicited in an infant held upright with the feet in contact with a surface. It can be seen months before the infant is able to stand, and adults, not knowing that stepping is a reflex act that later will recede, often assume that the child is advanced in motor skills. When the child is able to stand, although hand contact with some support may be necessary to maintain the upright position, intent will inhibit the reflex or permit it to function. If the child wishes to remain in one place, foot contact does not fire the stepping reflex; if the child wishes to move toward an object beyond reach, the built-in joint actions occur. There is no awareness of the joint actions; the child is aware only of having moved. Intent, a cortical activity, set off the pattern that resulted in lifting one foot and then transferring the weight to it. After the child has learned to stand and walk, the joint actions of the early stepping are modified with continued use. The early wide stride is narrowed; hip flexion of the swinging limb is decreased, and therefore the foot is not lifted as high; and the step is lengthened.

Once walking is well established, progression to running is easily made, since the nervous system no longer needs the assurance that the forward foot has made contact before the rear foot is lifted. Then the rear foot can give its final push before the front foot makes contact, and since both feet are in the air at the same time, a running pattern has been achieved. With practice, additional modifications can be made and a number of other patterns, such as the hop, skip, jump, and leap, can be developed. All are achieved without conscious direction of joint action; the child has a general idea of the desired pattern, and somehow the nervous system provides the necessary joint actions. The general idea of the new pattern may have come from observation of other performers, or perhaps the child may have produced the pattern and made efforts to repeat it.

Although desirable changes in the stepping pattern are unconsciously made by the young child, it is possible after a certain age to make them voluntarily. If they are consciously made, the teacher, at least, should have an understanding of the mechanics. For the instructor it is not enough to know that extension at hip, knee, and ankle are necessary when the body (that is, its center of gravity) is to be moved; there should be an understanding of the contributions that each moving segment makes to the desired action—the contributions that each makes to the force that will move the body.

For such understanding, three features should be kept in mind. First, whenever the toes are not free to move (as is the case when they are in contact with the supporting surface and are supporting the body weight), each segment proximal to the toes is moved by reversed muscle action. Metatarsophalangeal joint action moves the foot, not the toes; ankle joint action moves the leg, not the foot; knee joint action moves the thigh, not the leg; hip joint action moves the trunk, not the thigh.

Second, gravitational force is a major contributor to segmental movements in locomotor patterns. When the body's center of gravity is not directly above the ankle joint, gravity tends to initiate movement in that joint. If the center of gravity is in front of the ankle joint, gravitational force tends to flex the ankle. If muscles at the ankle contract and prevent such movement, gravity can raise the foot; if the action is moving the center of gravity forward, the heels will be raised; if the action moves the center of gravity backward, the fore part of the foot and the toes will be raised.

Third, locomotor patterns are pushing patterns—pushing against the supporting surface. Some segments will move in a direction other than that of the desired line of force. Counteraction to the undesired movements must occur. In addition, as a segment moves, it carries with it all segments proximal to it. As the leg moves (when the foot is fixed), it also moves the thigh and trunk; as the foot moves, it moves the leg, the thigh, and the trunk. Therefore the movement and position of a segment are determined not only by action of the joint at its distal end but also by the movements of

the segments distal to it. Before the movements of a segment can be described or explained, both the movement of the immediately distal segment and the angle of the segment must be described (measured).

Measurement of joint angle is familiar to students of movement; measurement of segmental position has not been widely used. This position is described as the angle that the line of the segment makes with a horizontal line and is known as the *angle of inclination*. The angle can be measured from the front or the back. If the segment is perpendicular, its angle of inclination is 90 degrees, whether measured from the front or the back; if the segment is inclined forward 45 degrees, the angle of inclination is 45 degrees measured from the front and 135 degrees measured from the back. Obviously the sum of the front and back measures will always equal 180 degrees. In describing angles of inclination one must know whether measures were made from the front or the back.

In summary, the main propelling force in the stepping-running-jumping pattern is derived from knee extension; to this is added the force of gravity, which rotates the entire body around the metatarsophalangeal joints. Ankle and hip extension keep the center of gravity in an advantageous position to move it in the desired direction.

MINI LABORATORY EXERCISES

1. Observe a walk, a run, and a jump and record the sequences, similarities, and differences in the actions.
2. Where film of these actions is available, project the images on a wall or digitizing surface and draw the body segments used in each motion, showing the differences.
3. Have the walkers, runners, and jumpers chalk their bare feet and then execute the motion so that the imprint on the surface can be seen.

STEPPING

Steindler has stated that walking ''is a series of catastrophies narrowly averted.'' First there is a falling of the body forward; then the legs move under the body and prevent such an accident from occurring by establishing a new base of support with the foot.

Walking is a type of reflex action. The reflexes, such as righting and stepping, displayed by the infant are the very foundation on which the walking movement is based. Reflexes are the first clues to later voluntary movement. The postural reflexes exhibited by the young child during the first months of life are evident during the standing and stepping actions induced by parents. They are the prelude to the walking action. The adult walking action is the very epitome of the harmonization of joint action and the synchronization of muscle action into a flowing movement. The action is beautiful to watch but extremely complex to analyze. It is a remarkable accomplishment, considering the design of the human body, which features a high center of gravity and a small base of support.

The first true walking steps begin between the ages of 10 and 16 months. The young child between the ages of 4 and 7 years usually is thought to walk with adult characteristics. Illness and consequent confinement for a long period of time may cause the walking act to be delayed or, in an adult, to have to be relearned.

Some of the phases of walking are altered in injured and permanently disabled persons. A continuous attempt is being made by biomedical researchers to develop artificial limbs that enable persons with a pathologic condition to walk as nearly normally as possible.

The bipedal position permits rapid initiation of the motion of walking. The center of gravity is easily displaced in the desired direction because (1) it resides high (at approximately the second sacral segment) over a small base of support and (2) the greater portion of the body weight is located in the trunk, head, and shoulders, rather than in the lower extremities. This inherently unstable situation necessitates close cooperation of the neuromusculoskeletal system in the act of walking.

That the center of gravity is located above the main joint of support adds to the instability. The human body is classified as having three effective joints and two effective segments (the lower limbs) for speed and is not considered to have the most effective leg joints and segments in connection with balance. Thus the human body is designed for rapid initial movement in walking and running but not for sustained speed.

There are two theories concerning the initiation of the step in walking. One involves the displacement of the center of gravity and then activation of both the step reflex and the righting reflex. The movement is termed a falling-catching act, as previously noted. The other theory is that the movement of the center of gravity to its highest position—which is reached when the foot rises onto the toes—activates the gastrocnemius and hamstring muscles. They contract with the pulling of the heel off the ground and, along with the gravitational action on the center of gravity, activate the step. Each of these theories has its proponents.

The various phases of walking (Fig. 10-2) may be broken down as follows:

Stance
Heel strike	0%
Foot flat	15%
Heel off	30%
Knee flexion	45%
Toe off	60%

Swing
Toe clearance	40%
Leg swing	
Heel stride	100%

The stance phase, composed of heel strike, foot flat, heel off, knee flexion, and toe off is approximately 60% of the walking cycle, and the swing phase, composed of toe clearance and leg swing, is 40% of the walking cycle. Some of these percentages are changed in the running and jumping aspects of motion.

The stance phase encompasses the heel strike, mid stance, and push-off. The swing phase includes the beginning of the acceleration of the leg, which involves the body weight's being centered over one foot while the other foot is pushing against the ground. The swinging of the non-weight-bearing leg and its deceleration in preparation for the heel strike make up the other portions of the swing phase.

Walking can be described as having two energy phases, a high- and a low-energy phase. The high-energy phase of walking occurs during the stance phase. This is explained by the fact that the descending leg is decelerated just before and at the time of heel strike, thus preventing injury to the heel. In addition, the shock of the heel as it strikes is absorbed by the lower limb and the entire body, which requires energy (Fig. 10-1). Since the shock absorption enables the body to be balanced during mid stance, the energy cost is high. The leg abductors are very active during this time. Finally, the push-off portion of the stance phase initiates the forward propulsion of the body and therefore is high in energy requirements.

The low-energy phase occurs during the acceleration portion (swing phase) of the walking cycle. The hip flexors and knee extensors help keep the heel from rising too high. Dorsiflexion of the toes at the midpoint of the swing in preparation for the heel strike prevents the toes from striking first. The hamstring muscles also expend energy in decelerating the leg during the latter stages of the swing. The question might then be raised: Why is this the low-energy phase? The reason lies in the pendulum action of the swinging leg, which takes considerably less energy than is expended at heel strike, absorption of shock, and push-off. Gravity is working in favor of the pendulum swing by pulling the leg mass down toward the ground. The momentum gained at push-off helps carry the leg through the swing phase.

It has been estimated that during a portion of the swing phase the lower leg reaches a velocity of 32.18 kmph (20 mph). In running this becomes 64.36 to 80.45 kmph (40 to 50 mph).

The most efficient walking is approximately at the rate of 70 steps/min for most individuals, but not for all. Amar has found that at just above 190 steps/min it is more economical, in terms of energy, to run than to walk. This is true until a speed of just under 250 steps/min is reached. The rise and fall of the body in a vertical direction is 5 cm (2 in), and the percentage of body weight alternates between 80% as one foot leaves the ground and 120% as the heel strike takes place at the time the foot descends. The path of the center of gravity is that of a sinusoidal, or smooth, curve; no sharp braking force is evident. There is side-to-side lateral and medial sway of about 5 cm (2 in). The physically disabled person has greater rise and fall in a vertical direction (as much as 10 cm [4 in]) than the normal individual.

In addition, there is backward force as the heel strikes the ground during the end phase of deceleration of the leg. When the foot is flat, there is a forward force as the push-off commences, as well as a torque as the foot twists about the hip joint. The axial rotation of the lower limb is such that it moves, in the swing phase, into internal rotation during heel strike, and then at push-off the external rotation takes place.

The muscles of the lower limb are busy firing in rapid order during the act of walking. Acting as stabilizers and shock absorbers, they contract over a short period of time and then become relaxed. They cause extension, flexion, and internal and external rotation. They help decelerate and accelerate, and yet they fire in milliseconds and then remain quiet a great portion of the time. During the last portion of the swing and the first portion of the stance phase, 20% of the major muscle action is in play.

The body weight is centered on the heel, and then it moves forward toward the lateral edge of

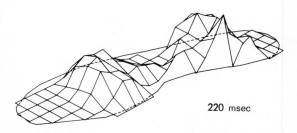

220 msec

Fig. 10-1. Pressure under foot during support phase of walking. (Courtesy Penn State University Biomechanics Laboratory.)

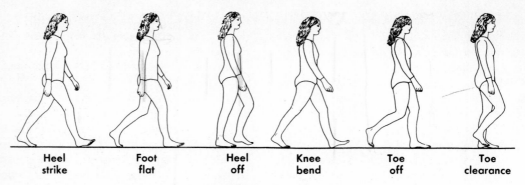

| Heel
strike | Foot
flat | Heel
off | Knee
bend | Toe
off | Toe
clearance |

Fig. 10-2. Walking stride of a woman.

the foot and diagonally toward the undersurface of the big toe. The effect of moving the body weight in such a manner enables the walker to offset much of the recoil effect.

DETERMINANTS OF WALKING

Saunders, Enman, and Eberhart have discussed the following six determinants of gait (walking):

1. *Pelvic rotation.* The pelvis rotates forward with the swing leg, and the center of gravity rotates forward on each hip as the step is taken. There is a total of 8 degrees of rotation, which reduces the drop of the center of gravity.

2. *Pelvic tilt.* The pelvis tilts downward during the stance phase of one leg, which tends to shorten the leg and keeps the center of gravity from rising too much.

3. *Flexion at the knee.* It is to be remembered that as the heel strike occurs during mid stance, the knee is in full extension. When the foot is flat, the knee begins to flex about 5 to 15 degrees; it then extends and flexes again at push-off. The purpose of this flexing and extending is to prevent the center of gravity from rising unduly.

4. *Foot and ankle motion.* The foot and ankle help take up shock and smooth out the path of the center of gravity at heel strike. The foot is in dorsiflexion at heel strike, and as

the heel-off and toe-off phases occur, the knee bends, smoothing out the path of the center of gravity. The foot, ankle, and knee work together as a dampener at heel strike.

5. *Knee motion.* There are two separate actions of the knee during walking. As the ankle rises during the heel-off and toe-off phases, there is flexion at the knee. The flexion at the knee serves as a shock absorber and reduces the degree to which the center of gravity rises.

6. *Lateral movement of the pelvis.* During walking, the lateral movement of the pelvis is 4.45 cm (1.75 in) at each step. The femurs are adducted and the tibias are in slight valgus, enabling the body weight to be transferred downward to a narrow base without too much lateral motion (5 cm [2 in]). (See Figs. 10-2 and 10-3.)

If walking starts from a stationary position, the first joint action to occur is ankle flexion. The reason is that there is a decreasing amount of tension exerted by the ankle extensors in the standing position when the center of gravity is in front of the ankle joint. When walking is initiated, the ankle extensors permit the center of gravity to move beyond the forward limit that is habitual in standing. The nervous system does not initiate a correction because one foot will be moved forward to receive the body weight. As the forward-moving foot is

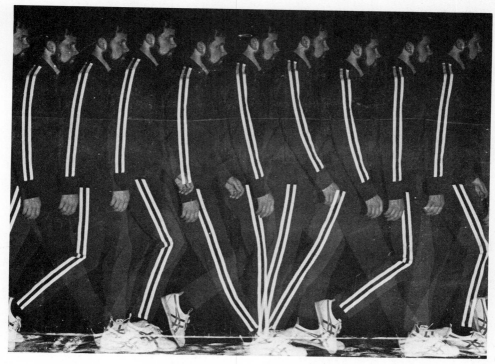

Fig. 10-3. Strobe photograph of walking, by a male, taken at 300 flashes per minute. Note change in foot position from being flat to being raised, with toes just touching floor.

placed on the walking surface, the momentum of the moving body and the push from the rear foot carry the center of gravity over the new support. As each new foot contact is made, joint adjustments in that limb use and facilitate the already developed momentum.

Joint actions of lower limbs

Joint actions of the lower limbs include those of the supporting limb and of the swinging limb.

Joint actions of supporting limb. Movement at the hip, knee, ankle, and metatarsophalangeal joints from the time the heel makes contact with the walking surface until the toes leave that surface is shown in Fig. 10-4. A graph such as this one presents detailed and exact information that if described verbally would require many times the space taken by the graph. Here one can see the

direction of each joint action, its degree in a given time, and the relationship between actions. Students should develop the ability to interpret such graphs and to visualize the joint actions and the body positions shown at each time interval. In the illustration they should see that the heel makes contact at 0 second in time; then for the first 0.15 second, the ankle joint is extending, thus bringing the entire foot in contact with the walking surface. From this point all joint actions will be reversed muscle actions: ankle flexion inclines the leg farther forward, knee action moves the thigh, and hip action moves the trunk.

Because after 0.15 second the center of gravity is in front of the ankle joint, gravitational force will flex it; this action is controlled by the ankle extensors, which lengthen. Hip and knee extension will be the result of contraction of the extensors at

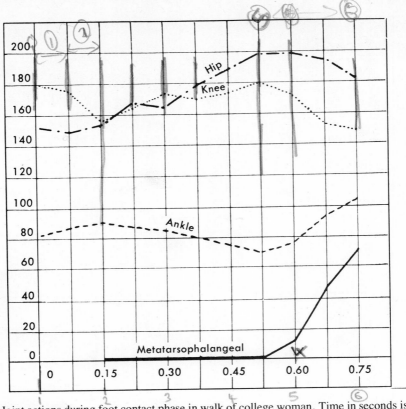

Fig. 10-4. Joint actions during foot contact phase in walk of college woman. Time in seconds is shown at bottom; angles between body segments are shown in degrees at left. Downward slope of lines indicates flexion, and upward slope indicates extension.

these joints. At 0.525 second the leg has reached the desired degree of inclination (not consciously determined), and the ankle extensors contract with force enough to resist gravity, which now acts on the metatarsophalangeal joints and raises the foot from the surface. At point 0.60 second the other (advancing) foot is making contact; then the center of gravity is moved over that foot by the forward momentum developed in the time from 0.15 to 0.60 second and by the final push with the toes and extension at the ankle of the rear foot. Note that the hip and knee are flexing in this final phase. Further explanation of the function of joint actions will be presented in the section on inclinations of the segments.

Joint actions of swinging limb. After contact the

rear foot must be swung forward to establish the new contact. The swing, occupying 0.45 second, is accomplished by hip flexion. From full extension it flexes 34 degrees, bringing the thigh ahead of the trunk. Just before contact the hip extends slightly (3 degrees), lowering the limb for contact.

The knee, which was flexed 50 degrees as the foot left the ground, continues to flex for a brief period—0.075 second. This action lifts the foot from the ground and also shortens the resistance arm for the hip action, thus reducing the energy needed for moving the limb forward.

The ankle joint, which was extended 115 degrees as it left the ground, flexes immediately, lifting the forepart of the foot to clear the ground. Flexion continues until the last 0.075 second be-

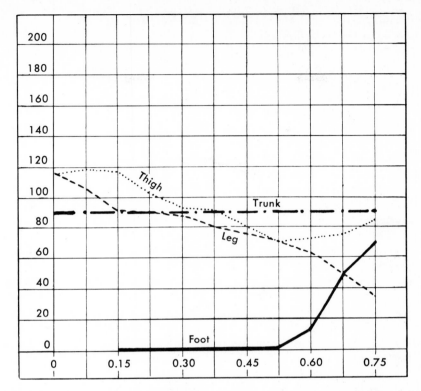

Fig. 10-5. Angles of inclination of body segments during foot contact phase in walking; joint angles are given in Fig. 10-4. All angles are measured from front horizontal except those of foot. Note constant inclination of trunk, resulting from adjustment of hip joints to thigh inclination. Time in seconds is shown at bottom; angles between body segments are shown in degrees at left.

fore contact. Then extension begins and continues until full foot contact is made.

Inclinations of segments of supporting limb. In all locomotor and balance activities, movement of any joint in the supporting limb changes the inclination of the segments above that joint. In standing, ankle flexion inclines the legs, thighs, and trunk toward the horizontal; extension moves these segments away from the horizontal. In most forms of locomotion simultaneous action is likely to occur in the joints of the supporting limb. This action may counteract the effects of distal joints or increase them. (See the discussion on locomotor patterns on land, in this chapter.)

The angle made by each segment with the horizontal in walking is shown in Fig. 10-5. The angles are those between a horizontal line drawn through the joint at the distal end of the segment and a line drawn through the segment. All angles are measured from the front except that for the foot, which is measured from the back. Foot measures shown begin at the time the foot is in full contact, and its inclination is therefore 0 degree until the heel is raised. At 0.525 second the heel leaves the contacting surface, and the angle of inclination changes from 0 degree to 72 degrees as the final push is made.

Leg inclination during full foot contact is

changed by ankle action only. As ankle flexion occurs, it is paralleled by the change in leg inclination. However, when foot inclination begins to change at 0.525 second, foot inclination and ankle action affect leg inclination. Fig. 10-4 shows that as foot inclination begins, the ankle starts to extend at the same rate as the foot inclines; the inclination of the leg remains constant. If ankle extension occurs at the same rate as foot inclination, the inclination of the leg remains constant. If foot inclination is greater than ankle extension, leg inclination will increase. These changes are shown in Fig. 10-5. From 0.525 to 0.75 second the ankle extends 36 degrees, and the foot inclines 72 degrees. During this time the leg is inclined forward 36 degrees.

Inclination of the thigh is determined by the inclination of the leg and by knee action. Knee extension moves the thigh toward the front horizontal; forward inclination of the leg moves the thigh in the same direction. From 0.15 to 0.525 second the knee extends 26 degrees, as shown in Fig. 10-5 as the leg inclines forward 20 degrees. The thigh during this time is moved 46 degrees toward the front horizontal. In the last phase of foot contact the knee flexes 50 degrees, moving the thigh away from the horizontal as the leg inclines 36 degrees. Thigh inclination during this period decreased 14 degrees.

Inclination of the trunk will be determined by thigh inclination and hip action. As the thigh inclines forward, the hip extends at the same rate, keeping the trunk at a constant angle. This is efficient mechanics, eliminating the effort that would be required if the trunk inclination changed.

Additional joint actions

The joint actions just described provide the major forces in propelling the center of gravity in walking. At the same time other joints contribute to the total movement. Among these contributions are rotation of the pelvis on the supporting femur because of medial rotation in the hip joint. These actions lengthen the stride. At the same time the swinging limb is rotated laterally at the hip to keep

the foot along the desired line of direction. The torso is also rotated by spinal action to keep the shoulders facing the desired line of progression. As the speed of walking increases, the rotation of the spine is aided by shoulder action, with the right arm moving forward as the left foot advances.

Variations in stride

Speed. The joint actions and segmental inclinations shown in Figs. 10-4 and 10-5 are those of a college woman walking at what she considered her average speed. As the speed of walking changes, the relative duration of the support and swing phases changes also. In slow walking the stance phase may be almost twice as long as the swing phase; in fast walking the stance and swing phases are likely to be equal. In slow walking gravitational force contributes less; the inclination of the leg decreases, and the length of the step is shortened. Whatever the speed the same joints are acting, and each will be making the same type of contribution. However, variations occur in timing, range, and speed of joint actions.

The number of steps per time unit varies with the speed of walking and the length of the lower limbs. Morton and Fuller report that a man 1.76 m (5 ft 8 in) in height took 100, 112, 122, and 130 steps per minute when walking 4.02, 4.82, 5.63, and 6.43 kmph (2.5, 3.0, 3.5, and 4.0 mph). A man 1.98 m (6 ft 0.5 in) in height, walking at the same speeds, took 92, 100, 108, and 115 steps per minute.

In studying the energy cost for 19 college women walking on a treadmill electrically driven at 3.2, 4.02, and 4.82 kmph (2, 2.5, and 3 mph), Baird found the optimal rate (ratio of the amount of work to the oxygen consumption) to be between 4.02 and 4.82 kmph (2.5 and 3.0 mph). A strobe picture enables the investigator to integrate time with body and joint positions (Fig. 10-3).

Stair walking. There is some alteration in the walking pattern used in going up and down stairs. In the ascending pattern there is more knee lift and more dorsiflexion of the ankle during the swing phase, resulting in greater action by the leg extensors. If the stairstep is higher than normal, the center of gravity must be forward of the foot-flat position before extension of the leg takes place. This would be especially true for elderly persons.

In the act of walking downstairs the center of gravity of the walker must be firmly held over the supporting foot. Flexion of the leg and dorsiflexion of the ankle are greater than normal, and there is also some flexion at the hip, followed by extension at the hip and knee. As one foot descends, plantar flexion occurs. The action of the muscles in the foot-flat position is a cooperative one in which the quadriceps, femoris, hamstrings, and gluteus medius, as well as the soleus, act during the supporting phase.

Further analysis of the locomotor pattern is described in Chapter 22.

MINI LABORATORY EXERCISES

1. Using a metronome, a stopwatch, or just a hand or drum beat, vary the walking pace. Observe and record limb and body differences.
2. Determine whether there are any differences in gaits of various persons wearing high-heeled shoes, clogs, skirts, and other types of attire.
3. Record differences in gait patterns between injured and normal individuals.
4. Compare the walking patterns of young children and adults.

REFERENCES

Amar, J.: The human motor, Dubuque, Iowa, 1972, W.C. Brown Co.
Baird, J.E.: Energy costs of women during walking, thesis, University of Southern California, 1959.
Morton, D.J., and Fuller, D.D.: Human locomotion and body form, Baltimore, 1952, The Williams & Wilkins Co.
Saunders, J.B., Inman, V.T., and Eberhart, H.D.: Major determinants in normal and pathological gait, J. Bone Joint Surg. **35A:**543-558, 1953.
Steindler, A.: Kinesiology of the human body under normal and pathological conditions, Springfield, Ill., 1955, Charles C Thomas, Publisher.

ADDITIONAL READINGS

Andriacchi, T.P., Ogle, J.A., and Galante, J.O.: Walking speed as a basis for normal and abnormal gait measurements, J. Biomech. **10:**261, 1977.
Broer, M.R., and Zermicke, R.F.: Efficiency of human movement, Philadelphia, 1979, W.B. Saunders Co.
Basmajian, J.V.: Muscles alive: their functions revealed by electromyography, ed. 4, Baltimore, 1978, The Williams & Wilkins Co.
Cavagna, G.A., and Margaria, R.: Mechanics of walking, J. Appl. Physiol. **21:**271-278, 1966.
Eberhart, H.D.: Physical principles of locomotion, proceedings of the International Conference of Neural Control of Locomotion, New York, 1976, Plenum Press.
Murray, M.P.: Gait as a total pattern of movement, Am. J. Phys. Med. **46:**290, 1967.
Smidt, G.L.: Hip motion and related factors in walking, Phys. Ther. **51:**9, 1971.
Wells, K., and Luttgens, K.: Kinesiology, ed. 6, Philadelphia, 1976, W.B. Saunders Co.

CHAPTER 11

Running

Running is a modification of walking and differs from the latter in two significant aspects. First, during one phase in running neither foot is in contact with the ground; second, at no period are both feet in contact with the ground. Although these differences necessitate differences in joint action, the same joints and segments are used in running as in walking. Differences in joint degrees and timing of actions can be anticipated. Since only one foot is on the ground at one time, it is possible to run relatively smoothly with one leg shorter than the other, whereas in walking this same condition would cause a limp. In addition, once speed in running has developed, the force of the forward momentum is greater and contributes more to forward movement of the body than during walking. The action of the swinging leg in running is greater in amplitude and velocity and is likely to contribute the most to the forward movement of the body.

Running is a bipedal action, and it is three dimensional in action just as is walking. All the determinants of walking are prominent in running. Pelvic rotation, pelvic tilt, lateral motion of the pelic, knee flexion, foot and ankle motion, and knee motion are present to a greater degree in running than in walking. In addition, there are greater flexion and extension of the legs and arms. A major difference is that whereas in walking there is an overlapping of the stance phases, in running there is an overlapping of the swing phases.

Often the factors that are important in speed running are considered less important in distance running. Proper mechanical positions and speed are essential to a sprinter; physiologic endurance, efficiency, and pace are all important to a distance runner. In races involving both speed and endurance the ability to utilize proper mechanics and to have sufficient endurance is paramount. Yet there is some use of both factors by the sprinter and the distance runner: (1) some element of endurance is necessary in a longer sprint race, and (2) at the end of a distance race the distance runner may need to become a sprinter and use correct mechanics to win the race.

It is believed that the mechanics of running have an effect on efficiency of performance. For example, it may be possible to delay the onset of fatigue by maintaining effective mechanical positions such as a high knee lift and an upright trunk.

A study of the animal kingdom reveals that the fastest runners and the longest jumpers have certain mechanical characteristics that enable them to excel. The cheetah has been clocked at 112.63 kmph (70 mph) and has reached a speed of 72.06 kmph (45 mph) in 2 seconds. It has a stride length of 7.7 m (23 ft), the same as a horse; yet its stride frequency is one and one-half times that of the horse, whose maximum speed is 64.36 kmph (40 mph). The cheetah's great flexibility in both sets of limbs, and especially in the lower back, enables it to have such a long stride. For speed running, great power in the legs and buttocks (gluteal, hamstring, and quadriceps muscles) is an asset. In addition, the location of bulky muscles so that they are close to the joint centers decreases the resistance arms and permits power and speed of movement to be combined. Therefore the heavy muscles are located proximally and the lighter ones distally.

In distance running the less body weight carried during the run, the more effective the runner. Height varies among individuals who are successful. Excessive height could be detrimental because of wind resistance, and most distance runners are at or below the population mean for height. Extremely short (several inches below the mean) individuals would have difficulty when a long stride is needed. Again, a light body weight (with low body fat) would be advantageous for the short individual, especially the runner with slow-twitch muscle fibers. In speed running, fast-twitch muscle fibers are essential.

STEP AND STRIDE

Since there is some disagreement among some of the scholars in defining step and stride, a definition of each will be given here. A *step* is that part of running action which commences at the moment when either foot terminates contact with the ground and continues until the opposite foot contacts the surface, whereas a *stride* consists of two steps during which there is a period of support and a period of flight. A stride is identified by the termination of contact of a foot with the ground and the subsequent contacting of the same foot with the ground—thus the involvement of two steps.

The stride may be divided into almost the same elements that were discussed in connection with walking, namely, foot strike, foot down, toe off, rear foot lift, and knee lift in front. There are two periods of support (one for each foot) and two periods of nonsupport for each stride (Fig. 11-1).

MECHANICS OF RUNNING

Stride length and running velocity. Many authors (such as Hoffman, Teeple, and Sparks) have shown that there is a positive relationship between step or stride length and running velocity. It must be kept in mind that speed of the run equals stride length times stride frequency. If a short-legged runner desires a fast pace, he or she will have to take more strides per unit of time than a longer-legged runner, whose stride should be longer. A combination of long stride and fast frequency is an indication of a fast runner. On the other hand, a runner desiring to run a long distance will run with a short stride and will depend on pace and lower stride frequency to conserve energy (Fig. 11-2).

In most instances leg length is associated with body height. The taller person has longer legs normally and therefore should be able to take a longer stride. In addition, a positive relationship exists between the force exhibited by the legs at push-off and length of stride. Furthermore, if there is a minimum amount of braking force at the *foot down* position, the runner can move faster in a forward direction.

Speed runners have the longest stride of all the runners. The stride length is approximately 4.87 m (16 ft) for men and 3.65 to 4.26 m (12 to 14 ft) for women. The top female sprinters have a step frequency of 4.48 steps per second, and the male sprinters, 5 steps per second.

It has been reported that to gain speed initially an inexperienced runner must increase stride length. However, after a stride of optimal length has been attained, the increase in speed becomes a matter of increasing stride frequency.

Arm action. The arms of the fast runner move in opposition to the legs and are 180 degrees out of phase with the adjacent leg, as in walking. How-

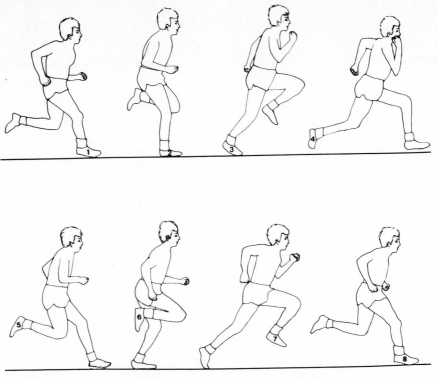

Fig. 11-1. Sprinter in action. *1,* Foot strike on outside border of foot near ball. *2,* Foot-down position with foot completely flat. Some sprinters would show heel not touching surface. *3,* Toes almost ready to leave surface (No. *7* shows supporting foot's toes just touching surface). *4,* Both feet are off ground (nonsupport). *5,* Rear foot lift (see Nos. *1* and *8*). *6,* Knee lift in front, almost complete. *7,* High knee lift and long stride potential. *8,* Foot strike as seen in No. *1.*

ever, as the speed increases, the arms move more rapidly in a flexed to partially extended position (Fig. 11-1). The arms move toward the midline of the body in the forward position and then to the rear, with the hands seldom going beyond the hips.

Aristotle (384-322 B.C.), who has been called the father of kinesiology, was able to observe arm action and its contribution to the running motion. More than three centuries before Christ, Aristotle wrote:

The animal that moves makes its change of position by pressing against that which is beneath it. Hence, athletes jump farther if they have the weights in their hands than if they have not, and runners run faster if they swing their arms, for in extension of the arms there is a kind of leaning upon the hands and wrists.

Center of gravity. The rise and fall of the center of gravity is greater in running than in walking (5 to 6.3 cm [2 to 2.5 in]), but the amount of force against the ground is nearly the same for running and walking, approximately two times body weight. Slow or unskilled jogging may produce greater vertical forces than running and may impose undue stress on some of the internal organs.

The jarring effect of jogging can be reduced by using rubberized insoles, which reduce the friction

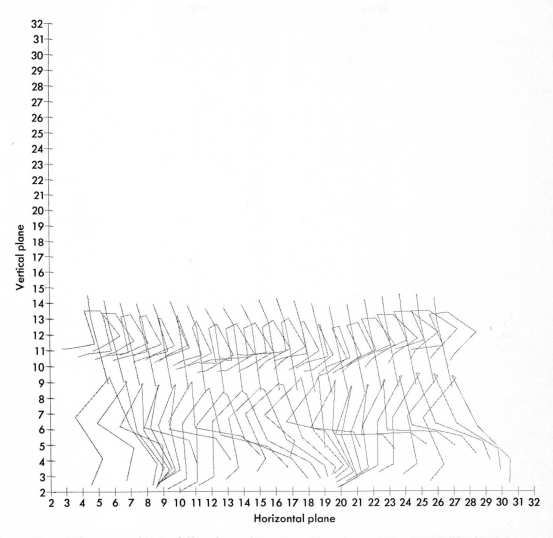

Fig. 11-2. Computer printout of film of marathon runner. Note short stride and small lift of body's center of gravity. (Prepared by James Richards.)

and force against the ground. They have a cushioning effect of up to 20% to 30% greater than does a regular shoe and can be a help to many who jog, including elderly persons.

Tension. To prevent tension from occurring in the arms and neck, the runner must learn to run explosively but in a semirelaxed manner; that is, the runner tries to run as fast as possible without unduly contracting the arm and neck muscles or other muscles extraneous to the action. This is termed differential relaxation. Runners use some of the following strategies to reduce tension: (1) Generate tension in the thumb with pressure against the forefinger to prevent the hand and arm from being the center of tension. (2) Roll out the lower lip and yawn while running, to keep the jaw and neck muscles from tensing. Tension usually begins in the neck, jaw, and arms and then proceeds to the torso and finally to the legs. The legs under tension may rotate so much externally that the stride of the sprint runner is decreased considerably and the speed is reduced.

Foot position. The contact of the runner's foot with the ground at foot strike is slightly different from that of the walker's foot, the degree of difference depending on the velocity of the run (Fig. 11-3). At high speed the contact is first made on the lateral edge of the ball of the foot. The heel is lowered, and a controversy exists as to whether it actually touches the surface. In middle-distance running, the first contact is made with the rear part of the ball of the foot. In the case of slower or distance running, the heel does come down so that the foot is flat on the ground at contact. In very slow running the heel strikes the ground first. The body weight moves forward after foot contact, the same as in walking. However, the contact time of the foot in running is much shorter than in walking, being slightly less than 0.01 second for speed runners and greater for other runners, depending on their body velocity. In walking, it is ±1.0 second, depending on speed.

Knee action. The knee lift (thigh flexion) should reach the level of the hip, and the rear "kickup" of the foot (flexion of leg during swing phase) should

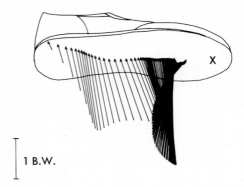

All subjects: 6 min/mile

Right foot

1 B.W.

Fig. 11-3. Computer graphics display of magnitude and direction of force across shoe during running. (Courtesy Penn State University Biomechanics Laboratory.)

again be nearing the horizontal. These conditions at the maximum are only true in speed running. Knee lift and rear kickup are not as pronounced in the distance runs.

The position whereby the heel is moved high and just to the edge of the buttocks during the running cycle is an advantage. The radius of rotation is decreased as the heel moves high and closer to the edge of the buttocks. This position is a characteristic of a fast runner.

Flexion at the knee occurs at foot down, and extension occurs as the toe-off movement takes place. There is some disagreement regarding the amount of extension present as the foot leaves the ground. Apparently, with the world's top sprinters, complete extension does not occur, because of the short time the foot is in contact with the ground (support time). Some researchers have found an increase in flexion at foot down as an increase occurs in running velocity.

Braking force. It has been hypothesized that if the foot of a runner is moving backward as it strikes the ground with a negative velocity equal to the positive velocity of the center of gravity moving forward, braking force would be zero. It is known that faster runners show a greater negative foot velocity than do slower runners. It appears that this diminution of the braking force aids in speed running. Most researchers agree that if the foot at foot strike is directly under the center of gravity, the braking force is reduced to a minimum.

Hip action. Considerable rotation at the hip occurs during the sprint action, and much less during long-distance running. The former motion results in a long stride and facilitates the development of greater stride frequencies. The reverse is desired in long-distance running.

Support and nonsupport time. It has been found that as the speed of running increases, the nonsupport time increases and the support time decreases. Most researchers have found that the respective times may be close to 50% for each. With distance runners the ratio is somewhat different, that is, 20% nonsupport and 80% support (for marathon runners). This ratio may be reversed with world-class sprinters in favor of increased nonsupport time (52% nonsupport and 48% support). It is just the opposite in fatigue situations; the more fatigued the runner, the more time is spent in support.

Trunk angle. The trunk angle, or upper body lean, during running has been a subject of debate for some time. There is some agreement that after the initial starting distance, which is 13.71 to 18.28 m (15 to 20 yd) in sprinting, there need be very little lean, or inclination. Many coaches are now advocating an almost upright position after an optimal running posture is attained.

It is known that sprinters do not accelerate after running 54.8 to 64.0 m (60 to 70 yd) from the start. They just try to maintain a constant velocity as long thereafter as possible. On the other hand, distance runners set a pace and may accelerate at times to obtain a better position among the other runners or to relive monotony or tension. In the latter instance they may lean forward to increase velocity, and then as they assume a more even pace, they become more upright.

Usually the researchers find a trunk lean of 5 to 7 degrees forward during speed running. A few have even found a trunk lean of a few degrees to the rear. In distance running the trunk lean is about the same as in sprinting. Depending on the wind or air resistance, the lean may be greater or less than upright. The important factor is that muscle effort should not be used to maintain body lean, and the respiratory muscles must be free to function.

TYPES OF TERRAIN

Curve running. Running a curve is relatively easy at a slow pace. As velocity is increased, the runner must make certain accommodations to negotiate the curved path effectively. For example, the center of gravity is moved laterally to the inside of the track oval (body lean toward curb), and a wider base of support is achieved with the feet spaced somewhat apart to give better balance. The runner may accelerate part of the way on the straightaways but must run under control at the initial entrance onto the curve; then the runner may accelerate on the curve. These accommodations are necessary because of centrifugal force. To overcome this force the runner initially pushes outward with the feet and leans the body toward the inside to reduce the radius of rotation and increase the lateral ground reaction forces; otherwise he would be forced toward the outside and would not be able to run the curve effectively. The greater the velocity of the runner, the greater will be the lean.

Grade running. Henson studied six cross-country male runners while they were running on a treadmill at 15 combinations of speed and grade. He found that

when increasing his speed on a downhill slope, the runner should do so primarily by increasing the length of his stride. This results in a more bounding type of movement but makes greater use of the pull of gravity as the runner moves farther down the hill with each stride as the flight phase becomes greater. The muscle contractions would be primarily eccentric contractions opposing the pull of gravity, which do not require the same amount of energy as concentric contractions in running on the level or up hill. Also, because fewer strides per minute are required in this bounding type of movement, the limbs are not required to oscillate as rapidly nor as frequently; thus additional energy is saved in accelerating and decelerating the limbs. When running up a long incline, the runner should shorten his stride and lean into the hill slightly as he slows the pace to avoid producing excessive oxygen debt. These techniques should aid the novice runner in making the most efficient adjustment to a hilly cross-country and result in maximum improvement of performance.*

JOINT ACTIONS

Joint actions of supporting limb. In Fig. 11-4 are shown the angles of the lower limb measured on a

*Henson, P.L.: Pace and grade related to the oxygen and energy requirements, and the mechanics of treadmill running, doctoral dissertation, Indiana University, 1976.

film of a male Olympic competitor as he neared the finish line in the 1500-m race. The time per frame for this film is based on the speed, which is assumed to be approximately 64 frames/sec. The support phase was therefore approximately 0.075 second. The runner landed with full foot contact, and the foot flexed immediately and continued to do so for 0.03 second. This action would be caused by the forward momentum of the body and consequent rotation at the ankle joint. At 0.03 second ankle extension begins, preventing further rotation at the ankle joint; the forward momentum cannot now rotate the body around the ankle joint, and its force must act at the metatarsal joints. This action

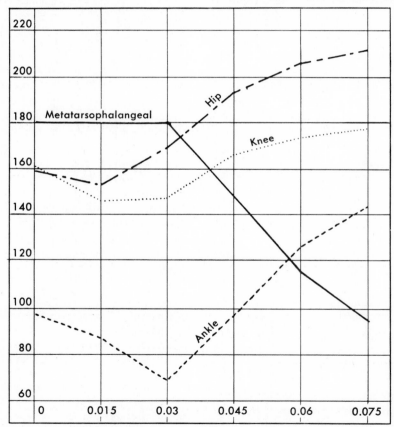

Fig. 11-4. Joint actions of supporting limb during foot contact in running. Time in seconds is shown at bottom; angles between body segments are shown in degrees at left. (Taken from film of male Olympic contestant.)

continues to the takeoff. Angle extension, as the foot (except for the toes) is lifted, moves the leg backward and upward from the positions to which it would be carried by the metatarsophalangeal action. The leg flexes at contact, easing the force of impact as the foot touches the ground. During the final 0.045 second the knee extends, carrying forward the entire body except the supporting leg and foot. This action is due to contraction of the knee extensors and the forward momentum of the body. The hip joint also flexes at impact and then begins extension to maintain the angle of inclination of the trunk.

It is interesting to compare the joint actions of the skilled runner with those of a college woman who had had no special training in running. In Fig. 11-5 are shown the joint actions of the woman as she ran at her top speed. The pattern of action is the same for the two runners; that is, the direction of joint movement is the same. The differences are in speed of action and in range and are shown in Table 11-1.

Comparison of information in Figs. 11-4 and 11-5 shows that except for the metatarsophalangeal joints, the range of movement for the man is greater, especially in the knee and hip joints. The speed of the man's actions is also greater in all joints; in the knee it is more than 8.8 times as great. Further comparisons can be made of the angles of inclination.

Joint actions of swinging limb. The joint actions of the swinging limb can be visualized from the positions shown in Figs. 11-6 and 11-7. The differences in segmental inclinations of both supporting

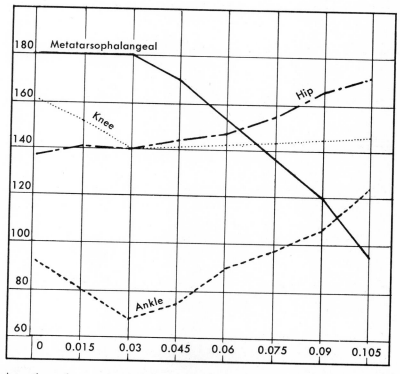

Fig. 11-5. Joint actions of supporting limb during foot contact in running. Time in seconds is shown at bottom; angles between body segments are shown in degrees at left. (Taken from film of college woman with no special training in running.)

Table 11-1. Comparison of joint actions of trained man and untrained woman in running

Joint action	Man			Woman		
	Range	Time	Velocity (degrees/sec)	Range	Time	Velocity (degrees/sec)
Metatarsophalangeal extension	86	0.045	1911	85	0.075	1133
Ankle extension	73	0.045	1622	56	0.075	746
Knee extension	32	0.045	711	6	0.075	80
Hip extension	59	0.06	983	32	0.075	426

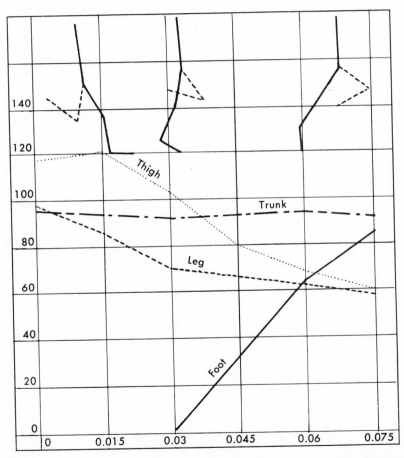

Fig. 11-6. Segmental inclinations of supporting limb during foot contact in running. Time in seconds is shown at bottom; angles between body segments are shown in degrees at left. (Taken from film of male Olympic contestant.)

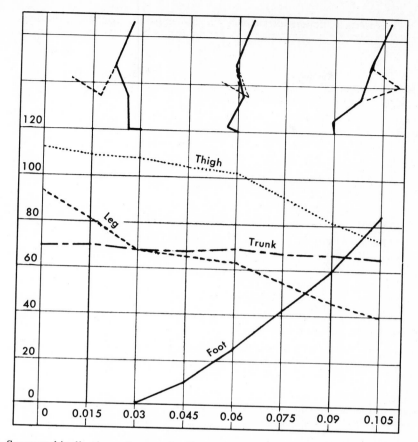

Fig. 11-7. Segmental inclinations of supporting limb during foot contact in running. Time in seconds is shown at bottom; angles between body segments are shown in degrees at left. (Taken from film of college woman with no special training in running.)

and swinging limbs are shown. The ensuing description is of the runner in Fig. 11-6. Those of primary interest are the hip and the knee. In the takeoff the rear limb is about to leave the ground, and the swing will begin with the extended hip and knee. During the period of no contact, this limb will reach the position of the rear limb shown at contact. During this time, which for the 1500-m male runner equals the support phase, the hip joint has not yet brought the thigh in line with the trunk, but the knee has flexed through almost 120 degrees, bringing the heel to hip level. At contact the hip flexes rapidly, bringing the thigh in line with

the trunk and then up toward the front horizontal at takeoff. During the first two thirds of support, the swinging knee flexes, bringing the leg closer to the thigh. This moves the center of gravity of the limb toward the fulcrum (the hip) and facilitates its flexion. The speed with which the thigh and leg are swung forward and upward (closer to the front horizontal) during contact adds to the projecting force. Observation of a vigorous kick will show that the swinging limb can move the whole body forward. (One film of an expert football punter shows that the body is moved forward more than 0.6 m [2 ft] with no observable action in the supporting limb.) According to Fenn and Fortney, better runners bring the thigh closer to the horizontal at takeoff.

From the position at takeoff the leading limb during flight prepares for contact by extending the hip, thus lowering the entire limb, and the knee is extended, thus increasing the length of the stride. In other film observations some runners have been seen to flex their knees just before contact; this action moves the foot back under the body and may decrease the possible backward push on contact, but it does decrease braking force and enables the runner to move his leg rapidly forward. In many cases the forward movement of the total body is greater than the backward movement of the foot because of knee flexion, which seems to be advantageous, since it rotates the distal end of the leg backward; as foot contact is made, ankle flexion rotates the proximal end of the leg forward. Thus the direction of leg rotation before contact is continued after the foot is placed on the ground.

Angles of inclination of supporting limb. The graphs in Figs. 11-6 and 11-7 show that to understand movement in running, one must consider both joint and inclination angles. The inclination of the trunk of both runners remains at an almost constant angle during foot contact, and yet the hip joint (which moves the trunk) has extended 59 degrees in the man and 32 degrees in the woman (Table 11-1). In both runners thigh inclination has equaled hip action. The graphs show that foot inclination is the same for both, approximately 85 degrees; leg inclinations differ, indicating a difference in ankle action. During foot rising the man's leg inclines 12 degrees and the woman's more than twice that amount. If the man is using better running mechanics, the primary cause of the woman's poor performance may be the small range of ankle extension. Do her extensor muscles lack strength, or does the reflex for ankle flexion fail to respond with sufficient strength? Leg inclination could explain the difference in thigh inclination. That of the woman is less. Greater thigh inclination combined with her leg inclination could be too much for balance. This comparison of good and poor performance illustrates the value and limitations of film in studying movement. A possible cause of poor performance has been suggested; its validity needs further testing.

Additional joint actions. It was noticed in reviewing the film of the male runner (Fig. 11-6) that the pelvis rotates to a greater degree in running than it does in walking. When the thighs are separated, the pelvis is rotated on the supporting femur. As one thigh is swung forward, the pelvis rotates forward on the same side, adding length to the step. Hubbard says that improvement in running is due to an increase in the length of strike, rather than to an increase in rate of movement. The comparison of the two runners described here suggests that both factors influence speed, as has been mentioned previously.

It can be seen that the arms swing in opposition to the legs. They aid in maintaining a forward position of the upper trunk, which would otherwise tend to face in the same direction as does the pelvis. The arm swing also affects the center of gravity of the whole body. At takeoff one arm is raised to the front and the other to the back. These positions raise the center of gravity of the total body, which reaches its highest point at takeoff. Shortly after contact, when the thighs are parallel, the arms are at the side of the body, with the elbow joints approaching extension. The arms now tend to lower the center of gravity of the entire body, which reaches its lowest point at this time. Modern sprinters are deemphasizing the backward extended movements of the forearms for a more rapid arm movement forward. This seems to be associated with increased leg action.

TRACK STARTS AND INITIAL SPRINTING PHASE

In running races it is desirable to move the body forward as rapidly as possible from the start. This is especially important in sprints, and most investigators have thought that the start is faster when executed from a crouching position. Yet some researchers (such as Ward) have found that top runners negotiate the first half of a 100-meter dash faster from a standing position than from a crouch-

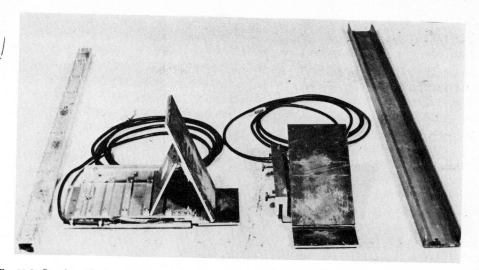

Fig. 11-8. Starting blocks and center rails used in Paul Ward's study of the stand-up start. (From Ward, P.: An analysis of kinetic and kinematic factors of the standup and the preferred crouch starting techniques with respect to sprint performance, doctoral dissertation, Indiana University, Aug., 1973.)

ing position. The height of the center of gravity is the same whether the runner is in a standing position at the starting line or has reached a point 13.7 m (15 yd) from the starting line after a crouching start.

It has been found through experience that the start is faster if blocks are provided for the push; they, too, increase the amount of push that can be directed horizontally (Fig. 11-8).

Since most sprinters use the crouching start because the results from the standing start are as yet not conclusive, the discussion here is stated in terms of the crouching start.

As the runner takes the crouching position, hands, feet, and rear knee are in contact with the supporting surface, with the rear foot supporting little of the body weight. The distance between the hands and the forward foot is short enough to force the spine to flex (arch); the value of this flexion will be shown later. In the "get set" position, which precedes the actual start, the rear knee is raised from the surface until the rear leg is inclined some 25 to 30 degrees as measured from the front.

(However, some runners completely extend the rear leg.) Both thighs are moved upward and forward by knee extension, thereby moving the trunk and the center of gravity farther forward. At the same time the spine flexes more; the head is held at the same height that it had in the first position.

As the trunk is raised, the rear foot pushes by sudden knee extension, which moves the thigh forward. Film has shown that the feet are moved slightly backward preceding the push. This push is of short duration because the limb must be moved forward quickly for the first step. Before the rear foot has left the block, extension of the front knee begins, moving the front thigh forward. Both knee actions are examples of reversed muscle action and are the primary sources of power for putting the body into motion. The leg of the front foot keeps a fairly constant inclination, adjusting its position to the movement of the foot. The trunk, which has been inclined slightly above the horizontal during the push of the rear foot, is raised somewhat as the rear foot is moved forward for the first step. Since the center of gravity is ahead of the supporting front foot, gravity will rotate the foot about the metatarsophalangeal joints. In general, the action is that described in the discussion on mechanics of the stepping pattern in this chapter. A noted coach has increased the height of the front block to decrease the amount of backward movement of the front foot and thus decrease the time that the foot pushes against the block.

The first five or six steps after the push differ from the steps of the run. There is only a short period in which both feet are off the surface. Because the center of gravity is so far ahead of the takeoff foot, little upward projection is given to it, and the succeeding step must be taken quickly to prevent it from falling below the desired line of flight. After the first step the trunk is gradually raised, thus increasing the amount of upward direction given to the center of gravity; with this change the steps can be gradually lengthened to equal those which will be used in the sprint stride.

During the striding action of the lower limbs the arms move in opposition to them. The upper arms are moved by shoulder joint muscles, and the forearms are held in approximately 90 degrees of flexion to shorten the moment arm of the shoulder levers.

At the starting signal the contacting segments leave the surface in sequence. According to Bresnahan, who observed 28 trained sprinters, all right handed, the order of breaking contact in all subjects was left hand, right hand, right foot, left foot. The average time between the signal and the left-hand break was 0.172 second and between the signal and the left-foot break 0.443 second. Bresnahan also observed one left-handed sprinter in whom the breaking order was reversed—right hand first and right foot last.

As the hands are raised, the spine extends, counteracting the pull of gravity on the upper trunk while the lower trunk is supported by the feet. As the spine extends, it moves the head and the center of gravity forward. In looking at film of this action

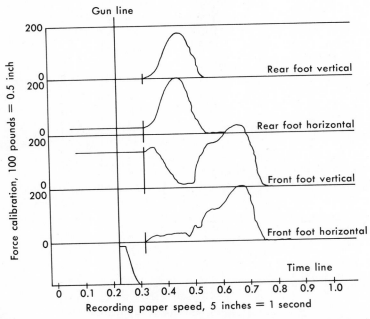

Fig. 11-9. Typical force graph for sprinter running 100-yard sprint from standing start (subject No. 103). (From Ward, P.: An analysis of kinetic and kinematic factors of the standup and the preferred crouch starting techniques with respect to sprint performance, doctoral dissertation, Indiana University, Aug., 1973.)

the viewer is reminded of Gray's statement: "By arching and extending its back, a galloping dog greatly increases the power and length of its stride."*

*Gray, J.: How animals move, London, 1960, Cambridge University Press.

The forces made against the blocks by runners using the standing and crouching starts are shown in Figs. 11-9 and 11-10 for comparison. Also in the crouching start note that the front foot in most instances, exerts force over a longer time but for

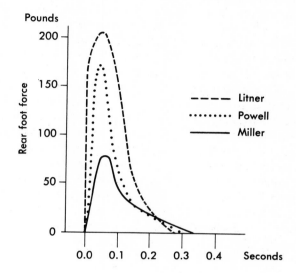

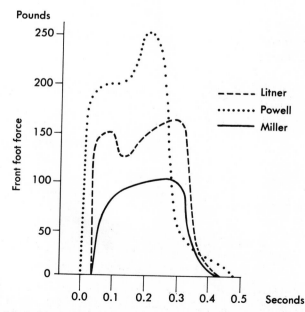

Fig. 11-10. Starting block force curves for three runners using crouching start. (From Barlow, D.A., Bates, B.T., and Vallière, A.: Unpublished study, Indiana University, 1973.)

less maximal force. (The impulse is greater for the front foot since multiplied by the time.)

The effect of foot spacing on velocity in sprints was studied by Sigerseth and Grinaker. The subjects were 28 male college physical education majors. In the crouching start the feet were separated 10, 19, and 28 inches, and times were checked at 10, 20, 30, 40, and 50 yards. At every distance the time for the 19-inch start was the lowest, but the records were statistically significant only when the means for the 19- and 28-inch starts were compared for the 10, 20, 30, and 50 yards.

Length of stride in speed running is dependent on several factors: (1) It is positively correlated with the ratio of leg length to body height, (2) it is directly proportional to the amount of force extended to propel the body into the air during push-off, and (3) it is inversely proportional to the amount of braking force at touchdown.

The following are certain starting mechanics agreed on by investigators Barlow and Cooper:

1. Block spacings vary from 27.9 to 38.1 cm (11 to 15 in), partially according to leg length. This arrangement enables the sprinter to attain a fast start.
2. In the set position the front knee joint angle should be near 90 degrees, since the sprinter remains longest over this leg before leaving the blocks.
3. The rear leg is near extension (varying from 140 to 170 degrees) to react to the gun signal as soon as possible and to apply nearly maximal thrust.
4. The head of the sprinter is relaxed and extended downward. It is the first body part to move to impel the body in the desired direction.
5. A sprinter usually takes about 0.11 second to react to the gun.
6. The time of exit of the rear foot from the rear block (mean time, 0.270 second) was less than Morris found for untrained sprinters (mean time, 0.343 second).
7. The mean time spent in the blocks by the front foot was 0.446 second, showing a greater time spent there by this foot.
8. The greatest horizontal force against the blocks was exerted by the rear foot. However, the front foot generates slightly more force over a longer time.
9. The first step by the best sprinter off the blocks was longer and closer to the ground.

In middle-distance running, Sparks found the following:

1. The best runners depend on their ability to consume and use oxygen efficiently. These same top runners supply more energy by the aerobic system and therefore produce less oxygen debt.
2. The better runners are more airborne during the race; that is, they are in the air slightly longer than on the ground. The reverse often happens as they become fatigued.
3. As the stress of the run becomes greater toward the end of the race, often the stride is shortened, and to keep up the pace the runner increases the stride frequency. The center of gravity is lowered, and the knee lift (knee flexion and extension) is decreased as fatigue sets in.

In distance running the same mechanical effects from fatigue can and often do occur. Stress tolerance and ability to consume and use oxygen efficiently may delay or even prevent the occurrence of mechanical faults. A strobe picture of a runner in action (Fig. 11-11) shows the leg and arm action in one plane clearly. The outward rotation of the foot is also depicted.

Several investigators, such as Sparks, have found that a fatigued runner exhibits most of the following:

1. Lower center of gravity of the body during air phase
2. Greater forward body lean
3. Lateral extension of the arms
4. Decreased leg lift
5. Shorter strides
6. Decreased step frequency
7. Wider base of support, with the legs rotated laterally (externally)

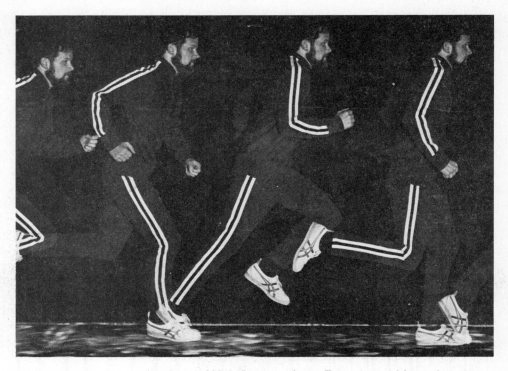

Fig. 11-11. Strobe photograph, taken at 300 flashes per minute. Foot, arm, and leg action are seen clearly in their sequential relationships. (Photograph by Phillip L. Henson, Biomechanics Laboratory, Indiana University.)

RACE WALKING

Race walking is a specialized walking technique usually found in a competitive situation in which the walker comes close to running. To be classified as a walking pattern, the action must be accomplished with one foot always in contact with the surface. It involves smooth upper body movement with exaggerated arm action. In addition, there are considerable pelvic rotation and pelvic tilt, as well as unusual lateral movement of the pelvis. All these movements are made with almost completely extended knees (locked). In the Olympics the walkers at each distance adhere to the movement principles mentioned above, with accentuation of the leg, pelvic, and arm actions.

CONCLUSION

The differences between an untrained and a trained runner are shown in Figs. 11-6 and 11-7. The trained one was finishing a 1500-m race as he was filmed. His joint actions differ from those of a sprinter. It must be kept in mind that any runner who is reducing speed increases the proportionate time of contact and decreases the number of steps per minute. In addition, the part of the foot that contacts the ground varies; it may be the heel, ball, or entire foot. (A carried object, such as a football or a hockey or lacrosse stick, affects the swing of the arms. The length of the limb and the distribution of weight also result in individual differences in joint action.)

It has been said by some that a sprinter inclines the trunk more than does the long-distance runner. Slocum and Bowerman question whether any good runner, regardless of the distance of the run, inclines the trunk forward beyond the vertical after the acceleration of the start. They also maintain that there is a backward tilting of the pelvis accompanied by flexion of the spine and that this so-called flat-backed position increases the ability to rotate the thigh laterally. (Lateral rotation of the thigh is needed to place the foot in the desired direction as the pelvis is rotated forward over the supporting hip.) The lower-limb actions of a sprinter and a distance runner are the same in general appearance, but there are differences in detail. The sprinter has greater hip flexion in the swinging limb and thus raises the flexed knee higher; the stride is also longer, there are more strides per second, and a smaller area of the foot contacts the ground. Other investigators (Sparks, for example) found trunk inclination to be 2 to 4 degrees forward of the vertical.

In reviewing publications on the direction of foot movement immediately before contact, Fortney found that authors did not agree on this direction but also that in most cases they did not make clear whether they referred to movement with reference to a fixed point in space or to a fixed point in the body. In studying film of eight elementary-school boys whose runs were photographed when they were in the second grade and again in each of the three following years, Fortney found that the heel moved forward with reference to a fixed point in space and that there was no apparent difference between runners classified as good and those classified as poor. However, she found that the heel moved backward with reference to a point within the body (the knee). Since the forward movement of the total body was greater than the backward movement caused by knee flexion and hip extension, the foot moved forward immediately before contact.

Other findings by Fortney point out differences between the good and the poor runners. At the beginning of the flight phase the good runners had greater flexion in the leading limb at the knee and the hip, the latter bringing the thigh closer to the front horizontal; at the beginning of the contact phase the good runners had greater knee flexion in the rear limb, bringing the heel closer to the buttock.

The path of the center of gravity of the body during the running stride has been studied by Beck. The subjects, 12 boys ages 6 through 12 years and representing the first 6 grades, were selected from their classmates as having the better time scores in a 27.4-m (30-yd) run. Beck found that regardless of age, all paths were wavelike, reaching the high point shortly after the body became airborne. After the high point the center of gravity moved downward through the next foot contact and for a short time afterward. The next rise began while the foot was in contact with the ground and continued through the takeoff, and the cycle was then repeated. With increased age there was an increase in the horizontal and vertical distances traveled by the center of gravity during each stride, and the stride also became longer. With age the percentage of the total stride time represented by foot contact decreased, and of course that of flight time increased. The horizontal velocity of the center of gravity increased with age; for the flight phase, however, the percentage of the horizontal velocity decreased, and for the support phase it increased.

MINI LABORATORY EXERCISES

1. Run in place without moving the arms. Then add arm action and observe the difference in response.
2. Divide into groups and record the number of step frequencies that each person can attain in 30 seconds while running in place.
3. Move the feet as rapidly as possible with no flexion at the knees in a type of running-in-place action. Keep a record of the number of movements made in 30 seconds.
4. a. If film of running is available, project it and draw contourograms of the following frames:
      (1) Toe off
      (2) Foot strike

(3) Greatest thigh lift

(4) Greatest flexion at the knee

  b. Compare these contourograms with the information presented in this chapter and assess the skill level and the speed of the runner.

5. Compare the segment action in jogging, distance running, and sprinting.

6. Run in sand, in water, on a slick surface, and up and down grade. Record the results.

REFERENCES

Barlow, D.A., and Cooper, J.M.: Mechanical considerations in the sprint start, Athletic Asia **2:**27, Aug., 1972.

Beck, M.C.: The path of the center of gravity during running in boys grades one to six, dissertation, University of Wisconsin, 1965.

Bresnahan, G.T.: A study of the movement pattern in starting the race from a crouch position, Res. Q. Am. Assoc. Health Phys. Educ. **5**(1) (supp.):5, 1934.

Fenn, W.O.: Work against gravity and work due to velocity changes in running, Am. J. Physiol. **93:**433, 1930.

Fortney, V.: Trends and traits in the action of the swinging leg in running, thesis, University of Wisconsin, 1963.

Hoffman, K.: Stride length and frequency in female sprinters, Track Tech. **48:**1522, 1972.

Hubbard, A.W.: Experimental analysis of running and of certain fundamental differences between trained and untrained runners, Res. Q. Am. Assoc. Health Phys. Educ. **10**(3):28, 1939.

Morris, H.H.: The effects of starting block length, angle, and position upon sprint performance, doctoral dissertation, Indiana University, Nov., 1971.

Sigerseth, P.O., and Grinaker, V.F.: Effect of foot spacing on velocity in sprints, Res. Q. Am. Assoc. Health Phys. Educ. **33:**599, 1962.

Slocum, D.B., and Bowerman, W.: The biomechanics of running, Clin. Orthop. **23:**39, 1962.

Sparks, K.E.: Physiological and mechanical alterations due to fatigue while performing a four-minute mile, unpublished paper, Indiana University, 1974.

Teeple, J.B.: A biomechanical analysis of running patterns of college women, master's thesis, Pennsylvania State University, Dec., 1968.

Ward, P.: An analysis of kinetic and kinematic factors of the standup and the preferred crouch starting techniques with respect to sprint performance, doctoral dissertation, Indiana University, Aug., 1973.

ADDITIONAL READINGS

Adrian, M., and Kreighbaum, E.: Physical and mechanical characteristics of distance runners during competition, Third International Seminar on Biomechanics, Rome, 1971.

Astrand, P.-O., and Rodahl, K.: Textbook of work physiology: physiological bases of exercise, ed. 2, New York, 1977, McGraw-Hill Book Co.

Barker, S.B., and Summerson, W.H.: The colorimetric determination of lactic acid in biological material, J. Biol. Chem. **138:**535, 1941.

Bates, B.T., and Haven, B.H.: An analysis of the mechanics of highly skilled female runners. In Bleustein, J.L., editor: Mechanics and sport, New York, 1973, American Society of Mechanical Engineers.

Deshon, D.E., and Nelson, R.C.: A cinematographical analysis of sprint running, Res. Q. **35:**451-455, 1964.

Dintiman, G.B.: What research tells the coach about sprinting (pamphlet), Washington, D.C., 1974, American Association for Health, Physical Education, and Recreation.

James, S.L., and Brubaker, C.E.: Running mechanics, J.A.M.A. **221:**1014-1016, 1972.

Jensen, C.R., and Fisher, A.G.: Scientific basis of athletic conditioning, ed. 2, Philadelphia, 1979, Lea & Febiger.

Slocum, D.B., and James, S.L.: Biomechanics of running, J.A.M.A. **205:**721-728, 1968.

Track and Field Quarterly Review, vol. 80, Summer, 1980 (entire issue on sprinting).

CHAPTER 12

Jumping

Jumping is one of the fundamental movements made by children after learning to walk and run. It is practiced by many of them to some degree at least until the teenage years and is a highly specialized activity of a few adults, such as Olympic competitors.

There are several kinds of jumps, such as the standing jump, standing vertical jump, long jump, high jump, and pole vault, as well as certain specialized jumps made in games and contests.

Jumping is a projection of the body into the air by means of a force made by the feet or hands against a surface. Often the jump is made after a run, and the takeoff may be made from either one foot or two feet.

The ability to project the body at an optimal angle at the takeoff is one of the factors determining the distance or height of the jump. Takeoff velocity is anther factor involved in the quality of jumps. Usually the force multiplied by the time of application (F × t = Impulse) determines the longest or highest jump. the best jumpers have the greatest impulse. In addition, they apply the force in the shortest time but have greater vertical force than the poorer jumpers.

Whenever a run precedes the jump, there develops a problem of redirecting some of the horizontal velocity into vertical velocity. Inevitably there is some sacrifice of one in an attempt to optimize·the other.

The path of the jumper who is in the air is that of

a parabola except in a purely vertical jump. The crossing of a bar or a landing for distance involves manipulating the center of gravity to gain advantages in its placement in the body or outside the body.

There is a rotational component connected with the takeoff in jumping. Most researchers (such as Bedi) consider the rotational component to be in a forward direction. Either using this force or counteracting it may aid the jumper.

A one-foot takeoff provides the greater forward momentum at takeoff but is the hardest to control in relation to timing a hit while the jumper is in the air, such as in a block in basketball. For distance, such as in the long jump, or height, such as in the high jump, the one-foot takeoff after a run is preferred.

The moving of the arms and legs while the jumper is in flight (airborne) does not add to the distance covered nor to the height of the center of gravity of the body. However, movement of the center of gravity within the body or outside of it can be accomplished by moving the body parts. Many of the leg, trunk, and arm movements are made for balance purposes and to project the center of gravity vertically or horizontally within the path prescribed to aid in the performance of the skill.

If the airborne jumper moves a part of the body in one direction, another part will move in the opposite direction. For example, movement of the head and upper torso forward and downward (clockwise) causes the feet and lower body to move upward and forward (counterclockwise). This action-reaction principle may be an asset or a liability, depending on its use. In addition, the timing of one movement to cause reaction in another is crucial to performance. One arm moving clockwise too soon may cause the performer's other arm to move counterclockwise, striking a crossbar and nullifying an otherwise effective action.

STANDING JUMPS (PUSHING OFF WITH BOTH FEET)
Standing broad jump

The standing broad jump is most frequently used in schools and colleges as one measure of motor ability and physical or motor fitness. It is a modification of the walking step—a modification that low-level performers frequently do not achieve effectively. These performers take off from one foot when they attempt to take off from both, in a reflex, or inherent, reaction to maintain balance.

Joint actions in takeoff phase. The following analysis of the mechanics of the jump is based on a film of a 12-year-old girl whose score ranks above the ninety-fifth percentile in a nationwide sampling of girls 12 to 17 years of age. The discussion is based on graphs of joint angles and segmental inclinations shown in Figs. 12-1 and 12-2. The lines in the illustrations begin at the time that the heels leave the ground and show that the propelling actions occur in the slightly more than 0.25 second from raising of the heel until the final thrust is made. For the first 0.18 second as the foot is raised from the floor, no action (or very little) occurs in the ankle joint, except for the slight flexion and immediate recovery at 0.09 second. This lack of ankle extension is noteworthy, since many authors attribute rising on the toes to ankle extension.

These graphs, like many others, show that, as the center of gravity of the body is moved downward by gravitational force, the foot rotating at the metatarsophalangeal joint is moved in an upward direction. This occurs only when the ankle extensors prevent ankle flexion. This apparent paradox—movement in an upward direction because of gravitational force—was also noted in connection with teeterboard action.

Once the leg has reached the desired angle of inclination, ankle extension parallels metatarsophalangeal extension from 0.135 to 0.21 second (Fig. 12-1), and by this means the inclination of the leg is kept almost constant (Fig. 12-2). In the final 0.03 second, ankle extension exceeds metatarsophalangeal action, and the leg is raised 10 degrees, adding to the upward thrust.

The knee flexes for the first 0.135 second, carrying the thigh downward and backward in reference to the knee. However, from 0.06 to 0.135 second the thigh is not inclined backward with reference to the horizontal because the forward inclination of the leg at this time exceeds knee flexion. At 0.21 second the thigh reaches the vertical, and after this point all joint actions increase in speed. Up to 0.21 second, thigh extension has lifted the thigh and the torso against gravitational pull; after that time both thigh extension and gravity are applying force in a downward direction. All joints (metatarsophalangeal, ankle, knee, and hip) react to this change in gravitational pull; all increase in speed. Here is an example of the marvelous capacity of a living organism to adjust to a situation; one can be assured that these adjustments are not voluntarily controlled. The nervous system reacts to balance and to the speed of the thigh; guided by the intended action, it provides the necessary joint movements.

The shoulder measures shown in Fig. 12-1 are

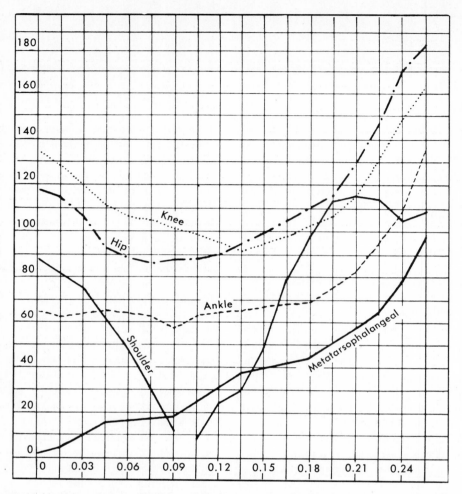

Fig. 12-1. Joint actions during takeoff in standing broad jump of highly skilled 12-year-old girl. Time in seconds is shown at bottom; angles between body segments are shown in degrees at left. For lower-limb joints, downward slope of lines indicates flexion and upward slope extension. Note lack of action in ankle joints until 0.18 second; also at this time all joints except shoulders increase speed of extension. All shoulder action is flexion.

those of the angle formed by lines drawn through the upper arms and the trunk. As the heels leave the ground, the arms are back of the trunk at an angle of 88 degrees. They are moved downward by shoulder flexion, pass the trunk between 0.09 and 0.105 second, and reach the height of their swing just before the thighs reach the vertical.

In this swing the arm movement affects the position of the center of gravity of the entire body, tending to move it forward and downward until the arms pass the trunk and then forward and upward.

In studying the standing long jump of 20 boys (five each at ages 7, 10, 13, and 16 years) who were selected as average jumpers, Roy found that

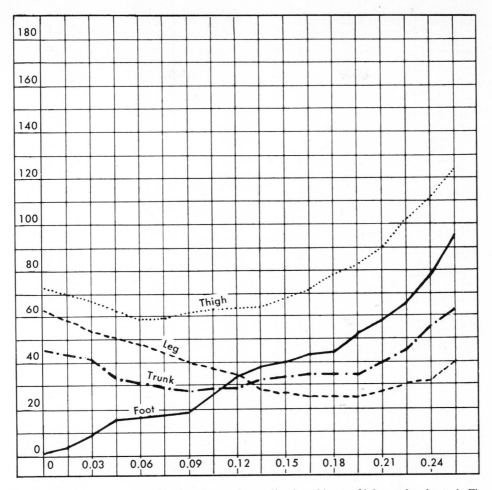

Fig. 12-2. Angles of inclination of body segments in standing broad jump of joint angles shown in Fig. 12-1. Note small range of movement in leg and trunk and large range of movement in foot and thigh. Time in seconds is shown at bottom; angles between body segments are shown in degrees at left.

the knee, ankle, and metatarsophalangeal joints reached peak angular velocity at takeoff except for one 10-year-old boy whose maximal knee velocity occurred 0.07 second before takeoff. Using measures derived from film and a force platform, Roy concluded, ''Kinematics of jumping are well established by the beginning of school age and re- main essentially constant through mid-adolescence for average performers.''*

Factors affecting the distance of the jump. The

---

*Roy, B.: Kinematics and kinetics of the standing long jump in seven, ten, thirteen and sixteen year old boys, dissertation, University of Wisconsin, 1971.

standing broad jump is customarily measured from the toes at takeoff to the point where the heels touch the ground in landing. This distance is determined by four factors: (1) the distance to which the center of gravity of the body is carried forward by the lean at takeoff, (2) the horizontal distance through which the center of gravity is projected during flight, (3) the distance beyond the center of gravity that the heels reach on landing, and (4) the time spent on the takeoff surface. Felton compared these factors as shown in the performances of five high-scoring college women, whose jumps averaged 2.19 m (86.22 in) and of five low-scoring ones, whose jumps averaged 1.08 m (42.78 in). At the time of takeoff the centers of gravity of the high-scoring group averaged 0.77 m (30.62 in) in front of their toes; for the low-scoring one the average distance was 45.9 cm (18.74 in). The heels of the high scorers landed 14.1 cm (5.56 in) ahead of the center of gravity, and the heels of the low scorers 9.14 cm (3.6 in) ahead. The degree to which the center of gravity is in front of the toes at takeoff is affected mainly by the degree of knee extension. The 12-year-old girl whose joint actions were shown in Fig. 12-1 reached a knee extension that was 16 degrees less than 180 degrees. In Felton's comparison of high-scoring and low-scoring women the average knee extensions were 165.7 and 141 degrees. The degree of extension may be due to the balance mechanism. The strength of the ankle extensors could also influence the amount of lean, for the tension in these muscles must move or hold all parts of the body above the ankle joint.

The position of the thigh at landing is the determining factor in the length of the reach with the heel. The more closely the thigh approaches the horizontal, the longer the reach. When the thigh is nearly horizontal on landing, the legs are almost vertical. This landing position enables the body momentum to carry the center of gravity over the stationary feet. In a running broad jump the horizontal velocity during flight is greater, and the legs can reach farther without the likelihood of the body's falling back of the contact point. The horizontal position of the thighs changes the position of the center of gravity and permits that point to approach closer to the ground before the landing contact is made. This increases the time of flight, adds to the horizontal distance gained during flight, and facilitates forward rotation of the body at the ankle, thus decreasing the possibility of falling backward. Observation of hundreds of films of children by one of us (R.B.G.) has shown that the position of the thighs at landing is a distinguishing feature between high-scoring and low-scoring broad jumpers.

The flight adds the greatest proportion to the distance of the jump. The range of flight is determined by the angle and velocity of the projection. Unlike those situations in which the takeoff and landing are in the same horizontal plane, a 45-degree angle is not the best to gain distance. Whenever the center of gravity is higher at takeoff than at landing, as it is in the standing broad jump, an angle of less than 45 degrees adds to the distance that the projectile will travel. The horizontal component of velocity becomes greater as the angle is decreased.

Measures of velocity and distance. A measure of the velocity of the center of gravity is rarely made; yet this is the most valid evaluation of the force developed in the takeoff. Halverson found an average velocity in the jump of kindergarten children to be between 1.8 and 2.1 m/sec (6 and 7 ft/sec), and the highest (for a boy) was 2.52 m/sec (8.28 ft/sec). Felton calculated the mean velocity of five high-scoring college women to be 2.47 m/sec (8.11 ft/sec) and that of five low-scoring women to be 1.72 m/sec (5.66 ft/sec). The highest velocity was 2.81 m/sec (9.22 ft/sec) and the lowest 1.53 m/sec (5.02 ft/sec). With horizontal and vertical scores from Roy's study, projection velocities of the center of gravity were calculated to be 2.71 m/sec (8.9 ft/sec) for age 7 years, 3.04 m (10.0 ft) for age 10 years, 3.20 m (10.5 ft) for age 13 years, and 3.93 m (12.9 ft) for age 16 years. The increase from age to age was due to greater horizontal velocity, whereas vertical velocity changed little, indicating that with age the center of gravity is lowered at takeoff.

Different scores for various age groups are fairly common. For example, in unpublished scores for elementary-school boys found in studies at the University of Wisconsin, the first-grade boys averaged 1.16 m (46 in), and the eighth-grade boys averaged 1.93 m (76 in). The scores for intervening grades fell between these; the score for each grade was higher than that for the grade below it. The shorter time spent on the takeoff surface, exhibited by the best performers, varied from 0.24 to 0.29 second.

Standing jump for height

The standing jump for height is widely used as a test item, and its successful performance adds to playing ability in many sports. Sargent was the first to propose the jump for height as a measure of motor ability. In 1921 he said, "I want to share what seems to me the simplest and most effective of all tests of physical ability with the other fools who are looking for one."* Since that time many investigators have found the Sargent jump test, or the "jump and reach," a valuable item in a test battery. For games in which an attempt is made to catch or to strike a high ball, the ability to jump is an asset. The receiver of a forward pass in football, the infielder and outfielder in baseball, the spiker in volleyball, and the basketball player who attempts to tip a ball toward the basket or to a teammate after a held ball will play more effectively if they can add to their reach by a jump for height.

Film comparison of joint actions in the broad jump and the jump for height of the same performer indicates minor differences in the action at the knee, hip, and shoulder. These actions are much like those in the standing broad jump (Fig. 12-1). The ankle joint action is an important key to the differences in the direction of the two projections. In the first third of the time between raising of the heel and final thrust, the ankle of one skilled performer (a college woman) flexed 10 degrees in the standing broad jump and 5 degrees in the jump

*Sargent, D.: The physical test of a man, Am. Phys. Educ. Rev. **26**:188, 1921.

for height. Since ankle flexion carries the center of gravity of the body forward and thereby increases the effect of gravitational pull (which pulls the feet, except for the toes, from the floor), the difference in metatarsophalangeal action at this time (15 degrees and 5 degrees) is to be expected. Beyond this point the ankle joints extended at the same rate until the final thrust, when the action in the jump for height exceeded that in the jump for distance. The first reached an extension of 134 degrees and the second an extension of 123 degrees. The leg in the first was closer to the vertical with reference to the ankle. Since the foot in the first third of the projecting time had been lifted farther from the floor in the broad jump, gravitational action was greater, and the foot rose more rapidly. At the final thrust in the broad jump the foot was at an angle of 78 degrees with the horizontal (measured from the back) and in the high jump at an angle of 44 degrees.

Since the inclination of any segment affects the inclination of all segments above it, in spite of the similarities of proximal joint actions in the two jumps the difference in foot inclinations results in differences in inclination of the remaining segments. In the observed actions the inclinations (measured from the front and with those in the jump for height given first) were as follows: leg, 91 degrees and 44 degrees; thigh, 102 degrees and 60 degrees; and trunk, 80 and 37 degrees (Fig. 12-3).

In the broad jump gravitational force adds to the final push; in the high jump it adds little or nothing. Without the aid of gravity the velocity in the jump for height would be slower.

Racing dive

The racing dive is an excellent example of the action of the lower limbs described previously in the discussion of mechanics of the stepping pattern. However, in this skill the projection force is directed almost horizontally, with little in the vertical direction. Therefore the directing segment, the leg, will be close to the horizontal in the force-producing phase. The dive is illustrated here by

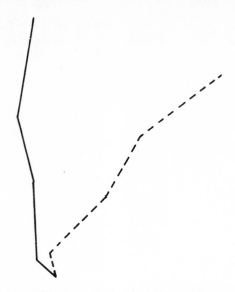

Fig. 12-3. Takeoff positions in standing jump for height (unbroken line) and in standing broad jump (broken line) of skilled college woman. Note that difference in inclination of body segments is due to difference in foot inclination.

tracings taken from film of a woman diver, a national champion (Fig. 12-4).

The diver stands at the edge of the pool with feet separated to bring them in line with the hips for an effective push. The eyes should be looking downward and forward at approximately 45 degrees. Next flexion of spine and head and forward raising of the arms with reference to the feet have moved the body's center of gravity forward, resulting in ankle flexion. This flexion is possible because the ankle extensor muscles have permitted it by lengthening contraction. The importance of streamlining is evident as the body readies itself to become a projectile in the air. The path of the center of gravity is determined at takeoff. The conservation of energy law could apply here (that is, energy can be neither created nor destroyed); thus the change is from potential to kinetic energy, resulting in the transfer of momentum, which is in fact the basic mechanical principle applied to the windup start technique (Fig. 12-4).

One of the newest racing start techniques is the grab start, whereby the swimmer holds onto the starting platform until the gun is fired and enters the water sooner than when using the windup start and at a lower angle. The swimmer gains in execution because the swimming action was started sooner. (See Fig. 12-5.)

Ankle extensors are contracting with sufficient force to prevent flexion at that joint; now gravitational force rotates the entire body around a fulcrum that is the point of contact between the feet and the edge of the pool. In addition, preparation has been made for the final application of force. The arms have moved backward; the knees have flexed; the hips have increased flexion, bringing the trunk close to the thighs; and the spine has flexed. The last action, like that described in the crouching start for running races, prepares for spinal extension, which will add to the power and distance of the body's flight.

Note that the change of inclination of the legs is due to changes in foot inclination, not to changes at the ankle joint. Application of final force is delayed until the legs are at, or close to, the desired direction. The beginning of the force-producing

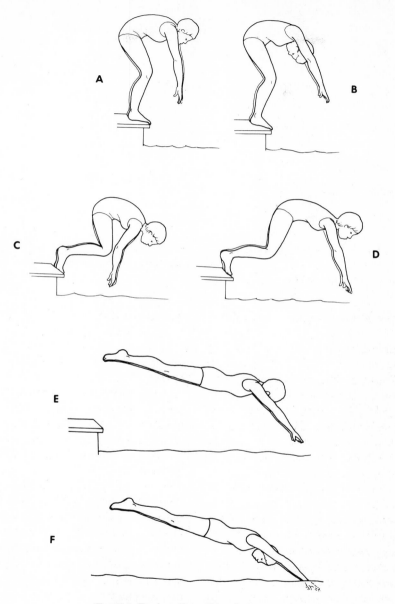

Fig. 12-4. Racing dive with windup start.

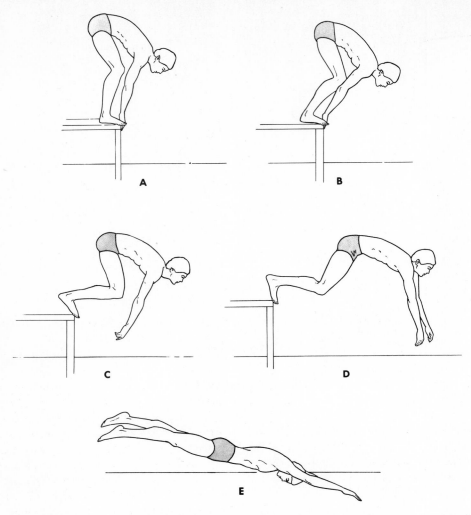

Fig. 12-5. Racing dive with grab start.

phase is seen—forward movement of the arms, facilitated by slight elbow flexion, spinal extension, and beginning knee extension. The knees and ankles have extended vigorously. In the last-named action, since the feet no longer support the body weight, ankle extension will move the feet; however, knee extension, because the feet resist a horizontal push, will be reversed muscle action and will move the thighs. During the forward, downward movement of the thighs, trunk inclina-

tion will be maintained close to the horizontal by hip extension, a direction technique.

Then head flexion can be seen, and it will affect the position of the center of gravity within the body. Gravitational force will respond by changing the inclination of the entire body. The upper part will incline downward and the lower part upward. At entry the inclination of the body is approximately 20 degrees; because this angle is small, the dive will be shallow, and forward momentum will

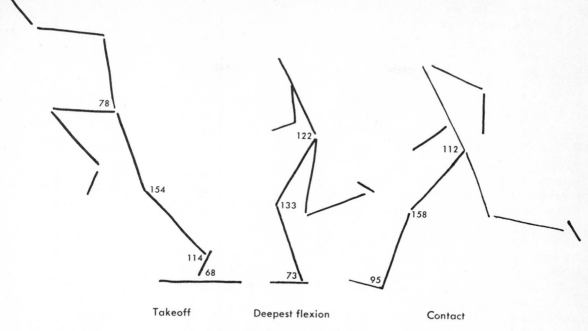

Fig. 12-6. Running long jump.

be much greater than downward momentum. The diver will glide until the momentum is equal to that of swimming speed.

The major propelling forces are knee extension, gravitational pull, and the final thrust from the feet and toes. The time spent on the starting surface is less for the better performers in relation to the time of entry.

RUNNING JUMPS—SINGLE-FOOT PUSH
Running long jump

The running long jump is a modification of the running stride. The differences can be seen by comparing the line representations shown in Fig. 11-6 with those in Fig. 12-6. On contact the center of gravity in the jump is seen to be farther back than it is in the run. After contact the jumper relies on the momentum of the run to carry the body mass forward by permitting the ankle joint to flex.

Adjustments to bring the center of gravity of segments closer to the fulcrum (the contact point)

are made by knee and hip flexion in the supporting limb and by hip flexion in the swinging limb. As the supporting limb reaches the point of deepest knee flexion, ankle extensors prevent further flexion at that joint, and the pattern described for walking, running, and the standing broad jump follows; that is, the heel is raised from the ground. At deepest knee flexion the center of gravity is almost over the foot and will be moved forward rapidly by knee extension of the supporting leg, hip flexion of the swinging limb, and shoulder flexion of both arms.

No action occurs at the ankle joint as the foot begins to rise; ankle extension begins as the center of gravity passes the metatarsophalangeal joints, but the range of this extension is approximately slightly more than half of the metatarsophalangeal action, and therefore the leg is inclined downward by foot action.

The takeoff tracing shown in Fig. 12-6 shows that the force of joint actions will be directed upward more than forward. This has been found to be

3.6 g (3.6 times the performer's body weight). If the jumper has not lost the momentum of the run, there will be a forward component acting on the body mass, and the resulting angle of projection will be between the horizontal and that suggested by the takeoff position. In the depicted jumper it was calculated to be 33 degrees. Bunn reports that Jesse Owen's angle of projection was between 25 and 26 degrees. Findings from recent studies show the takeoff angle to be even less, around 17 degrees for world-class long jumpers. This low angle indicates that the jumper is not able to transfer his horizontal velocity into a vertical thrust. His jump reflects reliance to a great degree on horizontal velocity. Angles of less than 45 degrees are essential for maximal distance, since the center of gravity at landing is lower than at the beginning of flight.

The movement in the air by the arms and legs is for balance and for the purpose of extending the lower limbs to increase the measured distance of the jump. The lower limbs could be carried in hip-flexed and knee-extended position if the hip flexors were strong enough.

The reach on landing can be longer than in the standing broad jump. A horizontal position of the thighs and a greater degree of knee extension will add to the measured distance. The trunk is hyperextended at midpoint in the flight and is then flexed to prepare for projecting the center of gravity forward at landing. If ankle flexion occurs immediately on contact, the horizontal component of the velocity of projection will carry the body mass forward past the feet. Hip flexion to raise the thighs before landing will also incline the trunk, bringing the center of gravity forward. The arms by swinging forward can aid in carrying the body over the landing contact. The knees are flexed to absorb the shock as landing is completed.

The flight of the center of gravity cannot be altered after the takeoff. The path is determined by the angle and velocity of projection and by gravitational force once the body is in the air. The only aids to distance that can be made during flight are positioning of the thighs and legs for the reach and of the trunk and arms for carrying the center of gravity forward on landing.

Bedi's investigation of the long jump revealed the following:

1. The jumpers in their run up to the board averaged 8.1 m/sec (26.6 ft/sec), with the best performers running the fastest.
2. The vertical force averaged 4133.64 N (930 lb), with the best jumpers exceeding this amount by more than 441 N (100 lb) of force.
3. The braking force was 3036.04 N (683 lb) on the average.
4. The largest impulses (force multiplied by time) were recorded by the best jumpers.
5. The best long jumper spent 0.11 to 0.12 second on the board, whereas the poorer one spent 0.13 to 0.14 second.
6. The jumpers all had a forward rotation at the takeoff, with a large horizontal braking force contributing to this rotational component.

Bedi believes that to jump farther the performers need to do the following:

1. The jumpers should reduce the horizontal braking force at takeoff to minimize the forward rotation and increase horizontal velocity at takeoff in an attempt to reduce wasted energy.
2. It is possible to perform a forward somersault in the air in order to arrive at touchdown with a better landing position, but more vertical force must be generated in the last few milliseconds that the long jumper is on the takeoff board.*

Triple jump

The actions of a triple jumper are similar to that of a long jumper, especially at the instant of the final takeoff. The triple jump involves more than a true jump. Once the triple jump was called the hop, step, and jump, which is more descriptive because it encompasses three movements. Whereas in the long jump (discussed previously) there is one flight period, in the triple jump there are three flight pe-

---

*Bedi, J.F.: Angular momentum in the long jump, doctoral dissertation, Indiana University, May, 1975.

riods. Couple these with not one, but three, takeoffs and three landings, and this event is an intriguing one to study.

The ratio of the distance of the three movements might be nearly even in the immediate future. Yoon found the ratio to be 7:6:7.

The triple jump is a beautiful motion when it is executed by an outstanding competitor. The rhythmic sounds made by the performer could be recorded and used by the beginner to facilitate improvement.

Some comments on the performance in this event are as follows:

1. The takeoff angle at each stage is low, 8 to 10 degrees.
2. There is a continuous compromise being made between horizontal speed and vertical lift, and the angle of takeoff is considerably lower than in the long jump.
3. The movements must be executed so that the movement is as nearly continuous as possible. The momentum of the jumper must not be decreased too much at each takeoff position; that is, the braking forces must be minimized.
4. There is a forceful downward extension at the hip, knee, and ankle joints of the takeoff leg at each position.
5. The center of gravity is maintained in front of the takeoff foot at the takeoff position.
6. The torso of the jumper is essentially an erect one so that the landing leg can be extended and the force of the foot against the ground can be exerted somewhat vertically.
7. The arms move laterally and backward and then forward together to counterbalance each side of the body for balance.
8. The landing foot first moves forward and then backward to ensure that the foot is moving backward faster than the body's center of gravity is moving forward. This enables the jumper to move to the next phase.
9. The landing shock is attenuated by the flexion at the hip, knees, and ankles. The arms move forward in extension, and the torso's

forward lean (flexion) enables the jumper to fall forward at landing.

Running high jump

The takeoff for the running high jump is much like that for the running long jump. The differences are those that keep the center of gravity higher to develop a greater vertical component in the flight. This is accomplished mainly by inclinations of the foot and the trunk. In the high jump the foot at the moment of thrust does not incline as far forward as it does in the long jump. As was shown in the description of the standing jump for height, the inclination of the foot will affect the inclinations of all other segments. As in the standing jump for height, ankle and hip actions serve to maintain the desired direction. The final force is derived from running momentum, from extension of the knee, and from the forceful swing of the free lower limb and the arms. Segmental inclinations of the foot, leg, thigh, and trunk are closer to the vertical and takeoff than in the long jump.

The jump must have a horizontal component to carry the center of gravity across the bar, and the skilled jumper will keep the proportion of this component as small as possible. One method by which this is accomplished is by a diagonal run to approach at a parallel with the bar. Space is thus allowed for lifting the free leg parallel with, rather than toward, the bar. Approaching from an oblique angle gives jumpers more latitude to accommodate for errors in spacing, so that they can vary position in crossing the bar.

The height of the center of gravity at takeoff is important. If a jumper is 1.82 m (6 ft) tall, the center of gravity in the normal standing position, according to Palmer's formula, would be 1.036 m (40.65 in) above the soles of the feet. In rising to the tip of the toes at takeoff the jumper could raise the center of gravity 17.78 cm (7 in). The position of the arms and the swinging leg could add another 20.32 cm (8 in), bringing the position of the center of gravity 1.41 m (55.65 in) above the ground at takeoff. How high would and could the velocity of the jump carry the center of gravity to enable the jumper to clear the bar at 2.28 m (7.5 ft)? If a superior jumper could raise the center of gravity another 0.76 m (30 in), the attained height would be slightly over 2.13 m (7 ft). Additional height is gained by manipulation of the body segments, which allows the center of gravity to pass under the bar.

This manipulation has been accomplished in various ways since the scissors jump was discarded in competition. One of these is the western roll, in which the trunk is lowered to the horizontal as it reaches bar height; one arm reaches over and is extended below the bar, and the rear thigh and leg

are also below the bar. From the high point the trunk rolls over as the rear limb extends, and the leading limb moves below bar level. A dive over the bar, with head and chest leading, has been developed. This method of jumping, coupled with the straddle roll form, in which the jumper goes over the bar facing downward, has enabled jumpers to continue to increase their jumping height.

When this style of jumping is used, the center of gravity is located to the rear before the takeoff (Fig. 12-7, *B*). The right (free) leg is swung forward with hip flexion and some knee flexion. As

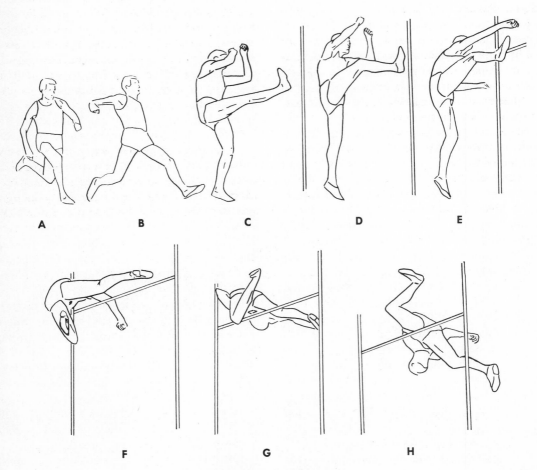

A   B   C   D   E

F   G   H

Fig. 12-7. Running high jump.

the leg starts upward, there is continued hip flexion, knee flexion, and then full knee extension at the top of the kickup *(C)*. Both arms are carried upward at the takeoff, with shoulder flexion and some elbow flexion *(D)*. The right arm has greater range of movement. The takeoff leg provides force and direction by hip, knee, and ankle extension *(D)*. The more vertical the takeoff, the steeper the parabola of flight. Present-day jumpers are emphasizing greater speed during the run, and at the same time they try to take off with an angle as close to 90 degrees as possible.

The roll, or turn, over the bar is accomplished by trunk rotation to the left (left-footed jumper). Neck and trunk flexion at the height of the jump enables the jumper to lift the lower limbs over the bar. As the trunk and lead leg cross the bar, the neck has been in slight rotation to the right. It is moved to the left, initiating total trunk rotation to the left, accompanied by left hip abduction and knee flexion. After crossing the bar the jumper continues to turn so as to land on the back.

One of us (J.M.C.) has stated his belief that the requirements for world record high jumping are the following (with the last three the most important):

1. Long legs, high center of gravity
2. Enough speed and strength at takeoff to give an upward thrust of considerable magnitude

3. Takeoff foot on the ground long enough for arms, swinging leg, foot, and toe to contribute transference of momentum
4. Style of crossing the bar like a tumble, so that the center of gravity does not actually cross over the top of the bar but goes beneath it

The Fosbury flop stype is shown in Fig. 12-8. The ease of execution and high lift of the hips (center of gravity) possibly make this mechanically best. (See Hay for greater detail.) The flop-style performer usually develops and utilizes greater horizontal velocity than other jumpers.

Ward has shown that force, action, and time aspects can be synchronized as shown in Fig. 12-9. Such a study involves using a force plate, three cameras, and an oscillograph recording device. The jumper shown here is a straddle roller. The shortest time on the ground at takeoff (0.15 second) and the most vertical thrust (4 *g*) have been recorded for the best jumper.

Pole vault

In the running high and long jumps the momentum of the run rotates the body over the supporting foot. The foot and lower limb serve much the same function as the pole does in the vault. During the run the pole is carried by the front arm in medial

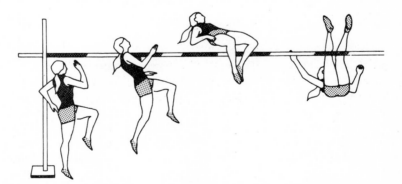

Fig. 12-8. Back flop style of high jumping. Note that jumper takes off from ground with her outside leg. Also note that jumper first executes a scissorlike jump and then twists to roll over bar on her back. This style is becoming more and more popular with women. It involves less lift and more flexibility than does straddle style. (From Wakefield, F., and Harkins, D., with Cooper, J.M.: Track and field fundamentals for girls and women, ed. 4, St. Louis, 1977, The C.V. Mosby Co.)

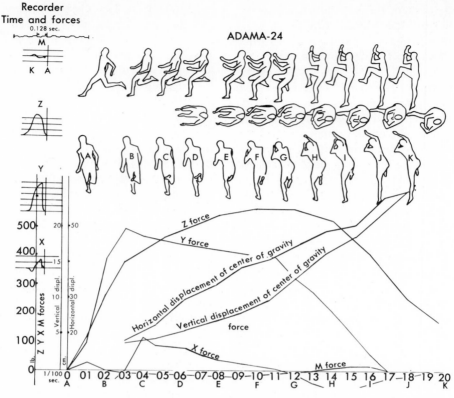

Fig. 12-9. Force-action-time relationships for jump of particular jumper, showing displacement of center of gravity and distribution of forces at takeoff. (From Ward, R.D.: An investigation into the use of computer integration of kinematics, kinetics, and cinematography data in motion analysis, dissertation, Indiana University, Aug., 1971.)

rotation, and the shoulder is adducted with some flexion. The elbow is flexed, and the forearm is pronated. In the rear arm there is some shoulder extension, and the elbow is also flexed (Fig. 12-10). A horizontal velocity is imparted to the pole by the run, and since the pole is raised upward and pointed downward in the final step, it will be rotated upward and forward, after contact with the box, by the horizontal velocity.

At the plant of the pole in the box, the right shoulder is laterally rotated and flexed. There is elbow extension. The left arm also has shoulder flexion and some elbow flexion (C). The left hand

momentarily releases the pole and then regrasps it. The tracings in Fig. 12-10 were taken from a film in which the performer used a glass pole.

As the pole is placed on the ground and the final thrust is made by extension of the thigh and plantar flexion of the foot of the supporting limb, the left elbow is extended and the shoulder is flexed. The right elbow extends to retain the grasp on the pole as it rebounds from its compressed position. Note that the hands are spaced well apart. Assisting the thrust of the lower limb is the rapid upward movement of the pole and of the swinging right lower limb.

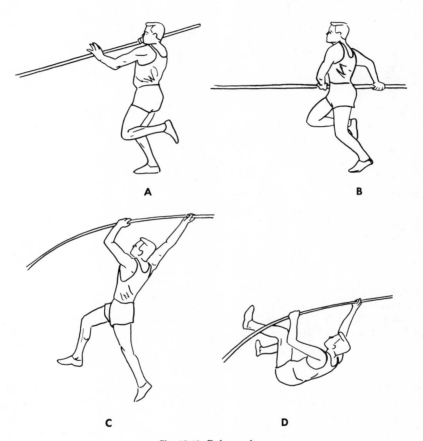

A

B

C

D

Fig. 12-10. Pole vault.

Continued.

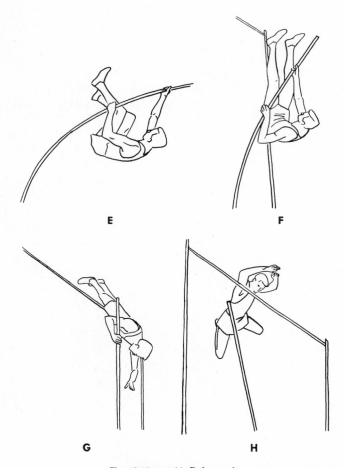

E F

G H

Fig. 12-10, cont'd. Pole vault.

At takeoff the supporting leg, according to Ganslen, is inclined 78 degrees, and since the trunk remains vertical, the thrust of the supporting joints can be assumed to be close to the vertical. As the pole rotates upward around its ground contact, the body rotates around the hand contact on the pole. The body rotation will be faster than that of the pole, and as the extended body passes the pole, its speed of rotation will be increased by flexion of the hips and knees.

For elevation of the lower part of the body above the hands, first the hips flex while the knees are flexed (Fig. 12-10, *E*); then the knee position decreases the amount of force needed to flex the hips by moving the center of gravity of the lower limbs closer to the fulcrum (the hip joints). As the thighs approach the vertical, the knees extend to bring the legs in line with the thighs *(F)*. The body's center of gravity is now close to the pole so that the vaulter is able to take greater advantage of the pole action. In *F* the trunk has begun to rotate to the left; pelvic rotation will follow, and the right leg will scissor over the left. As the jumper's center of gravity passes the pole, the pulling is converted into a pushing movement, which is achieved by shoulder flexion and elbow extension. This action is completed in one continuous movement, and the left hand is released from the pole first. The forearms are pronated as the release of each is accomplished. To project the legs as high as possible, the vaulter should keep the chin down toward the chest in preparing to go over the bar. The movement of the lower limbs downward after crossing the bar raises the trunk and arms. Elevating the arms still higher helps keep them from striking the bar as they go over. The vaulter must be sure to wait until the pole has almost reached the vertical position before executing the pull-up.

The higher the vaulter places the hands on the pole at the start, the faster the run will be, and the steeper the parabola of the path of the center of gravity in flight, the higher the vault should be.

Barlow, using rather elaborate electronic equipment, including force plates, special slow motion camera, force transducers, recording oscillograph, and necessary accessories, was able to secure kinematic and kinetic parameters of the pole vaulting of top performers. These data were analyzed by a computer and digitizing system.

Some of his findings are as follows:

Kinematic factors

1. The last stride of all vaulters was shortened.
2. The second to last stride was longer than either the third to last or the last stride.
3. The best vaulter (who was of world class) took longer strides throughout than any of the other subjects and shortened his last stride the least.
4. All pole plants of those who vaulted 4.87 m (16 ft) or higher were initiated in 0.423 second (mean time), compared with 0.408 second for the pole plants of those who vaulted less than 4.87 m.
5. Considerable deceleration over the final three strides occurred for those who vaulted less than 4.87 m.
6. The best vaulter accelerated longer in the run and decelerated less during the final strides.
7. Those who vaulted over 4.87 m attained a maximal velocity of 8.83 m/sec (28.97 ft/sec) during the second to last stride, whereas those who vaulted less than 4.87 m attained a maximal velocity of 8.30 m/sec (27.26 ft/sec) under the same conditions.
8. The average takeoff angle for the center-of-gravity projection of all vaulters was 21.9 degrees.
9. The angle of takeoff tended to increase as the height of the crossbar was elevated.
10. When the pole was perpendicular, the top vaulters had no vertical acceleration and the poorer ones had negative vertical velocity.

Kinetic factors

1. The average time on the force plate (of the takeoff foot) was 0.122 second.
2. The fastest time was 0.116 second for the top vaulter.

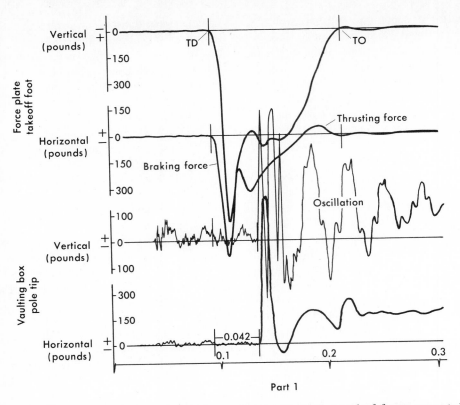

Fig. 12-11. Scale-reduced sample of typical recording oscillograph record of forces generated in takeoff and pendular phases of pole vault. (From Barlow, D.A.: Kinematic and kinetic factors involved in pole vaulting, doctoral dissertation, Indiana University, Aug., 1973.)

3. The peak vertical striking force at takeoff was an average magnitude of 3635.8 N (819 lb).
4. The top performers attained greater vertical force at takeoff than did those who were poorer vaulters.
5. The top vaulters supplied greater braking impulse at takeoff.
6. The vertical extension force tended to increase with the increased height of the crossbar (Fig. 12-11).

The findings of such a study reveal that the pole vaulter, in fact, does jump at the takeoff, attempts to generate considerable vertical force, and runs at close to top sprinting speed. Finally, by studying such data the researcher can find distinguishing factors characteristic of the better vaulters.

Hurdling

The high hurdler is a runner who vaults a series of hurdles. The run must be slightly modified on the approach to each hurdle. The shoulders are flexed and abducted and the scapulae elevated (Fig. 12-12, *A* to *C*). As the body's center of gravity is moved forward by the momentum of the run, the heel is raised (*B* to *D*). At the same time, the knee of the supporting limb extends. Considerable flexion of the hip of the lead limb takes place as the

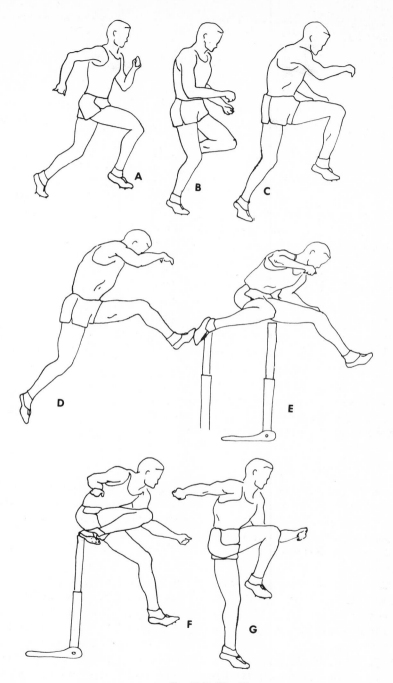

Fig. 12-12. Hurdling.

limb is swung forward with the knee extended. (Most hurdlers attempt to prevent the knee from extending completely to a locked position.) The skilled hurdler flexes the neck as well as the trunk so that the center of gravity will not go too high over the hurdle and contact with the ground will be made sooner. Note that the hurdler starts flexion of the trunk and neck before leaving the ground *(C)*. The rear leg *(D)* is brought forward by hip flexion. As the thigh is moved forward, it is abducted and rotated medially, bringing the flexed leg close to the horizontal *(E and F)*.

After the hurdle is cleared, the lead thigh extends to lower the foot, and the leg flexes, thus moving the foot backward with reference to the knee *(F and G)* and decreasing the possibility of backward push at contact. The rear thigh, after the hurdle is cleared, adducts and rotates laterally *(F and G)* to bring the foot in line for the next step. After contact, body momentum helps to extend the knee of the supporting limb.

The hurdler attempts to raise the center of gravity only high enough to clear the hurdle. Likewise an attempt is made to get the lead leg down as soon as possible so that the feet are in contact with the ground and the hurdler is able to run rapidly to the next hurdle. This involves an action-reaction phenomenon in that as the hip flexes, it aids in balance when the thigh is extended. The reason is that the extension of the thigh creates the action-reaction and brings about an extension of the trunk.

Steeplechase

The steeplechase is a type of endurance run coupled with a hurdling or jumping action. The mechanics used in running 3000 m are similar to those used in any run of that distance. However, scaling five hurdles or obstacles every 400 meters, with one located just before the water barrier, puts considerable emphasis on the endurance factor. Many performers in the past have jumped on top of the barrier and then attempted to clear or almost clear the water area. The other four hurdles are jumped over, or the performer leaps on top of the

barrier and then jumps into a running stride. The water jump is the one discussed here.

Many authors contend that a fast approach and rapid mount (if this is used), followed by a smooth takeoff, are the ingredients for success in this event. Formerly the steeplechaser usually tried to maximize the horizontal displacement and minimize vertical displacement. The jumper usually landed about 0.60 m (2 ft) from the forward edge of the water area in a stride position and accelerated from a flexed front leg (which reduces the body's moment of inertia) out of the water as rapidly as possible. Recently a runner from the University of Wisconsin has introduced a new technique whereby he jumps the water hurdle (rather than mounts the barrier and then jumps into the water) and lands just beyond the middle of the water hazard. A view of a film of his performance indicates that he landed sooner and was out of the water sooner than his opponents. His technique bears more scrutiny and research.

MINI LABORATORY EXERCISES

1. Use the Sargent (vertical) jump to determine the best vertical jumpers in class. Then list the reasons why some individuals jump higher than others.
2. Do a standing broad jump. Observe and analyze each jump.
3. From a standing position, do a sail, a hitch kick, and a hang as represented in the long jump. Determine how these movements influence the distance of the jump.

REFERENCES

Barlow, D.A.: Kinematic and kinetic factors involved in pole vaulting, doctoral dissertation, Indiana University, Aug., 1973.
Bedi, J.F.: Angular momentum in the long jump, dissertation, Indiana University, May, 1975.
Bunn, J.W.: Scientific principles of coaching, Englewood Cliffs, N.J., 1955, Prentice-Hall, Inc.
Felton, E.: A kinesiological comparison of good and poor performers in the standing broad jump, thesis, University of Wisconsin, 1960.
Ganslen, R.V.: Mechanics of the pole vault, Athletic J. **21:**20, 1941.
Halverson, L.: A comparison of the performance of kinder-

garten children in the takeoff phase of the standing broad jump, dissertation, University of Wisconsin, 1958.

Hay, J.G.: The biomechanics of sports techniques, Englewood Cliffs, N.J., 1973, Prentice-Hall, Inc.

Palmer, C.E.: Studies of the center of gravity in the human body, Child Dev. **15:**99, 1944.

Roy, B.: Kinematics and kinetics of the standing long jump in seven, ten, thirteen and sixteen year old boys, dissertation, University of Wisconsin, 1971.

Sargent, D.: The physical test of a man, Am. Phys. Educ. Rev. **26:**188, 1921.

Ward, R.D.: An investigation into the use of computer integration of kinematics, kinetics, and cinematography data in motion analysis, dissertation, Indiana University, Aug., 1971.

Yoon, Pat Tan Eng: The triple jump. In Wilt, F., and Ecker, T., editors: International track and field coaching encyclopedia, West Nyack, N.Y., 1970, Parker Publishing Co.

ADDITIONAL READINGS

Chistyakov, U.: The run of a high jumper, Track and Field, No. 8, Dec., 1966.

Elsheikh, M.: A three-dimensional model of the ideal technique in the broad jump, doctoral dissertation, Washington State University, 1975.

Ganslen, R.V.: Mechanics of pole vault, ed. 7, Denton, Texas, 1970, R.V. Ganslen, Publisher.

Pepin, G.: The long jump, Track Field Q. Rev. **76:** Fall, 1976.

Ramey, M.: It's a matter of projection: the long jump, Track Field Q. Rev. **76:**13, Fall, 1976.

CHAPTER 13

Fundamental concepts of throwing

Throwing includes a rapid acceleration of the trunk and arm segments, usually after a step and just before release of an object. Sometimes it involves a summation of the velocities of the body parts, all adding up to a crescendo at the time of release. At other times some body parts are moved for positional purposes to allow for the freedom of the body parts engaged in the primary action. In addition, an axis (pivotal point, fulcrum) around which the body rotates as the throwing action takes place is established so that the movement is effective.

ACCELERATION

Throwing a lightweight object such as a ball usually consists of accumulated accelerations of successive segments, especially of the upper extremity. This movement can be labeled concurrent motion; that is, all successive limbs move in the same direction. The result is much greater contraction of the large muscles such as the pectoralis major and the latissimus dorsi (which are actually arm muscles, in terms of action, even though they are located on the thorax and back). They attach to the humerus in the bicipital groove.

This type of high-velocity throwing calls for greater contractile length of the muscles of the throwing arm than of some of the lower-extremity muscles. The reason is that many of the arm muscles are biarticular in nature; that is, they usually move two joints in the same direction at the same time. This factor calls for proper timing of the action so that the thrower is able to be consistent. A slight error in any part of the movement is accentuated at the time of release. If accuracy rather than velocity is the objective, then the thrower uses the least number of segments possible. The pattern in such a case may be quite different because only a few segments are involved.

The movements involved in a high-velocity throw are as follows*:

1. The center of gravity shifts backward and then is displaced forward.
2. The performer steps forward with the leg opposite to the throwing arm.
3. The upper portion of the body is flexed after being extended (first acceleration).
4. The trunk rotates about its longitudinal axis to pull the throwing arm forward (second acceleration).
5. The scapula moves forward over the back (torso), as much as 15.24 cm (6 in) or more. This is one key to the ability to throw efficiently. A large scapula is considered an asset in high-velocity throwing.
6. The humerus acts in conjunction with the scapula as the former flexes on the latter over a range of 90 degrees.
7. The shoulder rotates internally around its

---

*Adapted from Gaul, J.S.: Throwing research proposal (unpublished), Rehabilitation Hospital, Charlotte, N.C., 1968.

long axis up to 90 degrees (another major acceleration).

8. The extension at the wrist at the end of the backward motion of the arm and the flexion at release together add another acceleration. (There is some controversy regarding this statement. Some researchers contend that there is no acceleration involved in the extension of the wrist and that the situation is only positional. Also, to speak of the "cocking," or flexing, and then extending of the wrist is misleading. It is the hand that does most of the movement, not the wrist.)

9. The fingers are extended first and then flexed to add a final acceleration.

AXES OF ROTATION

There are four axes (fulcrums, or pivotal points) of rotation often involved in high-velocity throws. They are the planted foot on the opposite side of the throwing arm, the hip rotation opposite the throwing arm, spinal rotation, and shoulder rotation of the throwing arm. The body as a whole rotates about one axis—namely, the foot—whereas the other body parts rotate about various axes such as a joint or joints. In the so-called overhand throw the throwing arm begins the action from an extended-arm position with the hand pointing downward. The arm moves in an angular path to the rear and upward. From this rearward, fully-extended position the arm translates upward and backward. Then the arm flexes and moves forward at the elbow to increase the angular motion, after which it extends laterally before release takes place. This latter action gives the opportunity for centrifugal force to be utilized. The lateral body lean in the opposite direction enables the arm to be extended upward (Fig. 13-1). The nonthrowing hand moves backward, aiding in the torso rotation

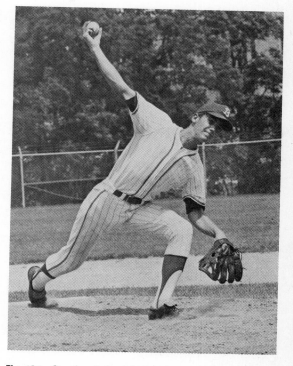

Fig. 13-1. Overhand throwing action. Note lateral body lean so that throwing arm can be extended upward.

and arm motion. Almost all throwing action has some or all of these segmental movements. Small, light objects are released in a plane lying parallel to the body and tangential to the movement. Heavy objects, such as in a shot put, are released in front of the body; otherwise, injury to the elbow would occur frequently. These objects are linked to the length of the moment arms.

The function of the arm in a throwing situation is to position the hand for the throwing action and to help develop efficient velocity of the hand. (The object is released with the same velocity that the hand has accumulated.)

For a better understanding of the upper limb complex and the amazing action that occurs during the throwing action, it seems appropriate to mention some anatomic and biomedical aspects.

A total of 28 bones in the arm-shoulder area are used in the whip-crack, flail-like action occurring during throwing. The scapula, humerus, radius and ulna, proximal row of carpals, distal row of carpals, metacarpals, and finally the phalanges are involved. In addition, the clavicle serves as a strut supporting the whole arm during the act of throwing.

The astounding thing about the shoulder girdle complex is its lack of stability, which results in great freedom of motion. In the upper swing of the arm the great range of movement is further enhanced by the broken hook structure involving the clavicle, acromion process, top of glenoid fossa,

and coracoid process. Furthermore, the scapula moves on the clavicle, and the clavicle moves on the sternum. The shallow depth of the glenoid fossa pushes the humerus farther away from the center of joint, promoting still more freedom of motion. The joint then has to rely on the rotator cuff muscles—the subscapularis, supraspinatus, infraspinatus, and teres major—as well as on other shoulder girdle muscles to preserve its integrity.

The spins and swings of the arm about its long axis, whereby acceleration is produced from a small radius of gyration, enable the arm to have great spinning motion. Its motion has been compared to that of a jackhammer.

The main muscles of the arm and adjacent region involved in throwing, as determined by electromyography, are the pectoralis major, latissimus dorsi, deltoid, trapezius, serratus anterior (magnus), rhomboids, and levator scapulae. The muscles acting on the scapula function as a force cou-

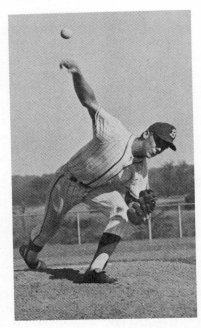

Fig. 13-2. Overhand throwing action. Note lateral extension of total arm and pronation of forearm and hand on forceful throw.

ple. One group produces an upward rotation, and another causes a downward rotation. This is similar to the action of a revolving door. The longer in length the scapula, the farther down the muscles attach, creating the possibility of a large force—hence one of the reasons some men can throw at the rate of 160.90 kmph (100 mph), whereas other men and most women throw at a slower rate.

There is usually a proximal-to-distal action of the segments during throwing. This means that the heavier parts initiate the movement, and the distal, lighter segments benefit by transfer of momentum and also are easier to move at the crucial point of release.

The hand is designed so that the grasping aspect is utilized in throwing. For example, there is opposition of the thumb, which is used only during the early stages of the throwing motion but is not evident at the release of lightweight objects. The skin of the hand on the palmar side is tight for grasping and flexibility, but on the back the skin is loose. The skin creases of the fingers are not located over the joints, allowing for greater flexibility. A natural pocket is formed by the thenar and hypothenar muscles and the metacarpals, and there is an increased angle of application of the profundus and superficialis when they are lifted upward to produce more effort.

All forceful throws from almost any position are characterized by medial rotation of the humerus and pronation of the forearm and hand (Fig. 13-2). The radius of movement of the forearm ranges from long to short to long, which gives the arm the longest moment arm and raises the possibility that the radius and the moment arm will be the same length. A throw of high velocity is likely to be the result.

It is possible for the thrower in certain situations to have lost contact with the ground and to be airborne before releasing the object. This is true in both shot putting and discus throwing. The object has by this time accumulated its own momentum and will continue unimpeded on its course, even though a foot is not anchored to the ground.

THROWING PATTERNS

Mechanics of underarm pattern. The underarm pattern is most frequently seen in skills that project an object by a throw. Its outstanding characteristic is movement of the arm, usually with extended elbow, by shoulder joint action. At the height of the backswing the arm is approximately at shoulder height; during the force-producing phase the arm is moved rapidly downward, and at release or impact it reaches a position that is usually parallel with or slightly beyond the line of the trunk.

The lever of this shoulder action includes the bones of the upper arm and forearm, the wrist and hand, and in the throw the portion of the phalanges up to the center of gravity of the projectile. If an implement is used, all the phalanges will be included, in addition to the length of the implement from grasp to point of impact. The resistance arm includes the same rigid masses as does the entire lever; the fulcrum is in the shoulder joint. The length of the moment arm at the time that the object is started on its flight will be the distance from the proximal end of the humerus to the point of impact or the center of gravity of the projectile. This line will be perpendicular to the axis and to the line of the applied force.

Various levers can be added to this primary action to increase the amount of applied force. Among the most common is that which moves the pelvis by rotation at the hip joint. This lever will include the pelvis, the spine, the right side of the shoulder girdle, and the rigid masses included in the shoulder-action lever. (This description and that which follows refer to a right-handed performer.) The resistance arm will include the same masses as does the entire lever. At release or impact the length of the moment arm will be the distance from the axis (a line passing through the hip joint that is rotating) to the point of release or impact. This line, perpendicular to the axis and to the direction of applied force, can be changed in length by the positions of the trunk and the arm. If the trunk is flexed to the right, the moment arm will be lengthened; if the trunk flexed to the left, the moment arm will be shortened. If the arm is abducted, the moment arm will be lengthened. In some underarm patterns that have been studied, although pelvic rotation occurred during the force-producing phase, it was not found to occur at the time of application of force. Thus if the linear velocities of moment arms acting at release or impact are determined and if the velocity of pelvic rotation is not one of them, then pelvic rotation makes no direct contribution to the force at that time. Most likely its contribution, made before the final phase, is reflected in the actions of the other joints.

Pelvic rotation is facilitated by a transfer of weight of the total body. In the preparatory phase the weight is transferred to the right foot, and the pelvis is rotated to the right; rotation can be more than 90 degrees from the intended direction of flight of the projectile. This range of rotation is not possible unless the weight is taken from the left foot. Pelvic rotation facilitates arm action. As the pelvis turns, it carries the torso with it until it, too, is at right angles to the intended line of flight. As the arm is raised upward and backward, it is abducting, instead of extending, as it would be if the torso were facing forward. The shoulder joint's abduction range is greater than its hyperextension range, and according to present knowledge a segment can be moved faster if its range of action is increased.

While the weight is on the right foot, the left foot can be lifted in preparation for a forward step. No evidence is available to indicate the most advantageous exact length of this step. Studies do show that good performers take longer steps than those who are less skilled and that the length of the step is a feature that distinguishes between good and poor performers. As the forward step is taken, some forward movement of the whole body occurs. This adds to the force that can be imparted to the projectile, but compared to that developed by hip and shoulder action it is small. The step alone is not an important factor in increasing force; the step accompanied by increased range of hip and shoulder action is important.

Rotation of the spine can add another lever to the pattern. In comparison to other possible levers that may be a part of the pattern, the spine makes a small contribution. Although the action occurs in many vertebral joints, the fulcrum can be considered to be located at the level of the sternoclavicular joint. The lever will include the right clavicle and the masses included in the shoulder lever; the resistance arm will include the masses of the entire lever. The length of the moment arm will be the perpendicular distance from the axis; it will pass through the upper spine to the point of release or impact. The length of the moment arm can be altered by changes of trunk or arm position, as described for the moment arm of pelvic rotation.

An important lever acts at the wrist joint, because the wrist can be the fastest of the acting joints and because the length of the moment arm can be greatly increased by an implement. For the throw the lever arm and the resistance arm include the bones of the hand and fingers to the center of gravity of the projectile; for the strike they include the bones of the hand and fingers and the implement, if one is used, to the point of impact. In a throw, depending on the size of the hand, the moment arm from the wrist to the center of gravity of the projectile could be 7.6 to 10.1 cm (3 to 4 in) in a child and 20.3 to 22.8 cm (8 to 9 in) in an adult.

The levers described in the preceding paragraphs, acting at shoulder, hip, spine, and wrist, are those most commonly used in a variety of underarm patterns. Whether more than one is used in the pattern will depend on the demands of the situation. Shoulder action will always be used, since it is the basis for the classification *underarm*. It is possible that in some situations other joint actions can be used efficiently, but such additions will not change the classification when the shoulder action is that described here.

Mechanics of overarm pattern. The overarm, like the underarm, pattern is commonly used in throws and strikes. Its distinguishing feature is shoulder joint action that rotates the humerus laterally during the preparatory phase and medially during the force-producing phase. Persons who cannot readily visualize these actions may be helped by going through the following movements: Hold the upper arm at the side in such a position that, when the elbow is flexed 90 degrees, the forearm will be horizontal and pointing directly forward. Keeping the upper arm at the side, move the forearm to the right 90 degrees in the transverse plane; the forearm will now point directly to the side. The joint action that brought about this change in the position of the forearm was lateral rotation of the humerus. If the forearm is now moved back to the original position, the action involved is medial rotation of the humerus.

These shoulder joint rotations can be made while the upper arm is in many positions. One position frequently used is described as follows: With elbow extended abduct the entire arm 90 degrees to the horizontal. Adjust the position of the upper arm so that when the elbow is flexed 90 degrees, the forearm will point directly forward. Move the forearm until it points directly upward. This will be accomplished by 90 degrees of lateral rotation of the humerus. Lower the forearm until it again points forward; it has been moved to this position by 90 degrees of medial rotation at the shoulder joint. This rotation of the humerus is the outstandng characteristic of the overarm pattern; this bone is usually abducted in the force-producing phase.

Present observations suggest that next to wrist flexion, medial rotation is the fastest joint action of the upper limb. Apparently there is a limit to the speed with which each joint action can be moved. Because the moment arm of shoulder medial rotation can be longer than that acting at the wrist joint, its linear velocity and therefore its contribution to the force imparted to a projectile can be greater than those contributed by wrist action.

In lateral and medial rotation of the humerus the axis passes through both the shoulder joint and the length of the humerus, whereas in the other actions at the shoulder the axis passes through the width of the humerus. The length of the moment arm in the rotating actions (lateral and medial) is the distance from the axis to the point of release or of impact. The line representing this distance must be perpendicular to the axis and also to the line of applied force. The moment arm will be longest when the forearm is perpendicular to the humerus; when the forearm is flexed either more or less than 90 degrees, the moment arm will be shorter.

With the elbow extended, medial and lateral rotation can be used effectively when an implement is held in the hand. If the arm is held at the side, the elbow extended, and a tennis racket held in the hand so that it is at right angles to the arm, the racket can be moved through 180 degrees in the transverse plane. In this action pronation and supination of the forearm will add to the range and the speed as the humerus is rotated.

Other levers that are commonly combined with arm action in the overarm pattern are the same as those described for the underarm pattern; they are brought into action by pelvic and spinal rotation and wrist flexion. Their resistance arms will be those described for the underarm pattern. The lengths of the moment arms for pelvic and spinal rotation are likely to be longer in the overarm than in the underarm pattern because the humerus is usually abducted.

According to Tarbell, the variety of forms of the overarm pattern that the upper limb can perform is characteristic of the versatility of this section of the body. This limb can apply great force and also act with extreme precision. In part this is due to the structure of the connection with the trunk. The humerus is connected to the freely movable scapula. The humeral head, which is almost half a sphere, fits into a cup of cartilage attached to the inner surface of the fossa on the upper distal section of the scapula. This attachment permits flexion, extension, and abduction of the humerus and the antagonistic joint actions. Variations are increased by movements of the scapula, which has no direct connection with the trunk. The scapula and clavicle are a functioning part of the upper limb and take part in practically all movements of the humerus, not adding to strength of action, but, rather, increasing range and versatility.

Mechanics of sidearm pattern. The sidearm pattern, like the underarm and overarm ones, is generally used in throws and strikes. Unlike the latter two the distinguishing feature of the sidearm pattern is not the type of shoulder joint action but the lack or limitation of action at this joint. The main action in the sidearm pattern is pelvic rotation, with the arm held fairly stable in an abducted position. The lever and the resistance arm for this action include the segments described for it for the underarm pattern. The moment arm for the pelvic lever can be one of the longest found in common activities. It extends from the axis passing through the left hip (for right-handed performers) to the line of applied force and includes the width of the pelvis, often the length of the whole arm, and part of the hand. The length of the moment arm is increased by the length of any implement that is used. With a tennis racket or a baseball bat the length of the moment arm could be 1.828 m (6 ft) or more in an adult.

Other actions that are commonly combined with pelvic rotation in this pattern are spinal rotation, wrist flexion, and often a small range of shoulder adduction. In wrist flexion and shoulder adduction the moment arm can be greatly increased when an implement is used.

Another outstanding feature of the sidearm pattern is the plane in which the movements are made (that is, the transverse); many movements of the underarm and overarm patterns are made in the sagittal plane.

The basic sidearm pattern, in which the shoulder and elbow joints are fixed, is rarely used in throwing light objects. Only when heavy objects are projected and in young, inexperienced children is the basic pattern likely to be observed. In a study of the sidearm and overarm throwing patterns of a highly skilled man and woman, the preliminary parts of the movements were found to be much alike. The differences were seen to be in the position of the arm and the degree and timing of elbow extension. The arm in the sidearm pattern was close to the horizontal as hip rotation began, and the elbow was more fully extended at release.

These arm positions would lengthen the moment arms for hip and spinal levels and shorten the moment arm for shoulder rotation. The hip action in both subjects contributed a greater proportion of the velocity in the sidearm throw than it did in the overarm pattern. The ball velocity for the man's sidearm throw was 3.657 m/sec (120 ft/sec) and for the woman's, 2.73 m/sec (89 ft/sec).

Continued study of the so-called sidearm throws of skilled performers has shown so much similarity in the overarm throw, especially those in which medial rotation of the humerus is followed by forearm extension, that some students have questioned classifying them as different patterns. Other observers believe that a distinguishing feature in the sidearm throw is a circular arm movement preceding release and that this is never seen in the overarm throw. Such observers say that the throw with the circular pattern should not be classified with the overarm throw. Further study of this feature is needed.

MINI LABORATORY EXERCISES

1. Put up a target and have class members throw at it, using underarm, overarm, and sidearm patterns and using only the arm segment. Record the differences.
2. Bring to the laboratory pictures of all types of throwing actions, preferably in sequence. Note segmental action.
3. Have a skilled performer demonstrate and explain his or her throwing action. Evaluate the statements with respect to what was demonstrated.
4. Contrast poor and skilled performances in a throwing action.

REFERENCE

Tarbell, T.: Some mechanical aspects of the overarm throw. In Cooper, J.M., editor: Proceedings of the Committee on Institutional Cooperation Symposium on Biomechanics, Chicago, 1971, The Athletic Institute.

ADDITIONAL READINGS

Broer, M.R., and Houtz, S.J.: Patterns of muscular activity in selected sport skills: an electromyographic study, Springfield, Ill., 1967, Charles C Thomas, Publisher.

Gollnick, P.D., and Karpovich, P.V.: Electrogoniometric study of locomotion and of some athletic movements, Res. Q. **35**:369, Oct., 1964.

Hay, J.G.: The biomechanics of sports techniques, ed. 2, Englewood Cliffs, N.J., 1978, Prentice-Hall, Inc.

Rasch, P.J., and Burke, R.K.: Kinesiology and applied anatomy, ed. 6, Philadelphia, 1978, Lea & Febiger.

Sanders, J.A.: A practical application of the segmental method of analysis to determine throwing ability, doctoral dissertation, Indiana University, 1976.

Track Field Q. Rev. **80:** Spring, 1980 (entire issue on javelin and hammer throws).

CHAPTER 14

Selected throwing skills

This chapter presents a number of analyses of selected throwing skills involving sidearm, underarm, and overarm patterns. There has been no attempt to include all the movements; only a representative sample has been discussed. In the sidearm example only the discus throwing is presented; however, many sidearm actions are in the striking pattern (Chapter 15).

DISCUS THROW

The discus throw is a type of sidearm throwing action. This throwing movement is used because it enables the thrower to attain the greatest possible distance with the discus. Factors influencing the flight pattern are height, velocity at release, and angle at release. In addition, the discus in flight is subject to aerodynamic factors and angle of attack (air resistance), which influence the distance traveled.

The velocity of the released spinning discus accomplished by top performers is 24.38 m/sec (80 ft/sec) or more, and the angle of release is approximately 35 degrees. The angle of attack, about 15 degrees, is the angle of the plane of the discus and the relative wind. The discus is thrown with a slight tilt so that the lift factor is greater than the drag factor. (See Chapter 5 for more information on lift and drag.) A head wind coming toward the performer at an angle of 45 degrees from the right (right-handed competitor) is the most advantageous wind, in terms of direction, for top performers.

If the radius of the throwing arm is long (externally extended) and coincides with the moment arm, great velocity is generated at release. Furthermore, the throwing arm is extended downward at the start of the spin and then is extended laterally and upward, utilizing centrifugal force at release.

The discus throw is an excellent example of the basic sidearm pattern, to which has been added a preparatory movement of the entire body. In the area (a ring with a diameter of 2.5 m [8 ft 2.5 in]) within which the body is permitted to move, the progression includes total rotation of the body one and one-half times, as well as movement from the back to the front of the space. Some of the world's best performers use all of the ring, starting well to the back and ending with the final step at the front of the ring. Some performers are now using two full turns.

The first step is taken with the left foot, which is moved toward the front of the ring and placed in line with the right foot. As the steps continue, they resemble those of a sprinter more than do those shown in Fig. 14-1. As the turns are made, the knees are flexed, and the right arm is held fairly close to the side; both positions lower the center of gravity and aid in balance. The arm position also moves the center of gravity of the rotating body closer to its axis and enables it to turn with greater speed. The speed of rotation during the stepping should accelerate and be as fast as possible and still allow the performer to maintain balance.

On the final step the right arm is abducted,

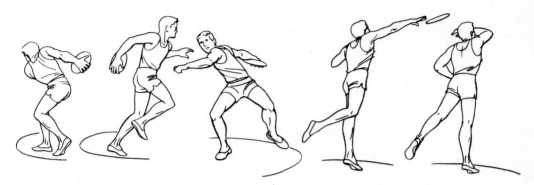

Fig. 14-1. Discus throw.

lengthening the moment arm of the pelvic lever, which can also be increased if the discus is held as close to the end of the fingers as possible and still be controlled. Adduction of the arm at release will start the flight well beyond the front of the ring. Wrist action in the final phase can be added to impart more velocity.

UNDERARM PATTERNS

Pitching underarm. In the basic underhand pattern the joints that move levers in the direction of the throw normally occur in the following sequence: hip rotation, spinal rotation, shoulder adduction and flexion, and wrist flexion. As the trunk is rotated backward, the arm is raised to the rear in a combined abducting and extending shoulder joint action; as the arm is moved forward, it is kept in the sagittal plane by a combination of shoulder adduction and flexion. The underarm throw and pitch are much alike in joint and lever actions. The moment arm lengths for this form of throwing were described in Chapter 13. However, observers will find many individuals modifications of the basic joint actions.

Normally the first forward movement is a step with the left foot. This necessitates first putting the weight on the right foot, facilitates pelvic rotation over that support, carries the left side of the pelvis forward, and increases the length of the step. As the left foot contacts the ground, the right arm usually reaches a horizontal position and is ready to begin its forward swing. For most effective action the upper torso would, at this time, be facing to the right with the shoulders in line with the direction of the throw. Women often fail to take advantage of this position. Instead they tend to keep the upper torso facing the direction of the throw and thereby decrease both hip and spinal actions, sometimes with complete loss of the latter. The major forward movement of the body is made as the left foot moves forward; there is rarely a slide on the left foot such as in bowling. At the time of release, forward movement of the body contributes little to the force of the throw.

A skilled woman's underarm throw is shown in Fig. 14-2. This is a windmill style of pitching in softball. Sling styles are also used to gain velocity in pitching. The performer in this illustration takes

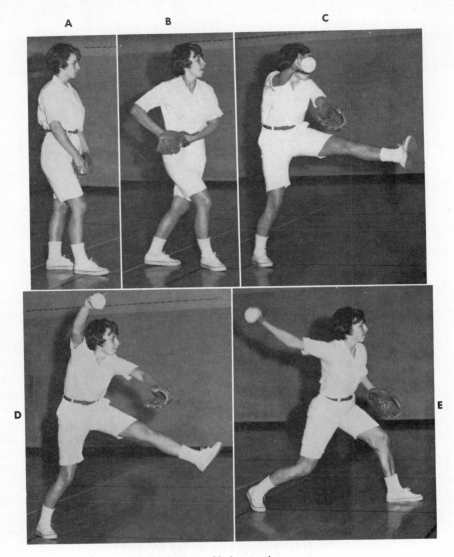

Fig. 14-2. Underarm throw.

a longer step than do most women; the step moves the total body except the right foot forward. The greatest part of that forward movement is seen to occur before the release phase; note the distance in which the head and upper trunk move with reference to the right foot from *C* to *F* and that these segments move a short distance with reference to

the left heel from *F* to release, which occurs between *G* and *H*.

The pelvis is rotated on the right femur when the right foot carries the weight (*C* and *D*). The range of pelvic rotation is limited somewhat by the position of the right foot, which is not turned 90 degrees from the intended flight of the ball. The

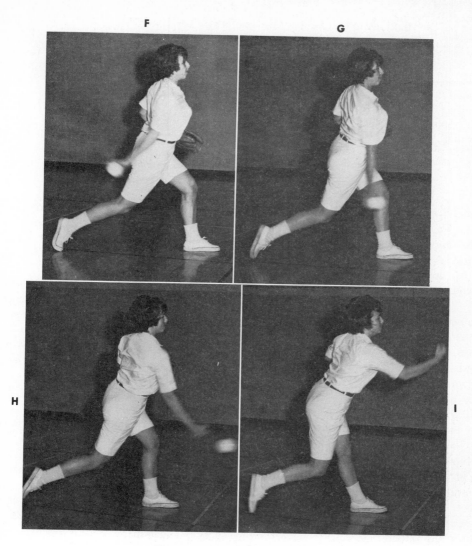

Fig. 14-2, cont'd. Underarm throw.

right-arm position, which is almost horizontal as the weight is taken by the left foot *(E),* is typical of most performers.

At release the contributing joint actions are left hip rotation, right shoulder and wrist flexion, and left ankle flexion. Note the hyperextension of the wrist in *F* and the flexion in *H*. The increasing speed of the ball can be seen in the change of the pictured image from *E* to *H*. Note that it is a circle in *E* and that in the succeeding pictures it becomes an oval that increases in length.

Medial rotation of the humerus and supination of the forearm will impart rotation to the ball. Film observations have shown that men frequently flex

Table 14-1. Lever contributions to ball velocity in underarm throw (pitch)

	Range (degrees)	Angular velocity (degrees/sec)	Moment arm length		Linear velocity	
			cm	ft	m/sec	ft/sec
Hip rotation	12	400	44.7	1.45	3.08	10.12
Spinal rotation	6	200	48.7	1.60	1.70	5.59
Shoulder flexion	22	733	76.2	2.50	9.74	31.98
Wrist flexion	30	3750	10.6	0.35	6.97	22.90

the elbow and use either lateral or medical rotation of the humerus to develop speed. In doing so they decrease the amount of shoulder flexion. Present information does not indicate whether rotation of the humerus develops more speed than does greater flexion of the shoulder with the elbow extended.

Measurements of the basic pattern provide insight into the potential contributions of each lever. Observations were made of the film of the skilled college woman pitcher. The measurements were made for two frames, including that showing the release; the time for all joint actions except the wrist was 0.03 second. The wrist action occurred in less than the time of one frame, and the time of the action was calculated to be 0.008 second. In the measurements given in Table 14-1 the range is expressed in degrees, the angular velocity in degrees per second, the moment arm length in centimeters (feet), and the linear velocity in meters (feet) per second.

The sum of the velocities is 21.5 m/sec (70.59 ft/sec); the ball velocity in the film was measured at 21.4 m/sec (70.26 ft/sec). Using the sum of the linear velocities as the total, one finds the contributions of the joint actions (expressed in percentages) to be as follows: hip, 14.3; spine, 7.9; shoulder, 45.3; wrists, 32.4. Shoulder joint action is the major contributor, as it was in the bowling performance discussed later in this chapter; wrist action in the throw with the lighter ball is more forceful.

Velocity measures of ball projections are not commonly made; however, they are a more valid measure of the force imparted by body levers than is a measure of distance. In measures made under the supervision of one of us (R.B.G.), two men, both pitchers on softball teams, had velocities of 32.91 and 33.22 m/sec (108 and 109 ft/sec); two women majors in physical education threw balls at 19.81 and 19.50 m/sec (65 and 64 ft/sec); and a teenage girl, an outstanding pitcher in a city softball league, delivered a ball at 24.68 m/sec (81 ft/sec). In addition, Joan Joyce, once the outstanding fast pitcher for women's softball, is reported to have thrown a ball at approximately 193 kmph (120 mph).

Hammer throw. The hammer throw is an underarm, two-handed throw unique in that a weight of 7.25 kg (16 lb) is attached to a wire string 117 to 121 cm in length. This increases greatly the arm length of the thrower. This sport is one of the few such activities in which centrifugal force is exceptionally high. Thus a relatively lightweight object such as a hammer can be propelled into the air rather easily by utilizing this force.

Two factors stand out as being important in gaining velocity at release and consequently greater distance in the throw: a long turning radius and an increased turning speed. Black has made this statement:

In an analysis of the Munich competition we found that the top throw by A. Bondarchuk of the USSR of 247′ 8″ [75.48 m] was achieved with a turning interval of 1.51 seconds. A further breakdown shows the increased body speed from one turn to the next. For example, the throw cited: First turn .645 (sic sec), second turn .36 (sic sec).*

The hammer is released at 26+ m/sec by the top throwers. Thus a decrease in turning time increases the final distance, provided that all other factors are held constant.

The thrower must keep in balance and control, gradually accelerating the hammer during the turns. There is torque between the upper and lower portions of the body. In a sense the hammer thrower hangs onto, or some say against, the hammer as velocity increases. The thrower makes three or four turns about the circle before the hammer is released.

There is an orbit, or path, established by the thrower as he turns about the circle, and there is a high and a low point of the hammer's path. A right-handed thrower flexes his right arm and then extends it as he regains a tighter hold on the handle. The left arm is kept straight (extended) throughout the movement. During this acceleration phase the plane of the hammer is relatively level. Any additional force, such as a pull inward, will decrease the radius and also prevent pelvis rotation (causing the hip to lead the movement).

As the thrower winds the hammer about the body, the center of rotation being the right shoulder, the degrees of rotation change from a low point of 280 to 290 degrees to a maximum of 320 to 325 degrees. These windups, or sweeps, have to be done with no loss of balance and with increased velocity of the hammer.

A "sit and stretch" action helps the shoulders relax and thus increase the radius. Doherty has stated that for every inch gained in radius there is a possibility for a 6-foot gain in distance. The flexing of the knees helps increase the length of the radius and also aids in maintaining balance by lowering the center of gravity.

The period of maximal acceleration is during the hammer's descent. The thrower at this time "sits"

---

*Black, I.S.: Russian and German techniques on hammer throwing, Track Field Q. Rev. **74**:204, Dec., 1974.

vigorously and thus increases the centrifugal pull. The "sit" is necessary to keep the center of gravity over the feet, especially the left heel (right-handed thrower).

As the thrower moves about the hammer ring, he attempts to increase the time of double support of the feet and to decrease that of single support. It has been shown that the hammer acceleration occurs only during the double support period. Double support is referred to as the "power" aspect and single support as the "gliding" phase.

The thrower must turn fast enough to stay ahead of the rotating hammer as he turns. Failure to do so causes a decline in acceleration, especially during the second and third turns.

To increase the torque in the body whereby there is a twist between the upper and lower portions, the thrower rotates the hips ahead of the shoulders during the turns. The hip lead over the hammer is anywhere from 45 to 90 degrees.

Hay has stated that the distance of the throw is primarily a result of four factors: velocity at release, height of the hammer at release, angle of release, and amount of air resistance. The latter factor has normally very little effect. The height of release is governed by the physique of the thrower and the position of the hammer. The release height should be at shoulder level.

The angle of release is considered to have the greatest influence on the distance of the throw. It is a result of the application of the horizontal and vertical forces at the moment of release. The best release angle for distance is between 42 and 44 degrees, since the hammer is released at shoulder height.

Two force couples act in the hammer throw. The first one is the outward, centrifugal pull of the hammer, which is countered by the inward, centripetal force exerted by the thrower. The latter involves the pulling of the thrower's weight through his center of mass downward. This force is opposed by the pushing of the ground upward against the thrower's feet. More centripetal force is needed to counteract the centrifugal pull as the speed of the turns increases. The Russians have conducted experiments measuring the strain on the handle of the hammer during the throwing action.

Relaxation of the shoulders helps increase the radius. There is a position of the central axis of rotation within the hammer-athlete lever system. To keep the system stabilized, the athlete must center the base of the axis over the left heel, thus increasing the smoothness of execution. The left heel is not only the center of rotation but the axis of the lever system.

Bowling. Among the least complex of the underarm patterns is the bowling delivery at the time of release. Obviously the major contribution to the velocity of the ball is the force derived from shoulder action. It is also apparent that hip and spinal rotation will be limited, since the bowler tends to keep the upper torso facing the lane, and the weight of the ball will limit wrist action.

Although each bowler's performance differs in detail from that of others, a general idea of the contribution of each acting lever can be gained from the following analysis. From a film showing the delivery of a man physical education major, observations disclosed that at the time of release spinal rotation and shoulder flexion occurred, but there was no hip rotation or wrist flexion. An unexpected action was elbow flexion.

To determine the contribution of each acting joint, researchers made the following measurements for the two frames preceding release: (1) the range of action of each joint (Table 14-2) and (2) the time during which this action occurred. The time per frame was 0.0158 second and for 2 frames was 0.0316 second, or approximately 64 frames/sec. The length of each moment arm at the time of release was measured from a side view. These moment arms were (1) for shoulder action (from shoulder to center of the ball), (2) for the elbow (from elbow to center of the ball), and (3) for the spine (a horizontal line from the upper spine to a vertical line passing through the center of the ball).

The sum of the linear velocities of the three levers is 7.8 m/sec (25.60 ft/sec). The velocity of the ball as it moved away from the hand was measured and calculated at 8.8 m/sec (29.11 ft/sec).

The difference suggests that a contributing factor was not included or that errors were made in measurement. Further study of the films showed that the torso moved forward during the two frames because of sliding on the left foot and flexion in the left ankle. The distance that the shoulder moved forward was measured at 44 mm (0.144 ft). The linear velocity of this movement would be 1.4 m/sec (4.56 ft/sec). The summed velocities were now 1.4 m/sec (30.16 ft/sec), or 0.32 m (1.05 ft) more than the measured velocity of the ball. The discrepancy is less than the 1.07 m (3.51 ft) before the forward movement of the body was observed; however, better techniques are needed to provide greater accuracy.

The film of a highly skilled woman bowler, whose season's average score in three leagues was 182, was studied by Anhalt; results are shown in Table 14-3. Measurements were made from a side view.

As shown in Table 14-3, the moving joints at release were the shoulder, elbow, and wrist. The sum of their linear velocities is 6.64 m/sec (21.81 ft/sec). The film showed that the body was moving forward at the same time at a rate of 1.4 m/sec (4.72 ft/sec). This, added to the lever velocities, totals 8.08 m/sec (26.53 ft/sec). The measured velocity of the ball in the film was 8.15 m/sec (26.74 ft/sec) after release. The degree to which the summed velocities agree with the ball velocity indicates the accuracy of the measurements.

In Tables 14-2 and 14-3 range refers to degrees, angular velocity to degrees per second, moment arm to length in centimeters (feet), and linear velocity to meters (feet) per second. The linear velocities were calculated using the formula given in Appendix D.

Increased velocity of the ball should be a goal for beginning bowlers; observations have not been extensive enough to set such goals with confidence. Casady and Liba recommend that women bowlers should impart to the ball a velocity that would send it from the foul line to the head pin in 2.5 to 2.75 seconds (7.31 to 6.67 m/sec [24 to 21.9 ft/sec]), and men bowlers in 2.0 to 2.5 seconds

Table 14-2. Lever contributions to ball velocity in bowling*

	Range (degrees)	Angular velocity (degrees/sec)	Moment arm length		Linear velocity	
			cm	ft	m/sec	ft/sec
Shoulder	14	443	74.67	2.45	5.770	18.94
Spine	6	190	31.69	1.04	1.050	3.45
Elbow	4	127	44.20	1.45	0.978	3.21

*Skilled man bowler.

Table 14-3. Lever contributions to ball velocity in bowling*

	Range (degrees)	Angular velocity (degrees/sec)	Moment arm length		Linear velocity	
			cm	ft	m/sec	ft/sec
Shoulder	12	400.00	75.59	2.480	5.27	17.31
Elbow	2	66.66	46.63	1.530	0.54	1.78
Wrist	11	366.66	12.95	0.425	0.83	2.72

*Skilled woman bowler.

(9.14 to 7.31 m/sec [30 to 24 ft/sec]). Randomly selected league bowlers, five from each of the following classifications, had the following average scores for the season: skilled men, above 190; average men, 150 to 160; skilled women, above 180; average women, 120 to 130. The velocity scores for these groups were as follows: skilled men, 8.65 m/sec (28.38 ft/sec), or 2.11 seconds for 18 m (60 ft); average men, 8.61 m/sec (28.26 ft/sec), or 2.12 seconds for 18 m; skilled women, 8.8 m/sec (29.12 ft/sec), or 2.06 seconds for 18 m; average women, 7.29 m/sec (23.94 ft/sec), or 2.50 seconds for 18 m. Since the expert does not deliver the ball with the greatest possible velocity but with only enough to make effective impact with the pins, the velocity of the highly skilled performer is one that the beginner can attain.

Both the man and the woman whose bowling delivery was studied (Tables 14-2 and 14-3) derived over 60% of their velocity from the lever acting at the shoulder joint. The bowler should strive to use this action effectively. It is frequently said that the arm should reach the horizontal at the height of the backswing. Shoulder hyperextension, when the body is erect, will not carry the arm to this height. By flexing at the hips, therefore, the bowler inclines the trunk forward. In this position, although the range of shoulder hyperextension is not increased, the arm, depending on the degree of trunk inclination, can approach, reach, or pass the horizontal. Widule found that, in the groups that she observed, the upper arms reached the following positions: skilled men, 185 degrees; average men, 180 degrees; skilled women, 199 degrees; average women, 163 degrees. (The horizontal is represented by 180 degrees; more than that means higher than the horizontal.) Inclinations of the trunk for these groups were 35 degrees for skilled men, 51 degrees for average men, 41 degrees for skilled women, and 54 degrees for average women. (If the trunk were erect, the inclination would be 90 degrees; the greater the forward inclination of the trunk, the smaller the inclination measure.) The height of the arm on the backswing depends on the degree of trunk inclination and the degree of shoulder hyperextension at the shoulder joint. At the height of the backswing Widule found the following measures: skilled men, 40 degrees; average men, 52 degrees; skilled women, 59 degrees; and average women, 37 degrees. (The greater the measure, the greater the degree of hyperextension.)

The length of the bowler's arm will also affect the linear velocity of that lever. In the measurements shown in Table 14-2, had the moment arm for shoulder action been 0.67 m (2.2 ft) instead of 0.74 m (2.45 ft), and had the angular velocity been the same (443 degrees/sec), the linear velocity would have been 5.18 m/sec (17.01 ft/sec). A difference of 7.62 cm (3 in) in length decreased the velocity almost 0.60 m/sec (2 ft/sec), or 1.93 ft/ sec.

The strength of grip has been shown by two studies (Curtis and Sabol) to be related to the speed of the swing. The nervous system evidently controls the speed, limiting it to the ability to hold the ball as it moves through the backward and forward arcs. The difference in strength of grip enables men to use a heavier ball than women normally use.

The contribution of the approach steps is not entirely shown in the forward movement of the torso at the time of release. As the ball is moved backward past the right leg by the arm, the approach steps are moving it forward. In the film study the ball was observed to move forward faster than it moved backward, so that during the backswing the ball was moving forward. This may be more easily visualized when compared to a person walking toward the rear of a railway car as the train moves forward. The person is walking backward but moving forward. As the bowling swing begins its downward, forward action, the ball already has a forward velocity, and the body levers add to this, rather than beginning from a zero velocity. The velocity of the approach increases with each step; the speed of the steps is usually kept constant, but the length of each increases over that of the preceding one.

If the velocity derived from body levers is to be fully used, there should be no downward direction in the ball's movement as it touches the floor. The arm should be a degree or two past the perpendicular at release, even if this means that the ball is released a few centimeters above the alley. The impact with the floor from this height will be slight and will be decreased by the roll given to the ball at release. Widule found that the upper arm had passed the perpendicular at release and also that the elbow was flexing. This action not only raises the ball slightly but adds to the velocity. (See Tables 14-2 and 14-3).

The analysis of the swing thus far has dealt with factors affecting the speed of the ball. The direction given to the ball is an important factor in the number of pins knocked down. In the distance that the ball travels from release to the pins, approximately 18 m (60 ft), a slight deviation from the exact line to the point of aim can result in a marked deviation as pin contact is made. For every 0.25 degree in direction, the ball will miss the point of aim by approximately 7.62 cm (3 in). A variation of 1 degree in direction would miss the point of aim by 30 cm (12 in); a ball started at the midpoint of the alley, if it deviated by 2 degrees from a perpendicular to the foul line, would end up in the gutter. Since slight deviations in direction have this marked effect on point of contact, the bowler must give careful attention to factors affecting accuracy.

Among these factors is the point at which the ball crosses the foul line. The starting position should be carefully determined with reference to this line, and the approach should be consistently straight forward. From the point on the foul line the ball should be directed along the selected line of direction. That line should be clearly visualized, and the arm should swing along this line even after the ball is released. (For additional details in achieving accuracy see Casady and Liba.)

OVERARM PATTERNS

When great speed and control are desired in a throw, often the overarm pattern is used. This uses the two joint actions that appear to have the highest speeds: wrist flexion and shoulder medial rotation. The sequence of joint actions can be seen in the football pass (Fig. 14-3) and in the baseball pitch

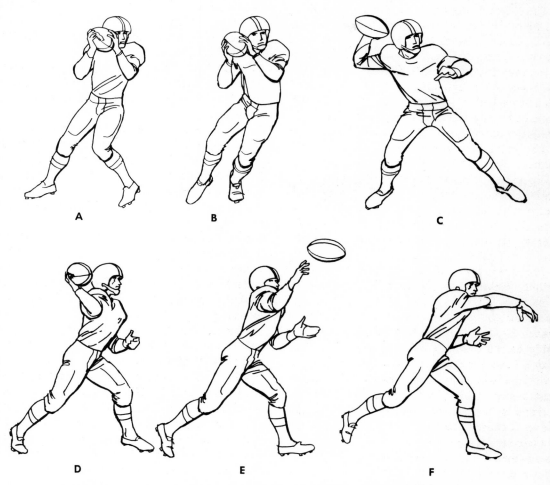

Fig. 14-3. Football pass. **C** and **D,** Lateral rotation of humerus. **E** and **F,** Medial rotation.

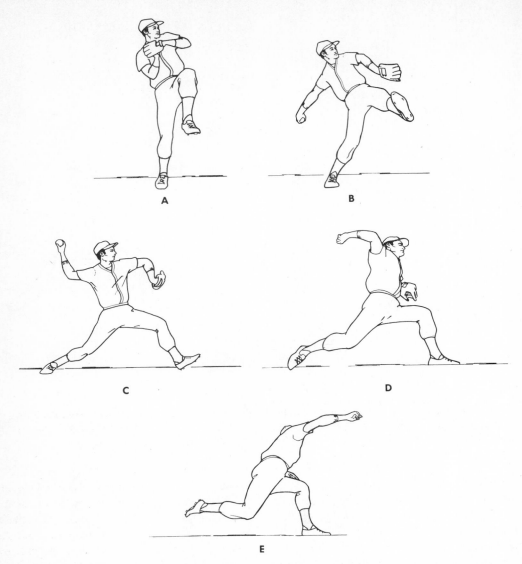

Fig. 14-4. Overarm pitch. **B** and **C,** Lateral rotation of humerus. **D** and **E,** Medial rotation.

(Fig. 14-4). Both show the step forward with the left foot, hip and spinal rotation, and medial rotation of the humerus. Apparently less wrist action occurs with the football throw than with the baseball pitch, which explains the greater velocity obtained with the smaller ball. Note in both series of pictures that, as the torso is rotated forward by hip and spinal actions, the humerus is rotated laterally. This timing is an important feature of complex movement patterns. The slower joints begin their

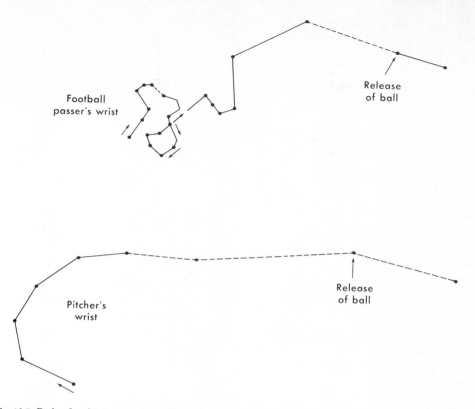

Fig. 14-5. Path of wrist (traced from film) of two throwers, one in football and one in baseball. Note that football thrower releases ball after height of wrist movement has been reached, and pitcher releases it just at height. (Biomechanics Laboratory, Indiana University.)

forward movement as the faster more distal joints complete their backswings. No appreciable pause between the backswing and forward swing of these faster-moving joints is necessary. The muscles responsible for the forward swing can begin contraction to stop the backswing. The combination of backward movement and beginning contraction stretches the tendons and connective tissue in the muscles, and thus the forward movement can be more forceful.

Note that in both throws the elbow extended somewhat before the ball was released, shortening the moment arm for shoulder medial rotation. Apparently, then, this action develops its greatest linear velocity before release, and this velocity must be used by the joints acting at release. However, elbow extension lengthens the moment arms for the hip and spinal levers and adds to the linear speeds of these levers at release. In both performances the right foot, as it supports the body weight during the backswing, is placed at right angles to the direction of the ball flight, which permits a greater range of pelvic rotation at the right hip.

Fig. 14-5 shows the path of the wrist in two throwing actions. The release of the ball by the pitcher is at the height of the wrist movement, but the football passer, because of the spin that must be imparted to the ball, releases it when the wrist is moving downward.

A physical education major, in analyzing his

Table 14-4. Lever contributions to ball velocity in overarm throw

	Range (degrees)	Angular velocity (degrees/sec)	Moment arm		Linear velocity	
			cm	ft	m/sec	ft/sec
Man						
Hip rotation	20.6	824	64.6	2.12	9.29	30.5
Spinal rotation	9.6	384	83.8	2.75	5.60	18.4
Shoulder rotation	38.5	1540	8.2	0.27	2.22	7.3
Wrist flexion	60.0	8571	14.9	0.49	22.34	73.3
Woman						
Hip rotation	20.6	735	70.7	2.32	9.08	29.8
Spinal rotation	20.9	746	67.7	2.21	8.77	28.8
Shoulder rotation	29.0	1036	10.6	0.35	1.92	6.3
Wrist flexion	42.0	5250	11.2	0.37	10.33	33.9

own football passes, measured the ball velocity as 18 m/sec (60 ft/sec) immediately before release. Shoulder medial rotation contributed 62%, spinal rotation 35%, and wrist flexion 3%. He had no hip rotation during the release phase.

Film study of the overarm baseball throw of a skilled man (a major league player) and a highly skilled woman gives indications of the contributions of the four levers of the pattern and also of individual adjustments in it.

Table 14-4 gives the range of movement in degrees at the time of release, the angular velocity in degrees per second, the length of the moment arm in centimeters (feet), and the linear contribution of each lever in meters (feet) per second. The time in which the joints moved through the given range was 0.025 second for the man except for the wrist, for which the time was 0.007 second. For the woman the time was 0.028 second except for the wrist, for which the time was 0.008 second. The high linear velocity for the wrist flexion shown in Table 14-4 has been questioned by later research, and the basis on which it was determined may be of interest to those who study film. Note that in the table the time for the measured range for the wrist is less than for the other joints. In the frame before release the angle at the wrist was measured; in the next frame the ball had been released and the wrist

angle had changed. The change was assumed to have occurred during the time that the camera shutter was closed, and this time, rather than the frames per second, was used to determine the velocity of the wrist joint. If this procedure is acceptable, the time cannot be longer than shutter time, and it could be less; in that case the angular velocity would be greater than was reported.

The sum of the linear velocities for the man is 39.50 m/sec (129.6 ft/sec); the ball velocity measured on the film was 39.90 m/sec (130.9 ft/sec). For the woman the sum of the linear velocities is 30.11 m/sec (98.8 ft/sec); the measured film velocity was 29.24 m/sec (95.93 ft/sec).

The wrist action in both performers is the greatest contributor to the linear velocity; the hip ranks second and shoulder rotation last. Both performers extended the elbow just before release, thus shortening the length of the moment arm of the shoulder lever. The measurements for this moment arm were shorter than those for the wrist lever, showing that the ball at release is less than 15.24 cm (6 in) from a line extending through the humerus. Shoulder action is likely to make its contribution earlier in the pattern.

In a study of the moment arm lengths in the overarm throws of high school girls, the best velocities were found to be developed by the girls who had the longest moment arms for the hip rotation levers and consequently the shortest moment arms for the shoulder medial rotation levers.

The tabulation of moment arm lengths shows that for the man the moment arm for the hip is shorter than that for the spine. This is due to a leaning to the left so far that the upper spine is to the left of the hip joint at release. The lateral flexion may be the cause of the small range of movement in the spine.

Certain limitations should be remembered regarding these reported contributions of joint actions to the velocity of the projected ball. In each case the measurements are those made for one subject and were taken during the release phase, so that they do not indicate joint contributions made in earlier phases. Furthermore, cinematographic methods have improved since the reported observations were made; current work questions the accuracy of the earlier methods of measuring joint actions. The doubtful measures are included here as an illustration of a procedure that can be followed with refined techniques to determine the contributions of body levers to ball velocity.

The most detailed and extensive current study of joint actions in the overarm throw is that reported by Atwater, who observed action in three planes, using side, overhead, and rear camera views. She included 15 subjects to provide opportunity for comparison: five skilled college men and five skilled and five average college women. Her observations include not only the release phase but also the 400 msec preceding the release. For the skilled groups that time period encompassed almost all the overarm pattern, including the backswing; for the average women only the later stages of the backswing occurred in the selected time. Displacement of the ball was measured in three planes, and the three velocities determined were combined algebraically into one "resultant velocity." Measured joint actions were related to ball displacement on the basis of observation and logic; moment arms and linear contributions of joint actions were not studied.

In observing displacement of the ball before its release from the hand, Atwater found that although the movement is primarily forward, vertical and lateral movement occur also. None of the subjects accelerated the ball continually, but all accelerated rapidly shortly before release, the men as much as 457.20 to 609.6 m/sec^2 (1500 to 2000 ft/sec^2); skilled women, 304.80 m/sec^2 (1000 ft/sec^2); and average women, 121.92 m/sec^2 (400 ft/sec^2). (See Fig. 14-6.)

In comparing joint actions Atwater found that all skilled subjects used essentially the same actions but that the range and speed were generally greater for the subjects who had the fastest ball velocities at release. Some of these differences can be seen in Fig. 14-6, which represents positions at times of approximately 0.070 and 0.025 second before release of the ball and 0.005 second after release. Note that in the lowest tracing for each subject the ball is behind the head and that this distance is greatest for the skilled man and least for the average woman. Differences in ball position at this time can be attributed largely to trunk position; the trunk of the skilled man is not yet facing the direction in which the ball is to be projected, whereas that of the average woman is facing slightly beyond that direction. To reach the positions shown in the top tracings the man's trunk moves through a greater range than do those of the women, and its rotation must therefore be at a faster angular velocity. Note also that the elbow of the average woman is flexed 50 to 60 degrees at release, whereas those of the skilled performers are almost completely extended.

The differences in length of stride are not as clearly seen in Fig. 14-6. Atwater reports considerable differences in the average stride length for the three groups: that of the skilled men was 1.18 m (3.87 ft); that of the skilled women was 15.8 cm (0.52 ft) shorter and that of the average women 47.8 cm (1.57 ft) shorter than that of the men. A similar finding related to stride is reported by Ekern, who studied the overarm throw of boys and girls selected as the better throwers from second, fourth, and sixth grades. Within that group she

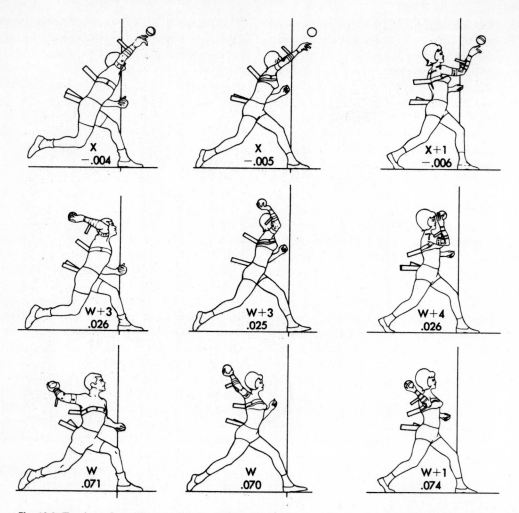

Fig. 14-6. Tracings from film study of overarm throw. Left, skilled man; middle, skilled woman; right, woman with average skill. (From Atwater, A.E.: Movement characteristics of the overarm throw, dissertation, University of Wisconsin, 1970.)

found that the better throwers, whose projected balls were fastest, have longer steps.

Fisk, in a review of the data in his study "The Dynamic Function of Selected Muscles of the Forearm: an Electromyographical and Cinematographical Investigation" made the following comments:

Preliminary analysis has been made of electromyographical data obtained from 12 subjects in the study. A great deal of individual variety in the function of the four muscles [mentioned in Fig. 14-7] during the performance of the overhand straight throw and the overhand curved throw was found. Conclusions drawn from the study indicate that the electrical response generated in

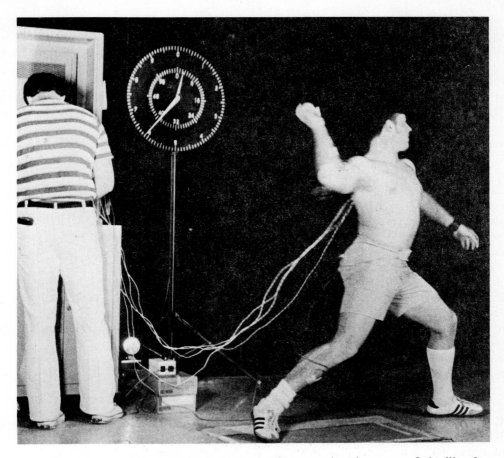

Fig. 14-7. Electromyographic apparatus used in study of overarm throwing pattern. Indwelling fine-wire electrodes were located in lateral head of triceps brachii, flexors carpi ulnaris and radialis, and pronator teres muscles. Subject as shown has started forward action of throwing arm. Also note that subject's rear foot is against force plate that could be used to obtain rear foot force during throwing action. (Calvin Fisk, investigator, Biomechanics Laboratory, Indiana University.)

the muscles took place during the final movements of the "laying back of the arm," just prior to when the elbow begins its forward movement and the wrist assumes its "cocked position." Once the forward movement of the arm begins the flexors diminish electrical activity. All four muscles were more active during the throws with spin than during the straight throws; therefore, it is assumed that greater muscular effort was required to perform the throws with spin. The onset of the maximal action potential response occurred earlier and endured longer for the throws with spin and occurred earlier and endured longer among the experienced performers. The contribution of the pronator teres muscle still remains partially unsettled; however, the results do suggest that this muscle contributes to the spin imparted to the ball at release when the throws with spin were performed.*

---

*Prepared by Calvin Fisk after a review of data from his doctoral dissertation, Indiana University, 1976.

The velocities of balls projected by the overhand throw have been measured more frequently than those of any other movement pattern. Among the reported velocities are the following:

1. Bob Feller's pitch, measured in 1946: 44.19 m/sec (145 ft/sec)
2. The throw of the winner of a city-wide contest in Philadelphia, an 18-year-old high school boy: 39.62 m/sec (130 ft/sec)
3. The mean velocity for 911 college women, reported in 1964: 13.59 m/sec (44.6 ft/sec); and for 1072 college women, reported in 1965: 12.95 m/sec (42.5 ft/sec)
4. The mean velocity of a group of high school girls, measured at the University of Wisconsin in 1959: 17.19 m/sec (56.4 ft/sec); highest velocity in the group: 27.64 m/sec (90.7 ft/sec)
5. Mean velocities for boys and girls, collected during 1956 through 1961 (with the mean velocities for intervening grades progressively higher)
   a. First-grade girls: 8.53 m/sec (28 ft/sec)
   b. Eighth-grade girls: 16.45 m/sec (54 ft/sec)
   c. First-grade boys: 10.66 m/sec (35 ft/sec)
   d. Eighth-grade boys: 22.86 m/sec (75 ft/sec)
6. Individual pitching velocities of seven men varsity pitchers (Slater-Hammel and Andres)
   a. For fast balls: 26.19 to 37.18 m/sec (86 to 122 ft/sec)
   b. For curve balls: 22.86 to 32.91 m/sec (75 to 108 ft/sec)
7. The mean velocity for 80 high school boys, reported in 1966: 20.84 m/sec (68.4 ft/sec)
8. Standards selected after personal observation and study of available data by Atwater in 1970 (see also data shown in Fig. 14-8)
   a. For skilled women: a range of 21.33 to 24.38 m/sec (70 to 80 ft/sec)
   b. For average women: 12.19 to 15.24 m/sec (40 to 50 ft/sec)
   c. For skilled men: 30.48 to 36.57 m/sec (100 to 120 ft/sec)

Shot put. Shot putting is a modification of the throwing action. It is a combination of overarm throwing and pushing because the rules dictate that the shot cannot be thrown as in many high-velocity throws (Fig. 14-9).

Dessureault found the following in his kinematic and kinetic study of poor and world-class shot-putters:

1. The entire action lasted 2.16 mean seconds.
2. The best shot-putters extended their bodies farther outside the rear of the circle and flexed the right knee more before beginning the move across the circle.
3. The shot-putters' mean displacement of the center of gravity was 1.52+ m (5+ ft) during the action.
4. The path of the shot followed a linear and slightly upward direction by the best performers and dropped vertically during part of the movement by the poorer performers.
5. The angle of release for the best performers was 38 to 41 degrees and was as low as 27 degrees for the poorer performers.
6. The majority of shot-putters lost contact with the ground and became airborne at release.
7. All performers had greater horizontal than vertical velocity at release.
8. The shot was released at a linear velocity of 13.52 m/sec (44.36 ft/sec) for the best performer; other velocities were less, the slowest being 9.14 m/sec (30 ft/sec).
9. The superior performers were in contact with the ground for a shorter time after the glide. (Mean time for all subjects was 0.296 second in the vertical plane and 0.287 second in the horizontal plane.)
10. There was a mean value of 278.14 kg (613.2 lb) of peak vertical thrust by the supporting foot and 1337.9 N (301 lb) of mean value by the front foot.

The shot-putter faces to the rear, as seen in Fig. 14-9, *A*, in preparation for moving across the ring. The weight is on the right foot. From position *A* the performer hops on the right foot to place it in

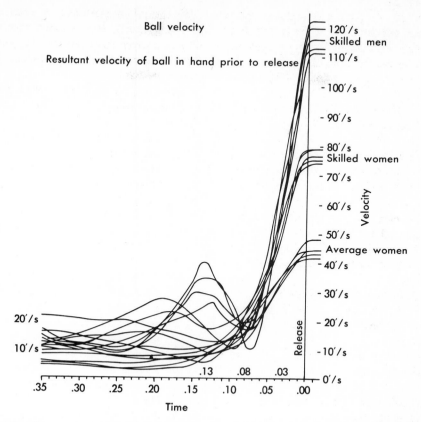

Fig. 14-8. Resultant velocities for overarm throw, calculated from measures taken from side, rear, and overhead views. At release, upper lines represent velocities of five skilled men, middle lines those of five skilled women, and lowest lines those of five average women. (From Atwater, A.E.: Movement characteristics of the overarm throw, dissertation, University of Wisconsin, 1970.)

the position shown in *C*. This action gives a forward movement to the shot, which should be used by adding to it the final lever actions (*C* to *E*). Knee flexion *(C)* is important for development of force. As the left foot makes ground contact (*D* to *E*), the torso can be moved rapidly upward by extension of the rear (right) thigh, and as the left foot takes the weight, the pelvis can rotate on the left limb. These two actions can accelerate the movement of the shot. Note that the upper arm is abducted to the horizontal in *D;* this position lengthens the moment arm for the lever moving at the left hip.

In the last phase of trunk rotation, shoulder adduction and flexion move the upper arm forward and upward. At the same time the elbow extends, moving the forearm forward and counteracting the upward movement of the upper arm. Final impetus is given by wrist flexion. Although these levers contribute to the force developed, as does the initial hop, the major contributor is the pelvic lever. The actions occurring from *E* to *G* are made to maintain balance.

Because the velocity of the shot is much slower than that of many objects that people project, and because its release point is higher than the landing

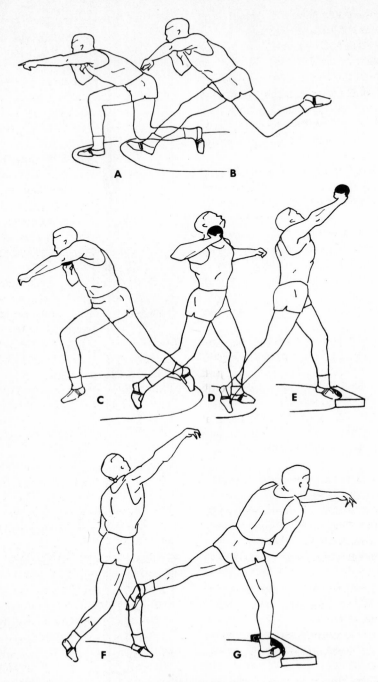

Fig. 14-9. Shot put.

point, the projection angle should be less than 45 degrees above the horizontal, as indicated by Dessureault's findings (reported previously).

Instead of a glide across the ring, some of the world's best shot-putters are utilizing a spinning action similar to that used by the discus throwers to attain higher velocity rates at release. A kinematic and kinetic study of this new method should be made to determine its potential and actual advantages and disadvantages.

Basketball shooting. The jump and set shots in basketball are types of overhand throwing actions. However, they cannot be classified as pure pushing or throwing motions, nor are they true high-velocity throws such as a baseball pitch. Thus, for want of a better way to classify this action, they might be termed soft, easy push-throws called "flips." Cooper and Siedentop have listed 20 principles of shooting as follows:

1. Shooters should always aim at a specific target.
2. Shooters should maintain constant eye focus on the target until the ball is released.
3. The ball should always be "wiggled" just before the release is begun so that good touch is obtained in shooting.
4. The shooter should not hold the body in a fixed position for a very long time before releasing the ball (especially the arms and hands).
5. In most instances the ball should be delivered with a reverse spin.
6. The better the shooter, the more intense the concentration on the act of shooting. In addition, the shots are not "sprayed." The missed shots are either long or short, not right or left.
7. Shooting is characterized by medial shoulder rotation, elbow extension, forearm pronation, and wrist flexion.
8. The longer the distance of the shooter from the basket, the more pronounced the forearm pronation.
9. The longer shots require that the ball be released at a higher angle (greater arch) to increase accuracy. To repeat, technically, the higher the arch of the shot, the more chance it has to go into the basket. However, there would be a compromise between the amount of force required to shoot the ball and the optimal angle (arch).
10. Longer shots require that additional parts of the body be used to add momentum to the hand.
11. The shooter should use as few levers as possible to avoid increasing the energy or work of any one lever beyond a moderate level. All movements should be made in one plane unless action is thereby restricted.
12. A 45-degree angle of release enables the player to propel the ball the longest possible distance.
13. Shots released at a greater height from the floor should be released with less arch.
14. Most shots should be aimed at a target (spot) just over the rim.
15. Every player must be able to rebound the ball off the board and into the basket when close to the basket.
16. Right-handed set shots should normally be delivered with the right foot forward.
17. The more backspin given to the ball, the farther from the basket it can be rebounded off the board.
18. The nonshooting hand should be used to support the ball until the last moment before release of the ball. However, the shooter should be careful not to "thumb" the ball with the nonshooting hand.
19. As a player moves up in competitive level, the delivery of the shots should be made with greater quickness to increase the opportunity to achieve success in scoring.
20. Although there are many styles of shooting a ball at the basket, it appears that there are certain basic patterns of mechanics that underlie all good shooting styles. For example, the eyes are focused on the target, the elbow of the shooting arm is pointed directly at the basket during release of the ball,

and the shoulders are squared and facing the basket. The latter is especially true on a jump shot taken from the outside corners of the court. It must be kept in mind that styles of shooting are affected by strength, height, weight, and previous learning experiences.

Gorton made a kinematic and kinetic study of top men and women basketball players executing a jump shot. Some of her findings are as follows:

1. The average time for the execution of the jump shot for both groups was 0.656 second.
2. The women had a longer preparatory period and the men longer transitional and thrusting periods.
3. The women released the basketball before they reached the peak of their height in the jump and the men just after the peak.
4. The women averaged a 77.7-degree takeoff angle and the men 80.0.
5. In both groups complete knee extension was not present at takeoff.
6. The trunk leaned backward at a mean angle of −3.25 degrees at takeoff and −2.8 degrees at release of the ball.
7. The mean angle of the trajectory of the ball was 48.9 degrees for the women and 39 degrees for the men.
8. At a distance of 4.57 m (15 ft) from the basket, the mean velocity of the ball at release was 7.55 m/sec (24.8 ft/sec) for both groups.
9. The men had a mean peak force against the force plate of almost 362.87 kg (800 lb) and the women almost 181.43 kg (400 lb). The peak force was 5 g and the lowest 3 g.
10. The braking force was greater for the men than for the women.
11. The vertical impulse was greatest for the men—187.5 per unit of weight for them, and 162.48 per unit for the women.
12. Both the vertical impulse and the horizontal impulse units were greater for the better jumpers.

The so-called "hanging in the air" jump shot has been theorized and then tested by Bishop and Hay. First, they hypothesized that it is possible that while in the air a player may move the body's center of gravity upward in relation to the trunk. This is done by manipulating parts of the body, such as the arms and legs, by moving them upward. A high vertical jump aids in attaining the desired height. Finally, the release of the ball on the downward path of the center of gravity gives an appearance of hanging.

Bishop and Hay found the following elements in this type of jump shot:

1. Ball release occurred after the peak of the jump.
2. Some arm and leg movement took place while the player was in the air, but not as much as expected.
3. There was a parabolic flight path.
4. There was flexion of the knees and the hips.
5. The extension of the knees as the player descended was not complete.
6. Finally, the hanging action did increase the time the performer was in the air (0.2 second because of the change of the center of gravity within the body).

The one-hand jump shot in basketball is a type of pushing-throwing action in which the actions of the upper limbs are unique in some ways but are generally in accord with most of the mechanics of throwing previously mentioned in this chapter. As the performer receives the ball (Fig. 14-10, *A*), preparation for the jump is being made primarily by flexion in the knees and application of braking action as noted by the movements of the feet, especially the right foot. In *B* the ball is being lifted upward by both hands and with flexion in the arms at the elbows. The propulsive phase of the jump is shown in *C*. The ball is now overhead, and the jumper is beginning to extend the legs. The eyes are focused on the target.

The jump shooter in *D* is now suspended in the air with the right elbow pointing in the direction of the target. Complete extension of the legs has been accomplished, but the two hands still remain in contact with the ball. The left hand remains in

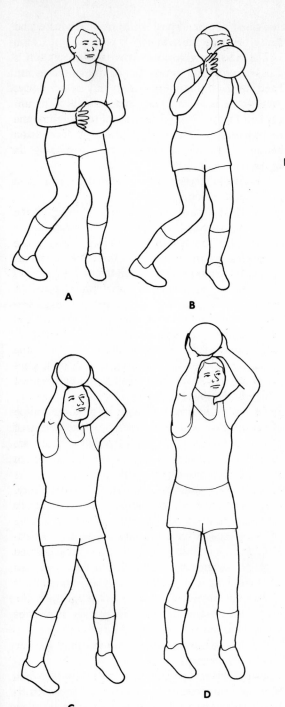

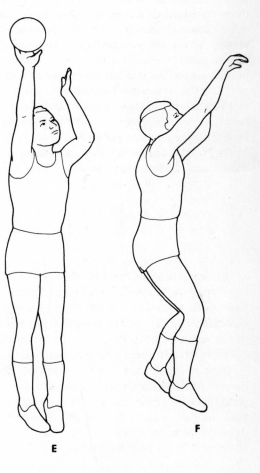

Fig. 14-10. Basketball jump shot.

contact with the ball as long as possible to help keep the ball balanced. The ball is near to being released with one hand. The left hand has relinquished contact with the ball *(E)*. A slight head flexion permits the shooter to "sight" with the dominant eye. The ball is normally released at the peak of the jump. Medial rotation of the shoulder and pronation of the forearm and hand is taking place during the follow-through *(F)*. This latter drawing was taken from a picture that is at a different angle from the other figures, to more clearly illustrate the action of the shoulder, forearm, and hand.

Basketball passing. Passing in basketball is the act of throwing or bouncing the ball from one player to another. It may be one of several types of throws, depending on the objective of the passer. A quick two-handed push pass is used when the players concerned are usually relatively close to one another. An "alley oop" pass is made by an outside player to a good jumper near the basket. A pass for distance may be overarm in nature but involves a compromise between vertical and horizontal velocity because the vertical velocity must be reduced as much as possible to reduce the time of flight. The following formula can be used if release and landing are at the same height:

$$T = t \text{ up} + t \text{ down}$$
$$= \frac{v \sin\theta}{g} + \frac{v \sin\theta}{g}$$
$$= \frac{2 v \sin\theta}{g}$$

Gravity is constant for any situation; v refers to magnitude (speed) of the velocity of the ball, and $\sin\theta$ is the sine of the angle of projection of the ball. Since sin 90 degrees is equal to 1, and sin 0 degree is equal to 0, the shortest time in the air occurs in the horizontal or negative angle of a pass.

There are many other types of throws, such as a bounce pass, which involves the angle of rebound and reflection as the ball strikes the floor. In this case the ball is spinning (backward or forward), causing some deviation in the reflection angle (making it smaller or larger). Others such as the

hook and one-hand pass will not be discussed because of space limitations.

The passing action involves medial rotation of the humerus and pronation of the forearm and hand, as in all throwing. A step may be used when great force is needed. Another element is the deception factor, which is practiced to a high degree in basketball. Cooper and Siedentop have listed certain principles of performance in passing the basketball, as follows:

1. Skilled passers make optimal use of peripheral vision.
2. Except in unusual situations, passes should be executed so that the ball is received at waist to chest height.
3. Except in unusual situations, passes should be accomplished so that the ball is delivered in a plane as nearly horizontal as possible.
4. The availability of vulnerable places to which a defensive player can pass the ball depends on the stance and the hand positions of the defensive player.
5. The closer a defensive player is to the passer, the easier it is to pass the ball without being intercepted.
6. A passer must be able to pass the ball as quickly and as forcefully as possible from any position at which the ball is received.
7. A passer should select a definite target spot before passing the ball.
8. Knee extension, shoulder medial rotation, and forearm pronation contribute to the force of the ball when it is thrown.
9. Increased ball velocity depends on one or more of three factors: greater range of motion, greater angular velocity of body segments, and larger number of segments.
10. The objective in passing is to get the ball to the desired teammate as quickly as possible without telegraphing the path of the ball to the defensive player. Quickness of delivery is essential.

Javelin throw. The javelin throw is similar to other types of overarm throwing actions in which the throwing objective is distance. A wide throwing stance is utilized just before release, and the body is projected into the air and follows in the direction of the javelin after release.

There is a run up to the throwing area to gain body momentum. The extreme stretching of the arm-throwing muscles aids in the throwing motion. The various axes of rotation—namely, the opposite hip, the spine, and the shoulder—increase the radius and moment arm at release (Fig. 14-11).

The angle of projection of the javelin is determined by the height of release above the ground, air resistance and the direction of the wind, and the velocity of the javelin at release. The javelin has aerodynamic qualities and is released at a lower angle than might be anticipated. Although many javelin throwers release the javelin at an angle of 42 to 50 degrees, the best throwers in the world release at 30 to 40 degrees.

The javelin thrower attempts to release the javelin with as much velocity as possible (27.43 to 30.48 m/sec [90 to 100 ft/sec]). The thrower often goes into the air one step before release. In other words, the thrower jumps, then plants the lead foot, and then follows through after release. Horizontal momentum is created during the run, and a braking force occurs at release, causing the momentum of the run to be transferred to the arm and

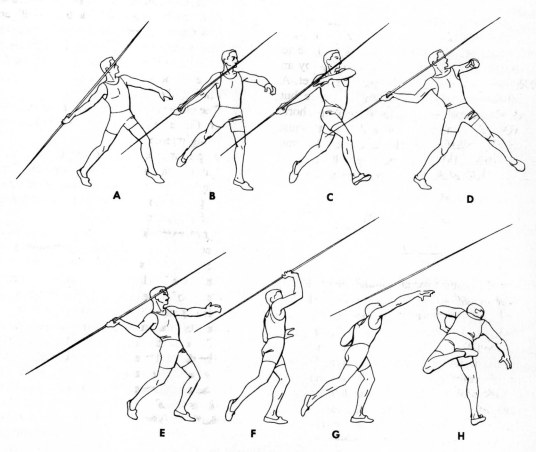

Fig. 14-11. Javelin throw.

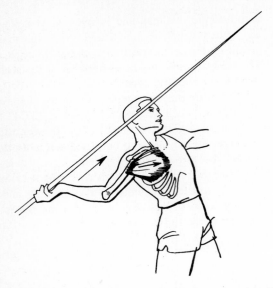

Fig. 14-12. Javelin thrower. Note position of pectoralis major.

javelin. The javelin must be pointed directly ahead and at certain angles of attack, depending on the direction of the wind. All the actions are related to aerodynamics and are affected by lift and drag, as discussed in Chapter 18.

The run is executed at a controlled speed and involves an acceleration in its last stages. Before the last step is taken, the body weight is on the right foot; with the final step the pelvis rotates at the right hip, adding to the length of the step. As the weight is shifted to the left foot, the humerus is rotated medially and the elbow is flexed (Fig. 14-11, *E*). The final force, added to the forward movement of the body, is derived from pelvic and spinal rotation, medial rotation and slight adduction of the humerus, and flexion of the hand.

Note the position of the pectoralis major in Fig. 14-12. This muscle is well suited for medial rotation of the humerus. In addition, the action of the latissimus dorsi should be visualized here, since it, too, is a medial rotator and its contraction would lower the humerus and pull it backward. The latter two actions are prevented from occurring by the pectoralis major. Acting together, these two mus-

cles are excellent rotators of the arm. Note that in the javelin throw the elbow is not fully extended during the final thrust, and the moment arm for medial rotation of the shoulder is almost at maximal length. In this skill medial rotation is a greater contributor than is wrist flexion.

MINI LABORATORY EXERCISES

1. Top performers in all the sports analyzed in this chapter should perform before the class, and the members should analyze the action through observation.
2. Analyze film, slides, or photographs of as many throwing actions as possible.
3. Calculate the velocities and accelerations of a throwing action similar to the procedure used in this chapter.
4. Ask a coach of a throwing activity to present ideas on performance of a skill. Evaluate these ideas in a kinesiologic framework.

REFERENCES

Anholt, C.: An analysis of levers contributing to the force in bowling, unpublished paper, University of Wisconsin, 1966.

Atwater, A.E.: Movement characteristics of the overarm throw: a kinematic analysis of men and women performers, dissertation, University of Wisconsin, 1970.

Bishop, R.D., and Hay, J.G.: Basketball: the mechanics of hanging in the air, Med. Sci. Sports **11**:274, Fall, 1979.

Casady, D., and Liba, M.: Beginning bowling, ed. 2, Belmont, Calif., 1968, Wadsworth Publishing Co.

Cooper, J.M., and Siedentop, D.: The theory and science of basketball, ed. 2, Philadelphia, 1975, Lea & Febiger.

Curtis, E.D.: The relationship of strength of selected muscle groups to performance in bowling, thesis, University of Wisconsin, 1950.

Dessureault, J.: Selected kinetics and kinematic factors involved in shot putting, doctoral dissertation, Indiana University, 1976.

Doherty, J.K.: Modern track and field, Englewood Cliffs, N.J., 1963, Prentice-Hall, Inc.

Ekern, S.R.: An analysis of selected measures of the overarm throwing patterns of elementary school boys and girls, dissertation, University of Wisconsin, 1969.

Gorton, B.: Kinematic and kinetic study of male and female basketball shooting, doctoral dissertation, Indiana University, 1978.

Hay, J.A.: The biomechanics of sports techniques, ed. 2, Englewood Cliffs, N.J., 1978, Prentice-Hall, Inc.

Sabol, B.: A study of relationships among anthropometric

strength, and performance measures of college women bowlers, thesis, University of Wisconsin, 1962.

Slater-Hammel, A.T., and Andres, E.H.: Velocity measurement of fast balls and curve balls, Res. Q. Am. Assoc. Health Phys. Educ. **23:**95, 1952.

Widule, C.J.: Analysis of human motion, LaFayette, Ind., 1974, Balt Publishers.

Widule, C.J., and Gossard, E.C.: Data modeling techniques in cinematographic research, Res. Q. Am. Assoc. Health Phys. Educ. **42:**103, 1971.

ADDITIONAL READINGS

Edwards, D.K.: The mechanics of pitching, Athletic J. **42:**40, March, 1962.

McCraw, L.W.: Comparative analysis of strength, arm length, and baseball throwing speed, paper presented at convention of the American Association for Health, Physical Education, and Recreation. 1974.

Morton, J.J., and Dudley, D.F.: Human locomotion and body form, Baltimore, 1952, The Williams & Williams Co.

Reiff, G.: What research tells about baseball (pamphlet), Washington, D.C., 1971, American Association for Health, Physical Education, and Recreation.

Siedentop, D., and Kaat, J.: Winning baseball, Glenview, Ill., 1971, Scott, Foresman & Co.

CHAPTER 15

Selected striking and kicking skills

Striking is the act of one object hitting another. For example, it may involve moving the hand or foot (in soccer, sometimes the head) in the striking action, as in throwing, or an extension of the arm, such as a bat or a racket, may be used. This type of implement will increase the radius of motion. The run or step made before an object is contacted increases the momentum of the foot or hand at contact because of transfer of momentum from a part to the whole.

Striking an object at rest, such as a golf ball or a soccer ball that is stationary, is somewhat different from striking a moving object, such as a baseball. Counteracting the momentum of a ball traveling at 144.81 kmph (90 mph) means that the mass times velocity of the bat must be greater than the velocity of the ball times its mass.

The stationary object must be struck with a force of sufficient magnitude to overcome its inertia. This involves the application of Newton's first law of motion. In addition, attainment of the maximal distance or maximal velocity in the flight of the struck object can be ensured if the striking implement contacts the object at a point tangential to the swing and through the center of gravity of the object. The takeoff angle of the struck object must be high enough to achieve maximal distance of flight if distance is the objective. Some of the struck objects have aerodynamic qualities, and the resistance to flight or form drag is decreased. The dimples in a golf ball help a golfer attain a greater distance in a drive. Both the number and depth of the dimples influence the distance of the flight.

The spinning ball traversing in the air is confronted with the Magnus effect (Chapter 5). For example, catchers in baseball know that a "pop" fly struck into the air behind home plate will curve toward the stands on the way up, and toward the infield on the way down. Consequently, to avoid missing the catch on the ball's return to the ground, they station themselves with their back toward the infield. In this position a catcher who slightly misjudges the flight path can block the ball with the body and then catch it. Likewise, a spinning baseball, hit to the outfield along or near the foul line on either side of the field, will curve toward the outside. Outfielders know this and play the ball accordingly.

Almost all of the research done with the use of cinematography reveals that the velocity of a badminton racket, a tennis racket, a baseball bat, and other striking implements decreases slightly at contact. In addition, there is a short period when the object struck is compressed, sometimes to as much as half its normal shape, before it rebounds. Furthermore, there is a period when the object struck adheres to the striking implement's surface before rebounding from it. The type of surface, the velocity of the implement, and the type of object determine the degree of compression.

There are other considerations that should be mentioned in relation to the striking action. For example, vibration of a compound pendulum occurs in various striking actions. If a bat is suspended from one end, its parts will vibrate at different rates. In a sense, pendulums of different lengths are involved, since the weight is distributed along the length of the bat.

Particles of the bat will vibrate more slowly near one end than elsewhere. A particle that will vibrate at the same rate as the undivided bat is located at the *center of oscillation*. The real length of the bat swinging as a pendulum is thought of as the distance between the center of suspension and the center of oscillation.

If the bat is struck at its center of oscillation with a sledge as it is suspended, it will swing evenly and without shocking or jarring the hands. If the bat is struck at any other point along its length, it will not vibrate smoothly and will therefore sting the hands of the striker. This center of oscillation is identical with the *center of percussion,* which is that point along a suspended object where a blow to it produces the least detrimental effect on the center of suspension. A ball can be hit with more velocity if it is struck at the center of percussion, called the "sweet spot" by performers. The location of the center of percussion varies according to the length and composition of the bat. The same is true with tennis rackets and other striking implements.

Richards and Barlow found that there were significant differences between wood and nonwood rackets in the variables of racket length, center of percussion location, and racket shaft flexibility, with the wood rackets being longer, having a center of percussion located closer to the throat, and being about one third less flexible.

BASEBALL OR SOFTBALL BATTING

The objective in baseball batting is to use a bat to strike a ball thrown with varying velocities by a pitcher. The bat is cylindric in shape and the ball is small and usually spinning as it is struck, making effective action difficult. The Magnus effect has influence, through air resistance, on the thrown and struck ball's flight. The stance of the batter and subsequent mechanical actions made by the batter determine the ability to hit the ball in a consistent manner.

The path of the center of gravity of an unskilled batter may show a drop of as much as 15.2 to 20.3 cm (6 to 8 in) during the swing. None of the skilled batters showed a drop of more than 7.62 cm (3 in). The skilled batters also turn their heads more to face toward the pitcher, to enable them to see the ball longer. The long radius and long moment arm aid the batter in achieving high bat velocity. Unskilled batters often pull the handle of the bat toward their bodies as they swing, reducing the length of the radius.

There is some "hitch," or backward movement, of the arms before they move slightly downward and forward. Depending on the height of the thrown ball, the path of the bat may follow the body's center of gravity or move downward and upward.

The rapid extension of the arms just before or as the step toward the pitcher is taken increases the speed of the end of the bat. Not only are the radius of swing increased and the moment arm lengthened, but centrifugal force comes into play to aid in bat velocity. The bat velocity has been calculated by Breen to be 0.19 to 0.23 second for the top hitters and 0.28 second for the poorer hitters. The velocity of the bat was calculated from the time the bat started movement toward the ball until contact with the ball was made.

During the swing the body weight of the above-average batter shifts forward, moving the center of gravity forward. The shoulder turn causes the bat-

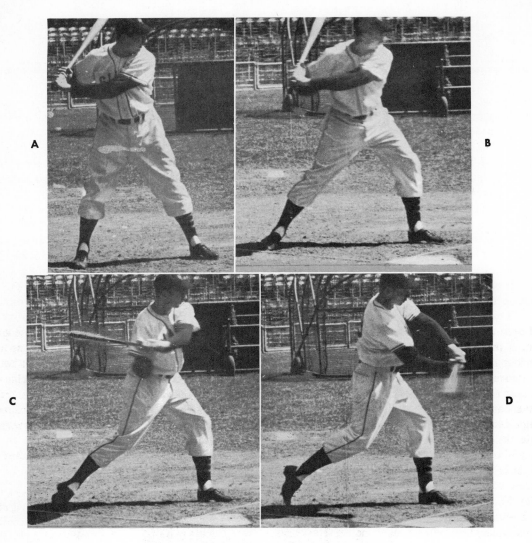

Fig. 15-1. Batting. (Courtesy Scholastic Coach.)

ter to be facing the pitcher as the ball is contacted. The rear foot is in plantar flexion, with only the toes touching the ground. Approximately 75% of the body weight is forward at the time of contact.

The head is held relatively stationary during the action. The eyes follow the ball until it is within 0.914 to 1.52 m (3 to 5 ft) of the plate. This is called "looking the ball into the catcher's glove," but in reality the eyes do not quite accomplish this task.

Hubbard found that batters reacted to the initial flight of the ball in 0.24 to 0.28 second. Breen found that the skilled batters started their swing when the ball reached half the distance to the plate and that unskilled batters started their swing sooner, or before the ball reached half the distance to the plate.

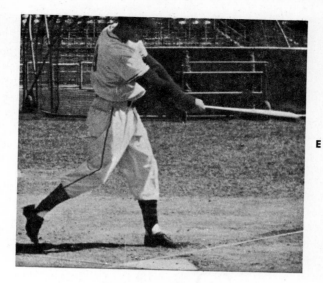

E

Fig. 15-1, cont'd. Batting.

The action used in batting normally is started from a position in which the performer has assumed a relatively wide base of support. Usually the stance is such that the feet are approximately 43.2 cm (17 in) apart. The step is 25.4 cm (10 in) as the ball approaches the plate (Fig. 15-1). The weight is mainly on the right foot, which is at right angles to the intended flight of the ball to permit freedom of pelvic rotation in the right hip. As the weight is transferred to the left foot, the pelvis is rotated at the left hip, turning through 90 degrees (B to D). The bat is moved forward in the transverse plane first by the turning of the torso (B and C) and finally by wrist action (C and D). The speed that the bat develops is shown by the blurring in D. A slight movement at the shoulder joints takes the upper arms forward and away from the trunk. The main contributing levers are those acting at the hip and wrist joints; the lengths of the moment arms for these levers have been greatly lengthened by the bat. Strong muscles acting at the wrist are important because they must hold the bat in the horizontal position, resisting gravitational pull, and move it with great speed in the final force-producing phase.

Note that the head is turned to the left in A and B to focus on the approaching ball. As the torso turns to the left, the head does not turn with it but remains facing toward the ball. Many coaches believe that if the batter's head moves to the left as the bat is swung, the left shoulder will be elevated, thus changing the path of the bat and reducing the possibility of contacting the ball.

After studying the film, Breen concluded the following:

(1) The center of gravity of the body follows a relatively level plane, thus indicating a level swinging of the bat. (2) Each hitter is able to adjust his head to a position from which he can get a better look at the flight of the ball for any given pitch. (3) The leading forearm tends to straighten immediately as the bat is swung toward the ball, immediately moving the end of the bat and resulting in faster bat speed. (4) The length of the stride is the same for all pitches for any single good hitter. (5) The body is bent in the direction of the flight of the ball after contact has been made, thus putting the weight on the front foot.[*]

*Breen, J.L.: What makes a good hitter? JOHPER **38**:36, April, 1967.

Another factor to consider in batting is the center of percussion, or "sweet spot." By way of further explanation, if one bat is suspended and then struck by another at its center of oscillation, it will swing as smoothly as a pendulum, without being jarred. A baseball batter can hit a ball with more velocity if the ball is struck at the center. (For additional information, see the discussion earlier in this chapter.)

BADMINTON

The stroking action in badminton is similar to other striking actions, such as in tennis, with some notable exceptions. It is also similar to throwing in many respects. The badminton racket and shuttlecock are much lighter in weight than the tennis racket and ball, and as a consequence the velocity of the shuttle is much less as it rebounds from the racket. The primary action is supination and forearm rotation in badminton strokes. The performer often jumps into the air to gain height to "smash" the shuttle.

The flight of the badminton shuttle does not follow a true parabolic path. The reason is that the shape and lightweight factors are such that the air resistance reduces the velocity of the shuttle very rapidly. A shuttle's horizontal momentum is diminished long before gravity has had its effect. This is most evident in a shuttle hit with great force; it produces an almost vertical drop after it has traveled a few meters.

Since the contact of the shuttle with the racket is relatively short, the angle of the face of the racket must be moved very rapidly in anticipation of the angle of descent of the shuttle. The velocity of the racket and shuttle determine the distance or height the shuttle will attain after being contacted.

Some of the strokes in badminton are done with the use of an immature throwing-striking pattern. For example, in some serving situations the foot that is on the same side as the striking arm (rather than the opposite) is placed forward. This is done when the server wishes to serve only a short distance or wants to have the feet in position for an unexpected return. If a long serve is desired, then the usual striking-throwing pattern would be used.

Because the rapid movement of certain body segments is necessary, the wrist (hand) and arm muscles bear the main propulsive responsibility. Transference of body weight from the rear to the front foot is possible when great force is desired. However, neither axes at the hip nor spin may be present when certain strokes are executed.

Hensley made a study of the badminton smash (Fig. 15-2) and drew the following conclusions:

1. The center of gravity of the body was found to move forward in a horizontal plane. This action would constitute an additional force which would be applied to the approaching shuttle.

2. The vertical movement of the center of gravity followed an "up and down" pattern. At the moment of contact, the center of gravity was moving upward near the apex of its movement. It is felt by the investigator

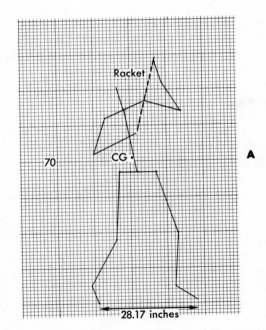

Fig. 15-2. Film analysis of a performer, showing the body and racket position while executing the badminton smash. (Prepared by Larry Hensley.)

that the most effective smash would be delivered immediately after the apex is reached and the center of gravity
has started downward. This factor would be important in
attaining the desired downward trajectory and velocity
of the shuttle.

3. The angle created by the upper arm and lower arm
at the point of contact was found to be 178 degrees, thus
supporting the theory that the most effective moment
arm is formed by an extended arm position. It is also
noted that the shuttle was contacted approximately 12.55
inches [31.9 cm] in front of the body. This again supports the theory that the shuttle should be contacted in
front of the body (about one foot) for the most desirable
results.

4. The main contributor of force to the stroke was the
medial rotation and pronation of the humerus and forearm. There was a great amount of forearm rotation
which is supplemented by wrist flexion immediately pri-
or to contact. This forearm rotation is a characteristic
action of all overhead throws.

5. The maximum velocity of the racket was attained

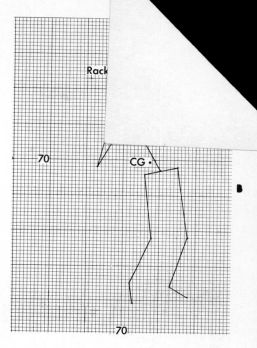

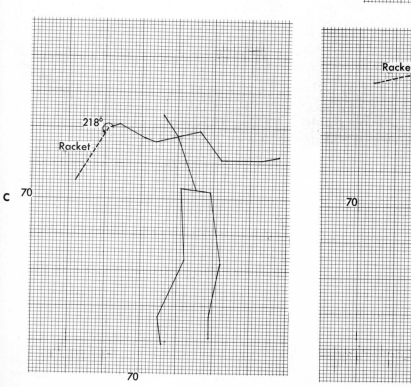

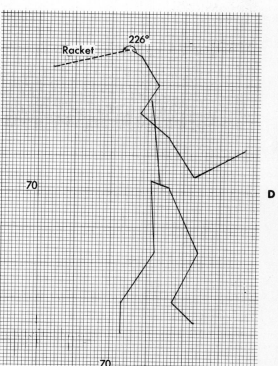

Fig. 15-2, cont'd. Film analysis of a performer, showing the body and racket position while executing
the badminton smash.

Continued.

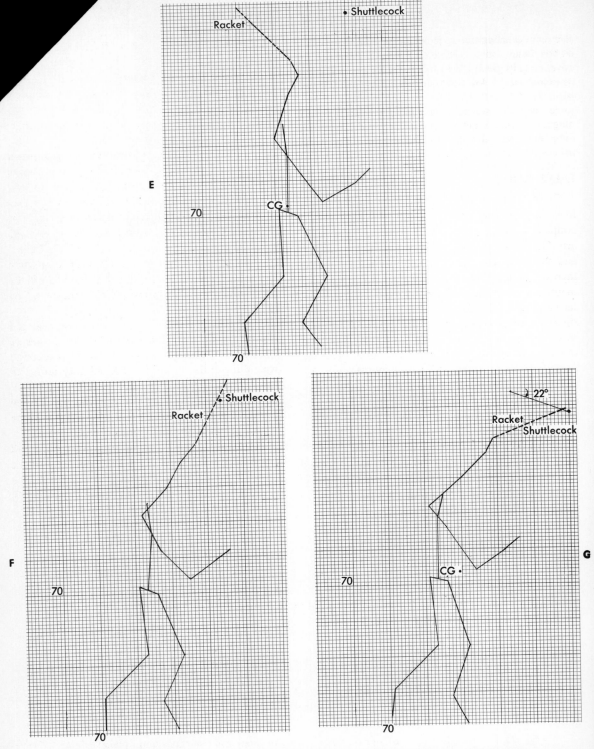

Fig. 15-2, cont'd. Film analysis of a performer, showing the body and racket position while executing the badminton smash.

at a point immediately after the racket had reached its highest point and had started downward. The racket, traveling at its greatest velocity, then contacted the shuttle immediately below this highest point. This again supports the theory that in order to achieve the greatest force, the racket should contact the shuttle upon beginning its downward motion. This would cause the shuttle to be contacted at the greatest feasible height, thus creating the potential for the best downward trajectory.*

TABLE TENNIS

Table tennis is classified as a striking activity involving all the elements of a striking action, coupled with the slight increase of the length of arm. There is a collision of two objects, the paddle and the ball. The ball is much lighter in weight than the paddle. The difference between the momentum of the paddle (the mass of the paddle times its velocity) and of the ball (the mass of the ball times its velocity) determines the direction of the resulting motion; it is in the direction of the greater momentum, that of the paddle. This is an application of the law of conservation of momentum.

The angle of incidence and reflection must also be considered. The angle of reflection is usually greater in connection with spinning balls, such as occurs in table tennis. The surface of the paddle, which varies somewhat with the type used, affects the action of the ball. The more irregular the surface, the greater the coefficient of friction. Thus the rebound from the surface can be executed with more spinning action.

As the ball is returned to the table surface by a strike, in accordance with Newton's first law, it tends to move at the same speed and in the same direction it assumed after being struck. However, the table resists the force of the ball and creates an equal and opposite force on the ball. Because of the frictional component, there is a decrease in the horizontal velocity. The vertical component is in accordance with the momentum of the ball and the striking angle. There is some decrease in vertical

velocity (V_y) in connection with the coefficient of restitution.

The speed and direction of contact of the ball with the paddle determines whether backspin, top spin, or sidespin is the result. If spin is desired, the ball is not struck by the paddle traveling in a completely linear direction. There are often two velocities in connection with top spin. One is the forward velocity in the horizontal direction, and the other is the horizontal velocity in a backward direction as a result of the spin. If the backward horizontal velocity is greater than the forward horizontal velocity, the friction that occurs when the ball strikes the table tends to increase the horizontal velocity. Thus the table tennis player applies top spin when it is advantageous to have the ball bounce off the table with great horizontal velocity and at a low angle of trajectory.

In certain situations, such as in a smash, the player may try to strike the ball at the center of percussion. This will cause the ball to rebound from the paddle at the greatest velocity and with little or no spin. Normally the opponent's shot should be contacted just before the top of the bounce. At this point the pull of gravity and the vertical momentum are neutralized.

Lopez found that the maximum speed of the ball struck by a defensive player in a backhand stroke was only 12 m/sec (39 ft/sec), compared to the speed of a smash reported to be 18.2 m/sec (60 ft/sec) by other investigators. From her comparative study of the backhand stroke of male and female subjects, she drew the following conclusions (Figs. 15-3 to 15-6):

1. The subjects had their knees flexed during the stroke.
2. The backswing of the subjects' paddle was close to the waist.
3. The forward swing of the subjects' paddle was upward and forward across the body.
4. The trunk angle during the stroke was less than 90 degrees.
5. The left arm was flexed and close to the body during the stroke.
6. The subjects stood sideways to the table.

Text continued on p. 284.

*Hensley, L.: Mechanical analysis of selected characteristics of the badminton smash, unpublished report, Indiana University, 1975.

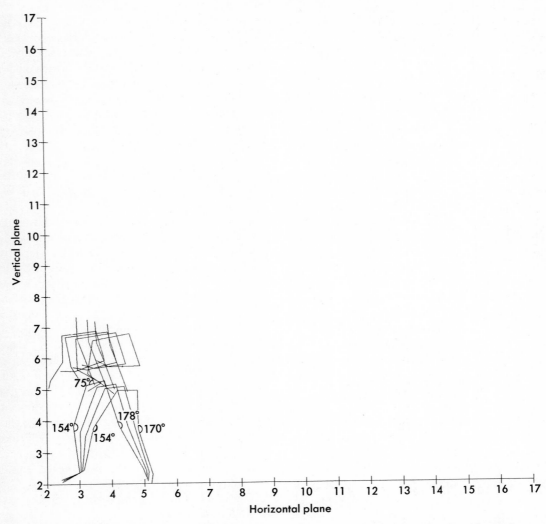

Fig. 15-3. Computer printout of film of backswing (male subject). Backhand stroke in table tennis. (Courtesy Jacqueline Lopez.)

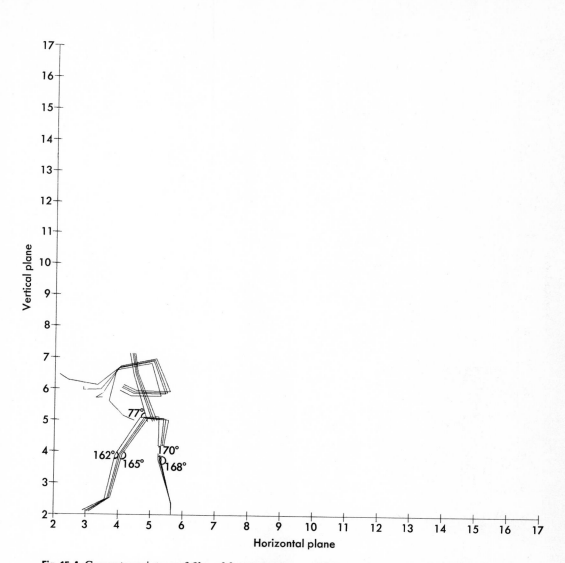

Fig. 15-4. Computer printout of film of forward swing and follow-through (male subject). Backhand stroke in table tennis. (Courtesy Jacqueline Lopez.)

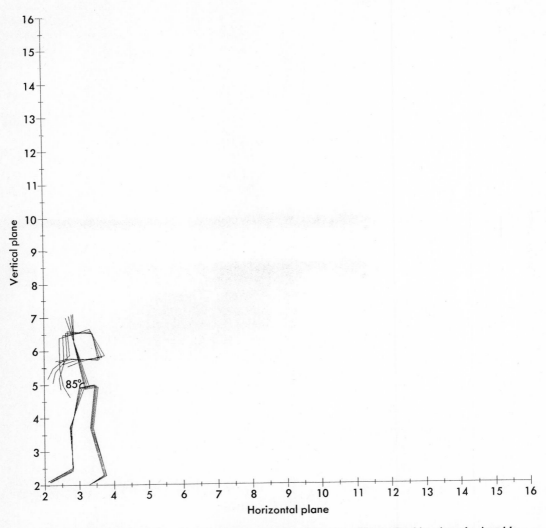

Fig. 15-5. Computer printout of film of backhand drive (female subject). Backhand stroke in table tennis. (Courtesy Jacqueline Lopez.)

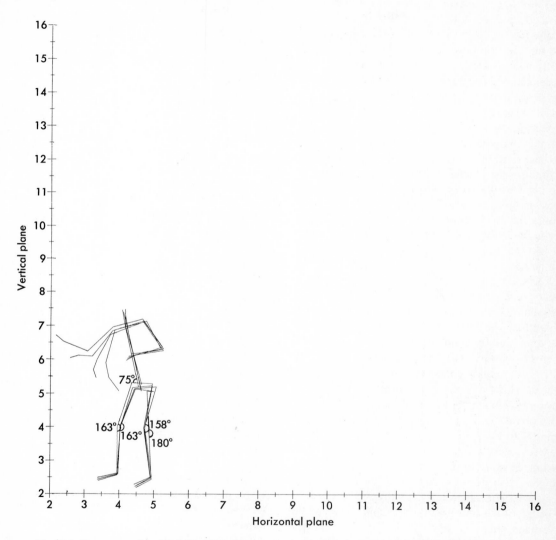

Fig. 15-6. Computer printout of film of forward swing and follow-through (female subject). Backhand stroke in table tennis. (Courtesy Jacqueline Lopez.)

TENNIS SERVE

The tennis serve is an overarm type of striking movement. At the beginning the trunk is rotated to the right (in a right-handed player) with the weight shifted to the rear foot. Note that in Fig. 15-7, *B*, as also shown in the pictures of the football pass and the overarm pitch, the right foot is placed at a right angle to the intended flight of the ball. This placement and the flexion of the left knee and lifting of the left heel permit greater rotation of the pelvis at the right hip joint. From full extension the right shoulder *(C)* is abducted and laterally rotated, and the elbow is flexed (*E* and *F*). At the peak of the backward movement the back is hyperextended with the wrist extended. Note the continuation of the head of the racket downward as the player's body moves forward (*E* and *F*). As the player moves the racket toward the ball, the right shoulder is medially rotated and the elbow is extended (*G* and *H*). The trunk and pelvis are rotated to the left *(H)*.

The tilting of the torso to the left (*G* and *H*), which here is due to abduction at the left hip, is frequently seen when height of reach is desired. This raises the right shoulder girdle and increases the length of the moment arm for spinal rotation.

In the tennis serve, medial rotation of the humerus is a major contributor to the speed of the racket. However, as in the overhand throw this action makes its major contribution before the impact phase. The humerus is laterally rotated in *F;* from *F* to *G* it has rotated medially close to 90 degrees. Here medial rotation imparts speed to the racket. From *G* to *H* the elbow extends to achieve height. Also during this time (*G* to *H*) the wrist makes its contribution by flexing. Except for the position of the upper arm, the tennis serve and the overhand pitch are much alike. The moment arm for wrist action is lengthened by the racket, and here, as in the golf swing, wrist action will be of major importance. Plagenhoef states that racket speed is no more important than firmness of grip.

The velocity of the ball and the height of impact will determine the angle at which it should be di-

rected to clear the net and to land in the service court. Gonzales, whose serve was measured electrically as 50 m/sec (164 ft/sec), is reported to have the fastest of measured serves. Kramer's serve was measured as 46.6 m/sec (153 ft/sec). These velocities will permit the ball to be directed below the horizontal. Stan Smith's serve has been reported to travel at the rate of approximately 60.6 m/sec (199 ft/sec).

A beginning player, before attempting to direct the ball downward, should develop such a velocity in the serve that when the ball is projected horizontally, it will clear the net and land in the service court. If the impact is 2.4 m (8 ft) above the ground and the projection is horizontal, gravitational force will bring the ball to the ground in 0.704 second ($8 = 16.1t^2$). In this time the horizontally directed ball must travel approximately 17.6 m (58 ft); its velocity would be $0.704x = 17.6$ m (58 ft), or $x = 25$ m/sec (82.4 ft/sec). If the impact is 12.2 m (40 ft) from the net, the ball will clear the net in 0.485 second, and gravity will have moved it downward 1.15 m (3.79 ft). Thus the net is cleared by 37 cm (1.21 ft). These figures indicate that a beginning player should develop a velocity of at least 24.4 m/sec (80 ft/sec) before attempting to direct the ball downward, unless the height of impact is considerably more than 2.4 m (8 ft). The average college woman can develop this velocity.

A velocity of 30.5 m/sec (100 ft/sec) has been measured in the better tennis players among college women. If impacted at a height of 2.4 m (8 ft) and directed downward at an angle 3 degrees below the horizontal, the ball will clear the net by 10.6 cm (4.2 in). That angle allows little margin for error and shows the importance of the height of impact.

These calculations were made without consideration of air and wind resistance and ball spin. If a player is able to develop a ball velocity well over 30.5 m/sec (100 ft/sec), the stroke should impart spin to the ball. Plagenhoef reports that five men whose serves he studied had ball velocities of ap-

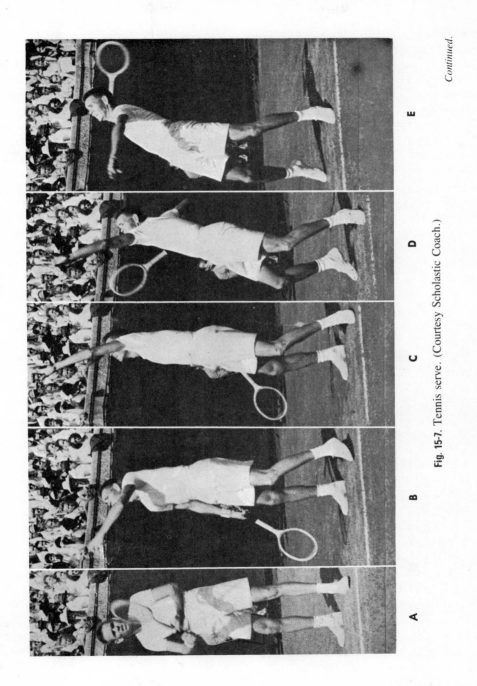

A   B   C   D   E

Fig. 15-7. Tennis serve. (Courtesy Scholastic Coach.)

Continued.

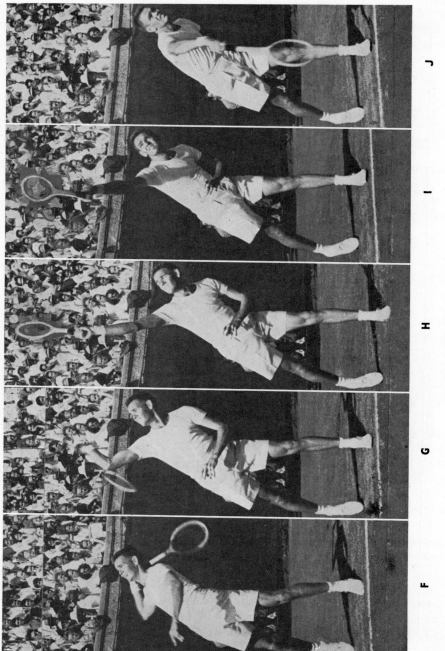

Fig. 15-7, cont'd. Tennis serve.

proximately 44.5 m/sec (146 ft/sec), or 160 kmph (100 mph). For these projections the rackets were moving at approximately 36.5 to 37.8 m/sec (120 to 124 ft/sec), showing that as reported for golf, the ball can move with greater speed than does the striking implement. This phenomenon is a result of the duration of force application (Impulse = Ft), or the work (Fd) on the ball while the ball and the racket strings are in contact with each other.

Smith did a comparative study of the kinematic and kinetic parameters of the flat and slice serves in tennis and found the following:

1. The mean backswing time in the serve was 1.62 seconds and composed 92% of the serving time.
2. The temporal analysis revealed that the mean total serving time was approximately 1.74 seconds.
3. The center of gravity of the racket reached a mean linear velocity of 33.6 m/sec (84+ ft/sec), with the flat serve being slightly faster.
4. The mean ball velocity for the flat serve was 43.8 m/sec (143.9 ft/sec) and for the slice serve 40.5 m/sec (133 ft/sec).
5. The mean angle of projection was different for each serve: 6.67 degrees for the flat serve and 8.00 degrees for the slice serve.
6. The ball was tossed approximately 0.76 m (2.5 ft) before contact was made with the racket.
7. In the kinetic analysis the vertical peak force, corrected for body weight, was 480 N (108.2 lb) for the flat serve (2.79 N [0.629 lb] per kilogram of body weight) and 521.8 N (117.4 lb) for the slice serve (3.05 N [0.686 lb] per kilogram of body weight).
8. The peak force before racket contact with the ball occurred at 0.046 second for the flat serve and at 0.051 second for the slice serve.

GOLF STROKE

The golf stroke is an underarm striking pattern similar to throwing, with modifications in the shoulder action. It might be called a *reversed underarm pattern,* since for the right-handed per-

former, the left arm is the guiding force, and in the downward swing the left shoulder action is abduction rather than adduction. The skill also differs from the usual underarm pattern in that both arms are active. Although the right arm does contribute to the force, it is used mainly to support the club except for the wrist action. Broer and Houtz have classified this skill as a sidearm pattern. However, we justify its classification on the basis of the movement of the left arm from a horizontal position above or at shoulder level at the height of the backswing (Fig. 15-8, *C*) downward to a position parallel with the trunk axis at impact (Fig. 15-8, *E*). The observations of Broer and Houtz show greater activity in the muscles of the left arm, supporting their statement that this arm action contributes more force than the right. This concept is subject to debate, as indicated above. The sequence of joint action is the usual hip rotation, spinal rotation, and shoulder action, with the wrist coming into action last. No step is taken, since the feet do not move from the starting position, but the weight shifts to the right foot on the backswing and back to the left foot on the forward swing. This shifting of weight increases the range of hip rotation (Fig. 15-8). At the height of the backswing, hip action is seen to have rotated the pelvis almost 90 degrees and spinal rotation to have turned the upper torso more. As the weight is transferred to the left foot, medial rotation in the left hip turns the pelvis toward the line of ball flight. In the skilled performer, forward hip rotation will begin before the shoulder and wrist have completed the backward movements. As the pelvis rotates forward, it will carry the arms downward. Shoulder action begins approximately at the time that the arm has reached the horizontal; wrist action will be delayed until the arm approaches the vertical (Fig. 15-8, *D*).

The moment arm lengths of hip and spinal levers must be measured from pictures taken with a camera placed in line with the flight of the ball. The moment arms are illustrated in Fig. 15-9. Depending on the length of the club and of the performer's arms and on the amount of spinal flexion, the mo-

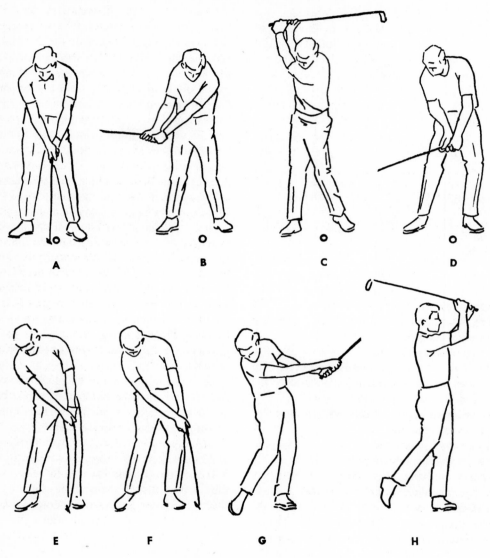

Fig. 15-8. Golf swing.

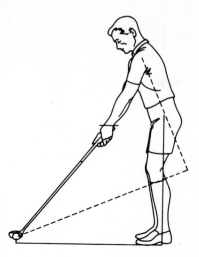

Fig. 15-9. Moment arm lengths in golf swing. Length for hip action is shown by unbroken horizontal line from hip axis to center of ball. Axis for spinal action is shown by broken line passing through spine; moment arm length is shown by broken line from this axis to ball.

ment arm length for hip action will be 0.9 to 1.2 m (3 to 4 ft). These factors will also affect the length of the moment arm for spinal action, which will be greater than that for the hip. The angular velocity of the hip and spine will be considerably less than that of the shoulder. A rough approximation of the linear contributions of the acting joints would be 70% for the wrist, 20% for the shoulder, and 5% each for the hip and spine.

Because extreme accuracy is necessary in golf, Cochran and Stobbs recommend that the movement pattern be made as simple as possible; they believe that the important levers are those acting at the shoulder and wrist joints. They say that the difference between good and poor golfers may lie in the simplicity of action and the ability to generate power in the acting muscles.

Full swings of the various clubs will have the same lever actions and the same proportion of linear contribution to the speed of the club head at the time of impact. In comparing full swings with the driver and with the No. 7 iron as made by five women golfers (handicaps 4, 5, 7, 9, and 12), Brennan found that the same joint actions were used in the two swings. In the degree of joint action in the forward swing and backswing she found only one significant difference in the mean measures. Although the degree of pelvic rotation in the backswing did not differ, with the driver the pelvis had rotated 7.2 degrees farther at contact than with the iron. The length of the club will affect the length of all moment arms and also the path of the club head; as the club is shortened, the path will become shallower and shorter. Photographs of a No. 2 iron and a wood swung by Bobby Jones show velocities of 40.23 and 43.28 m/sec (132 and 142 ft/sec), respectively, at the time of impact. The shorter distances obtained with shorter clubs result from the lower linear velocities of the levers as well as from the higher angles of projection.

Lever action in striking activities cannot be evaluated by comparing the summed linear velocities of acting levers to the velocity of the projectile. In throwing, the distal end of each lever is the center of gravity of the object to be projected. As each lever moves, this center of gravity is moved, and at release its velocity equals that of the contribution of the levers. In striking, the projectile is moved by body levers only during the brief period of contact.

The velocity of the golf ball can be greater than that of the club head at impact. Cochran and Stobbs report that a top golfer can have a club velocity of 2722.2 m/sec (8800 ft/sec), of 160.9 kmph (100 mph) and that the ball velocity will be 3621 m/sec (11,880 ft/sec). The difference is due to the smaller mass of the ball and also to the facts that the ball is flattened on impact and that during the 0.0005 second of contact the elastic ball pushes away from the club. These authors state that contact time is the same for almost all shots, even that of a putt—less than 1 msec.

The swing of a good golfer is so fast that detailed movement analysis can be made only with some device to aid vision. In the film of a professional golfer, Cochran and Stobbs found the time from the start of the swing to impact to be 0.82

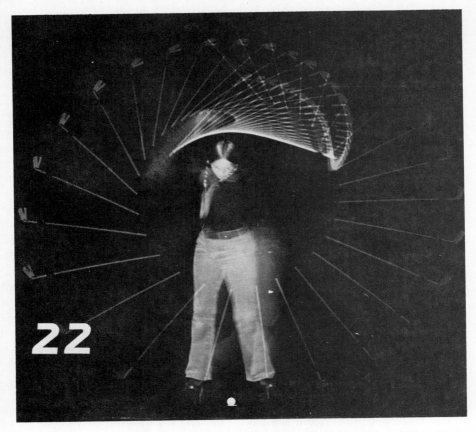

Fig. 15-10. Strobe picture of woman's golf swing, showing use of No. 5 iron. This action was photographed in frontal plane from top of downswing through follow-through. As downswing commenced, images of club were close together and then farther apart, indicating increase in velocity. (Courtesy Jan Sanner Merriman.)

second and that from the start of the downswing to impact to be 0.23 second. The downswing was more than two and one-half times as fast as the backswing. (See Fig. 15-10).

A study by one of us (J.M.C.) of the kinematic and kinetic aspects of the golf swing revealed the following:

1. The line of gravity was midway between the two feet at the beginning of the downswing.

This means that the force for each foot was the same.

2. The weight shift was such that 75% occurred on the front foot and 25% on the rear at impact (mean shift).

3. After impact there was a continued shift of some weight toward the front foot with most clubs, the greatest being with the high-lofted club and the least with the driver.

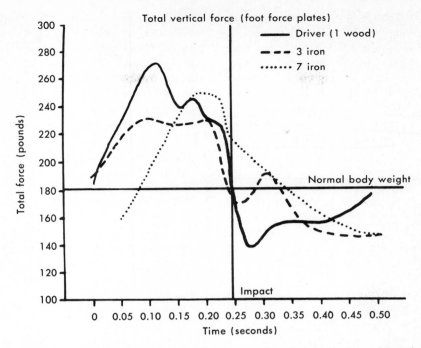

Fig. 15-11. Total vertical force during golf swing, measured by foot force plates. Note that body weight varies from approximately 1221.06 N (275 lb) (drives) during downswing to 621.3 N (140 lb) just after impact. During follow-through, golfer shifts body weight forward unusually far while using No. 7 iron.

4. After the impact position was reached, the performers using the highest-numbered club had a force distribution between the feet of a little more than 75% on the front and nearly 50% front and rear with the driver.

5. There was some change in the force distribution at the end of the follow-through, in that the shift was almost up to 80% on the front foot with the high-lofted club and nearly 70% with the driver.

6. The total vertical force exerted from the downswing to just at or before impact was from 133% of body weight (for the high weight) with the high-lofted club to 150% with the driver.

7. The total vertical force decreased with all clubs as impact occurred.

8. The total force exerted in the vertical direction was reduced to 80% of the total body weight, indicating that the centrifugal force of the club had pulled the body upward (Fig. 15-11).

Film measures of the swings of an average golfer, a college woman, found the average swing time with a No. 5 iron to be 1.41 seconds and with a No. 9 iron to be 1.34 seconds. The downswings were three times as fast as the backswings. Drives from the tee made by two highly skilled women golfers as they participated in a tournament were measured with a stopwatch and were found to average 0.64 (Berg) and 0.85 (Suggs) second. The swing of a highly skilled college man, measured on film, took 0.77 second; the downswing was twice as fast as the backswing. Films of Bobby

Jones showed that the backswing was completed in 70 frames and the downswing in 30 frames. His downswing was two and one-third times faster than his backswing.

KICKING

The kicking action is a striking pattern, used to apply force with the foot. It is a variation of running and thus is a modification of the walking pattern. The kick differs from the walk and the run in that force is applied with the swinging limb rather than with the supporting one. In the final force-producing phase the primary action is knee extension. The lever and the resistance arm include the leg and the part of the foot between the ankle and the point of impact. The length of the moment arm is approximately the distance from the knee to the point of impact.

Although little or no hip action occurs in the final phase, this joint makes an important contribution in the earlier force-producing phase. As the thigh is swung forward by hip flexion, it carries the leg and foot with it. During this time the knee flexes—an action that moves the foot backward. Film tracings show that in spite of the knee action the foot moves forward during this phase. Thigh action in this pattern contributes to the forward movement; in bowling, this is similar to the contribution of the approach steps, which move the ball forward as the arm is swinging back. The leg, then, will have not only the velocity developed by knee extension but also that developed by hip flexion, even though the latter action does not occur at impact. Immediately after impact the hip again flexes and moves the entire limb speedily upward in the follow-through. Unless one has studied slow motion on film, the pause in hip action is not likely to be observed; hip action is often thought to be continuous.

Another valuable lever can be added to the kick by pelvic rotation, which can be acting at the time of impact. This lever is used most frequently by performers who have had training in soccer and is effective when the ball is approached diagonally. The lever and the resistance arm of this action include the pelvis, the thigh, the leg, and the part of the foot between the ankle and the point of impact. The length of the moment arm, which is perpendicular to the axis passing through the left hip (if the kick is made with the right foot) and to the line of force, will be approximately equal to the width of the pelvis.

Ankle action is used mainly to position the foot for the impact.

Punting in football. Studies of punting skills used in football have shown that the major contributor at the time of impact is the lever acting at the knee joint; the hip joint makes its major contribution before impact. The pattern is illustrated in Fig. 15-12, where from A to B the thigh can be seen to have flexed; from B to C the inclination of the thigh has changed little if any. After C the thigh flexes rapidly, carrying the entire limb forward and upward.

From 90 degrees of flexion in A the knee extends; it has contacted the ball before C. Film studies show that impact is likely to be made before the knee is fully extended; this and the rapid flexion at the hip after contact protect the knee joint. Rotation of the pelvis can be seen from A to C.

Observations have shown differences in hip action at the time of impact. Some performers have no hip action; some have slight flexion, and others have slight extension. These facts suggest that, at impact, hip action is an adjustment to the position of the ball relative to the supporting foot. If this is true, studies should be made to determine whether a particular exact position of the supporting foot relative to a stationary ball will result in greater velocity and accuracy. The drop of the ball with reference to the foot should also be studied. Whether the foot is contacting a stationary or a moving ball, the eyes should be focused on it. Therefore the performer approaching the ball should flex the head and upper spine (Fig. 15-12, A to D).

When a step or a run precedes the kick, forward movement of the body can contribute to the force of impact. The placement of the final step differs

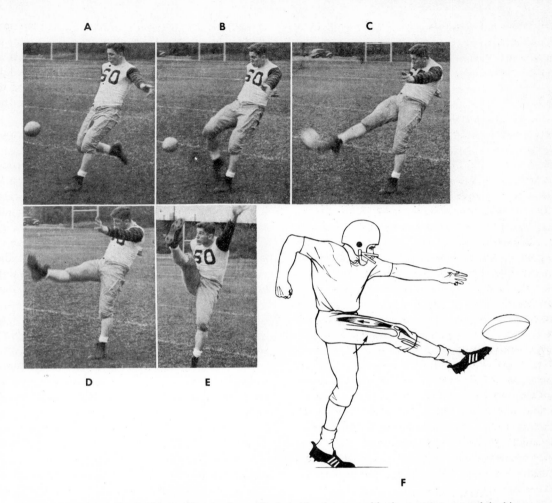

Fig. 15-12. A to **E**, Football punt. Note backward body inclination to enable the punter to extend the hip and knee. The head is held in one plane until contact. **F**, Drawing indicating body position and muscle action in punting. Note adjustment made for balance. (**A** to **E** courtesy Scholastic Coach.)

from that of the running step. In the latter the knee flexes just before the foot makes contact with the ground, so that the foot is brought more directly under the body's center of gravity; in the kick the foot is placed well ahead of the body's center of gravity (Fig. 15-12, *A*), so that the body can be carried forward by ankle flexion, thus adding its forward movement to the force. More important is the greater range of pelvic rotation that this foot placement permits.

Similarities in thigh and knee actions are reported by Glassow and Mortimer, who studied film of an untrained 9-year-old boy punting a ball and of a man, an experienced player, executing a placekick. The greatest degree of knee flexion was the same for the two performers, slightly more than 90 degrees; the rate of knee extension at impact was also the same, approximately 1280 degrees per second. The man, whose leg is longer, will have a longer moment arm for the lever acting at the knee and therefore greater linear velocity for this lever. Hip flexion, moving the thigh forward and slightly upward, occurred in both man and boy while the knee was flexing and continued, as the knee extended, until just before impact. Both performers extended the thigh a few degrees just before impact. This lowering has been observed in several studies; it does not add to the force of impact but is probably an adjustment to the ball position.

Much greater knee velocity for the kicks of three highly skilled Australian men is reported by Macmillian. The average velocity for each man was 1521.3, 1788.6, and 2008.7 degrees per second immediately before contact. During the same time the average foot velocity was 23.3 and 23.7 m/sec (76.5 and 77.9 ft/sec). The maximum ball velocities were faster than those of the impacting foot; they were 27.2 and 25.0 m/sec (89.2 and 82.0 ft/sec). This phenomenon was mentioned in the discussion of golf and tennis in connection with racket and ball velocity.

The velocity of the force as it strikes the ball, coupled with the angle of release, determines the distance attained. A high vertical velocity and a high angle (60 degrees) bring about a high-lofted kick. Conversely, a high horizontal velocity and a low angle (40 degrees) will cause the ball to traverse a longer distance. A high angle is used with the wind and a low angle against the wind.

The ball is spinning as it leaves the foot. The reason is that the leg and foot move internally toward the middle of the body on the follow-through. At contact the foot cuts across the underneath side of the ball, causing the spin. The ball is struck when it is off the ground just a few centimeters. The ball rides on the foot for a few centimeters.

Alexander and Holt found that before contact the superior punter's kicking foot had a linear velocity of 25.3 m/sec (83 ft/sec). The punters in his study struck the football with the kicking leg flexed at the hip (a maximum of 77 degrees). The ball was dropped so that it struck the foot at an angle of 25 degrees across the forepart of the foot

to produce the spinning action or spiral during its flight. The foot contacted the ball at approximately 38.1 cm (15 in) above the ground and rode on the foot for milliseconds. The more horizontal the drop, the more effective the punt.

Soccer kicking. Soccer kicking is primarily done as an instep striking action. The biarticular muscle action at the hip and knee consists of flexion and extension. The nonkicking foot is placed alongside the ball before the kicking leg is swung. Whittaker and Fabian studied the instep kick and recommended that the nonkicking foot be placed alongside the ball. Then the kicking leg should swing forward from the hip, and the knee should simultaneously bend so that the heel is well back. When the knee comes in line with the ball and the eye, the leg should straighten. The top of the instep or shoelaces should meet the ball, the toe being extended or pointed downward. The body should be over the ball. The power of the kick comes from the knee joint, not the hip, and is in almost direct relationship to the preparatory bend of the knee. The muscles of the leg should be relaxed until the kick is started; then the muscles act strongly until the ankle contacts the ball. The toe does not come into contact with the ball. A simple instep kick will have a backspin and will remain low in flight.

The instep gives the kicker the more stable kicking surface because the whole foot, rather than the toes, is the striking area. Plagenhoef has reported that the side-approach soccer kick produced greater ball velocity than did the straight-ahead approach. He found that the side-approach instep kick produced a ball velocity of 28.9 m/sec (95 ft/sec), whereas the velocity after straight approach with the instep and toe contact was 25 m/sec (82 ft/sec).

If the kicker wishes to have a low trajectory made by the struck ball, the nonkicking leg is placed opposite the side center of the ball. If the objective is to elevate the ball, the nonkicking leg is placed 10.16 to 15.2 cm (4 to 6 in) to the rear of the ball. The body leans backward so that the hip can be extended at contact. The velocity of the leg swing and that of the pelvic rotation culminates in a resultant of the magnitude and direction of all the applied forces. The kicked ball's path of flight is the result of the launch angle, the launch velocity, and the aerodynamics of the ball in flight. The angle of inclination of the striking foot and the major axis of the ball and boot also make a contribution.

Abo-Abdo found that the mean linear velocity of the soccer ball was 19.5 m/sec (63.85 ft/sec) and of the kicking ankle 17.6 m/sec (57.86 ft/sec). He supported the concept that the velocity of the ankle and foot depends on the velocity of the thigh and knee and the linear velocity of the body's center of gravity.

Abo-Abdo drew the following conclusions from his study:

1. From the initial leap through the follow-through, the head to trunk angle progressively increased the degree of forward flexion until the kicking foot began descending to the ground. Then the degree of forward flexion decreased. The trunk moved closer to the ball during the kicking action and was in back of the ball.

2. From the initial leap through the follow-through, the right thigh to trunk angle was first greater than 180 degrees (thigh was hyperextended behind the trunk) and then less than 180 degrees (thigh was flexed in front of the trunk) as the kicking leg moved forward in the kicking pattern. The forward motion of the kicking leg was started after the leap and before the nonkicking foot touched the ground.

3. As the right foot left the ground on the initial leap, the right thigh to fore leg angle began to decrease in size. This flexion continued until after the nonkicking foot had landed; then the fore leg began extending forward for foot contact with the ball and follow-through. As the kicking foot returned to the ground, the degree of flexion increased again.

4. At the time of contact with the ball, the position of the knee of the kicking leg and the focus of the eyes with respect to a vertical line through the center of the ball were as follows: (a) the knee of the kicking leg was in front of the center of the ball and (b) the eyes were focused on the back of the center of the ball.

5. From the initial leap through the follow-through, the fore leg to kicking foot angle was one of extension. The angle decreased at the time of contact with the ball, increased immediately after the ball left the foot, and decreased again at the highest point of the follow-through.

6. The placement of the nonkicking foot in relation to the center of the ball was alongside the ball. The nonkicking foot remained in approximately the same position throughout the kicking pattern. In the follow-through movement the heel of the nonkicking foot was not raised off the ground.

7. From the initial leap through the follow-through, the left thigh to fore leg angle progressively increased in the degree of flexion until, at the moment before contact, this angle started to extend from the position of the foot at contact until the highest point of the follow-through. Although the increase in flexion at the knee joint of the supporting leg appears to indicate that the center of gravity was lowered throughout the progression of kicking, the reverse was found to be true. The center of gravity was progressively raised throughout the kicking action and reached its highest point just before impact with the ball. This increase occurred because the body was raised by its rotation over the supporting leg, and the increased flexion at the knee joint of the supporting leg was not enough to lower the body's center of gravity before contact. Immediately after contact was made with the ball, the displacement of the center of gravity decreased during the movement from impact to follow-through. (See Figs. 15-13 and 15-14; Table 15-1.)

MINI LABORATORY EXERCISES

1. At a corner of a room, bounce a ball onto the floor so that it rebounds against a wall. Mark with tape or chalk the position of release of the ball, the site of landing on the floor, and the height of impact against the wall, using the second wall as discussed in Chapter 5. Connect the marks with sticks, chalk, string, or

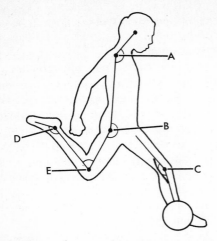

Fig. 15-13. Body angles in the soccer kick. Angles include *A*, head to trunk; *B*, right thigh to trunk; *C*, right foreleg to thigh; *D*, right foot to foreleg; *E*, left foreleg to thigh.

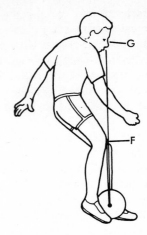

Fig. 15-14. Knee of the kicking leg and eye angles measured from a vertical line from the center of the ball at the time of contact with the ball in the soccer kick. Angles include *F*, knee of kicking leg to center of ball, and *G*, eyes to center of ball.

Table 15-1. Body angles of subject during three phases of soccer instep kick

Body angle*	R shoulder	R hip	R knee	R ankle	L knee
At placement of nonkicking foot	137	195	100	121	140
When kicking foot contacted ball	125	160	139	125	121
At highest point of follow-through	112	153	152	115	117

Adapted from Abo-Abdo, H.: A cinematographic analysis of the instep kick in soccer, unpublished report, Indiana University, 1979.
*Body angles are expressed in degrees.
R, right; L, left.

other materials and measure the angle of rebound and angle of incidence.
2. Varying the angle of bounce and the amount of spin to the ball, repeat the procedures given in step 1.
3. Compare your results and draw conclusions.

VOLLEYBALL SERVICE

All three basic patterns (underarm, overarm, and sidearm) of striking or projecting a ball can be used in executing the volleyball service. Although many players have been able to produce consider-able spin using the underarm and sidearm services, the overarm service is the most effective type of service if the objective is to cause the receiver to be at the greatest disadvantage. The greatest disadvantage occurs when the ball travels with the fastest possible speed, thereby forcing the receiver to respond in the shortest possible amount of time. However, some analysts may argue that a flat and fast serve is easier to handle than a floater, which causes directional difficulties. Since the height of the impacting of the ball by the server is greatest in the overarm service, this type of serve can be executed with the flattest trajectory. For example, a served ball traveling 13 m/sec will land near the opponent's baseline almost 20 m away if hit from a height of 2 m. The sidearm service, hit from approximately 1.3 m, must be projected at a greater angle and with a greater speed to land at the same spot. The angles and speed would be even greater for an underarm service because its probable height of impact is 1 m.

Based on the law of gravitation—that is, that all objects fall at the same rate—the overarm service will have the shortest air time and cause the receiver to make decisions and move more quickly than if the other two services were used. In addition, lever systems and muscles utilized during the overarm service have the potential to create the greatest horizontal speed. Thus the ball will be descending at a faster rate and a more horizontal angle, which is more difficult to receive, than in the sidearm and underarm services. For example, if the served ball is descending at a 30-degree angle, the arms of the receiver would need to be more vertical than horizontal. In terms of perception, this position is more difficult, and attenuation, by moving the arms in the same direction as the incoming ball, is also more difficult.

Since the underarm pattern essentially is a planar movement, players usually are able to achieve high levels of accuracy with this service. Persons with long arms can produce high speeds at the end of their lever, the hand. This speed can impart a high speed to the ball. The introduction of spin to the ball is another variable that must be considered by the receiver. Being unaware that the ball has spin will cause the receiver to be unsuccessful in achieving the correct angle of the arms to the ball.

The sidearm service offers a longer moment arm for the execution of a high-speed service. Since deviation is in the horizontal direction, accuracy is not usually achieved to the same level with this service as with the other two. In addition, placement of the ball to all areas of the court is not easily done without changing the body position

and thereby informing the opponent of the placement of the ball.

All three services can be executed with spin of some type and also without any spin. Since the volleyball is not perfectly symmetric with respect to weight, this latter type of flight will not maintain a parabolic curvature of flight or a predictable modification because of spin but will "wobble" or "float." The flight path depends on the ball's center of gravity, which may be to the right or left of the geometric center of the ball, and above or below it.

HANDBALL

Handball involves a type of striking motion and as such is similar to throwing. The movements are quite varied, depending on the shot desired at the moment. There are overhead, underhand, and sidearm motions. Most top players use a type of sidearm stroke in most situations. There is even a punch stroke to the ceiling. The wall and ceiling hits constitute still other variations. The following principles are especially emphasized in regard to handball strokes:

1. A nearly stationary head is maintained at the time of contact with the ball to avoid causing the path of the arm swing to change after it has been initiated.

2. The back leg is turned externally so that pelvic rotation takes place as the kill or pass shot is executed. This is especially necessary in sidearm strokes.

3. The point of contact is tangential to the motion of the arm and is therefore just medial to the inside of the front foot.

4. The motion is primarily elbow, wrist, and hand action, not a true shoulder swing.

5. The game as performed by top players is predicated on the execution of a successful serve. This is done with a sidearm motion that causes the ball to attain great velocity at a low angle of trajectory, 1.2 to 1.8 m (4 to 6 ft) above the floor. This angle keeps the opponent from having an easy return shot.

6. A great deal of pelvic rotation (hip rotation)

occurs during strokes made in returning a service.

FIELD HOCKEY

Field hockey is a game involving linear and angular motion. It also involves a change of direction while the player is running and striking with a weapon, a curved stick (Fig. 15-15). There are both men's and women's versions of the game. In the women's version an attempt has been made to prevent injury by prohibiting the player from elevating the head of the stick above the level of her shoulder.

In the linear running aspects of the game, the performers must learn to use the same mechanics as sprinters, with the exception that the hockey performers run under control, often at about 90% maximal speed. This control is necessary because it enables the player to change direction at a moment's notice.

The curved or angular running feature, which occurs frequently, involves moving the body's center of gravity laterally toward the inside portion of the curve and then accelerating after "setting" into the curve.

All these movements are made while the player is carrying a hockey stick. The additional weight of the stick, combined with its length and design, requires the player to have considerable skill in wielding the stick effectively. The ability to move the stick into a striking position while in a running stride is a feat that takes years to learn.

The striking aspects are identical with those mentioned previously in this chapter. The curved stick increases the length of the lever arm, raising the possibility that greater ball velocity can be developed than would be possible with a straight stick.

Skills that must be mastered for efficient and competent play include achieving maximal ball height and a low angle of trajectory, delivering a rolling ground ball, and receiving a ball coming at great velocity (Chapter 21).

Klatt studied the temporal and kinematic characteristics of the penalty corner shot, or hit-out, and found that the hit-out drive should be executed in approximately 1 second or less. She found that the optimal speed of the hit-out was probably 14.8 m/sec (48.65 ft/sec) (at 90% maximal speed). The hit-out involves high-velocity action, as long a traversed distance as possible, a short time interval, and a direction of the ball that will aid the receiver in returning the hit toward the mouth of the goal. Klatt used computer simulation to determine the following optimal actions by the defensive and offensive performers:

1. Develop a consistent speed and angle on the hit-out; the direction should be such that the ball is received directly in front of the goal mouth.
2. Have the receiver sprint into the circle to receive the ball, decreasing the time of the hit-out and increasing the angle open to the goal.
3. When the skill level is sufficient to merit use of the hand stop, utilize a hand stop to receive the hit-out.
4. Designate a "corner team" of three players; the corner team must practice independently of the whole team as well as with it.
5. Position the defensive team so that no one crosses the visual path of the goalkeeper on the defensive rush. Send two defensive players out on the shooter, one on the stick side and one on the non-stick side.
6. The goalkeeper should come out in direct line with the reception, moving out from the goal as far as possible to decrease the open angles.*

MINI LABORATORY EXERCISES

1. Use a softball on a batting tee and attempt to contact the ball at the center of percussion.
2. Observe several outstanding performers of the class as they demonstrate striking activities. Discuss their actions in class.
3. Construct two pendulums of varying weights and radii and have them collide with varying velocities. Discuss the results in class.

*Klatt, L.A.: Kinematic and temporal characteristics of a successful penalty corner in women's field hockey, doctoral dissertation, Indiana University, 1977.

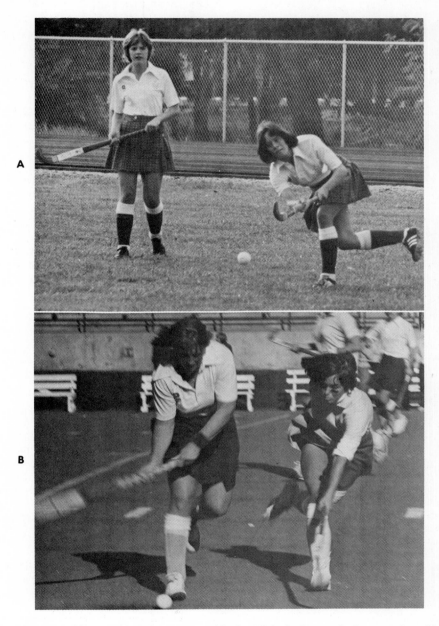

Fig. 15-15. Note the differences in balance and positioning of the body parts in the execution of **A**, the push pass, and **B**, the drive.

Continued.

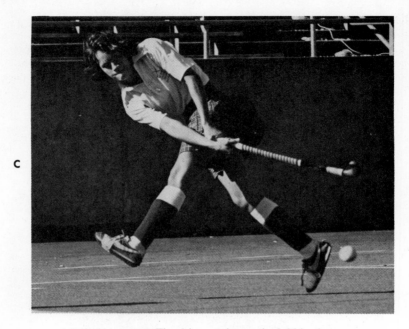

Fig. 15-5, cont'd. C, The drive on the run in field hockey.

REFERENCES

Abo-Abdo, H.: A cinematographic analysis of the instep kick in soccer, unpublished report, Indiana University, 1979.

Alexander, A., and Holt, L.E.: Punting: a cinema-computer analysis, Halifax, Nova Scotia, 1974, published by the authors.

Breen, J.L.: What makes a good hitter? JOHPER **38**:36, April, 1967.

Brennan, L.J.: A comparative analysis of the golf drive and seven iron shot with emphasis on pelvic and spinal rotation, thesis, University of Wisconsin, 1968.

Broer, M.R., and Houtz, S.J.: Patterns of muscular activity in selected sports skills, Springfield, Ill., 1967, Charles C Thomas, Publisher.

Cochran, A., and Stobbs, J.: The search for the perfect swing, Philadelphia, 1968, J.B. Lippincott Co.

Cooper, J.M.: Kinematic and kinetic analysis of the golf swing. In Nelson, R.C., and Morehouse, C.A., editors: Biomechanics IV, Baltimore, 1974, University Park Press.

Glassow, R.B., and Mortimer, E.M.: Soccer-speedball guide, Washington, D.C., 1966, American Association for Health, Physical Education, and Recreation.

Hubbard, A.W., and Seng, C.N.: Visual movements of batters, Res. Q. **25,** March, 1954.

Klatt, L.A.: Kinematic and temporal characteristics of a successful penalty corner in women's field hockey, doctoral dissertation, Indiana University, 1977.

Lopez, J.: Kinematic study of the badminton backhand, doctoral dissertation, Indiana University, 1979.

Macmillian M.B.: Unpublished material, Monash University, Victoria, Australia, 1970.

Plagenhoef, S.: Patterns of human motion: a cinematographic analysis, Englewood Cliffs, N.J., 1971, Prentice-Hall, Inc.

Richards, J.G., and Barlow, D.: Mechanical considerations in tennis racquet selection, paper presented at a convention of the American Association for Health, Physical Education, and Recreation, New Orleans, 1979.

Smith, S.L.: Comparison of selected kinematic and kinetic parameters associated with flat and slice serves of male intercollegiate tennis players, doctoral dissertation, Indiana University, 1979.

Whittaker, T., and Fabian, A.H.: Constructive football, London, 1950, Edward Arnold (Publishers), Ltd.

ADDITIONAL READINGS

Gowitzke, B.A.: Biomechanical principles applied to badminton stroke. In Terauds, J., editor: Science in racquet sports, Del Mar, Calif., 1979, Academic Publishers.

Gowitzke, B.A., and Waddell, D.B.: Technique of badminton stroke production. In Terauds, J., editor: Science in racquet sports, Del Mar, Calif., 1979, Academic Publishers.

Groppel, J.L., and Ward, T.: Coaching implications of the tennis one-handed and two-handed backhand drives. In Terauds, J., editor: Science in racquet sports, Del Mar, Calif., 1979, Academic Publishers.

CHAPTER 16

Gliding locomotion using devices

Although the term *skiing* originally meant to glide on snow by means of a pair of slender boards of wood known as skis, the definition has changed with the advent of water skis, single and double, and the dry land, cross-country, skateboard type of skis. In addition, one might consider surfboarding and skateboarding to be forms of skiing, since each resembles the single-ski technique of waterskiing. However, since both skateboarding and the dry land, cross-country type of skiing use a form of roller skate, there is a need for a clear delineation between skating and skiing. For ease in biomechanical analysis, one might place in two categories those forms of locomotion which utilize some type of device to produce a gliding motion: sliding friction devices and rolling friction devices. The latter category may be divided into (1) devices that roll as a result of a gliding of the body and (2) devices that roll because of the turning of pedals by the person. Examples of locomotion with sliding devices include downhill skiing, cross-country skiing, waterskiing, surfboarding, and ice-skating (including ice hockey). Examples of locomotion with rolling friction devices include roller skating, skateboarding, and dry land, cross-country skiing. Examples of rolling friction devices in which pedals are used include unicycles, bicycles, and tricycles.

Compared with other sports in America, skiing, skating, and cycling have not been thoroughly analyzed, but there has been some research. The water, snow, and ice media have not always proved to be convenient places for research. However, with the advent of controlled wave-making surfing areas, artificial snow, indoor ski hills, and indoor ice rinks, data collection on these media is not only easier but can be standardized. An increase in research concerning the biomechanics of winter sports and cycling has occurred because of the interest in understanding Olympic performance for the purpose of improving performance at various levels. For example, skiers have been filmed, force transducers have been attached to the skis, and electrodes for electromyographic recordings and electrogoniometers for angular displacement recordings have been attached to their bodies. Although the winter and summer skating, skiing, and cycling skills are not taught nationwide in the public school curriculum, they are important lifetime sports. They are unique in that gliding is not a common movement of humans. Because of this general unfamiliarity with these movement patterns by the majority of the population, the emphasis in this chapter will be on the application of biomechanical principles to the learning of these activities and to the role of the environment in successful performance.

CYCLING
Bicycling

Muscle forces. Movements of the legs during bicycling cause the pedals to move a gear that turns the wheels of the bicycle. The bicyclist varies the handlebar and seat-post (saddle post) positions to obtain the most effective position for force production and for decreased surface resistance of the trunk. These two effects are accomplished by adjusting the seat post so that it is equal to a near extension at the knee when the leg is in the "down position" (pedal at lowest point in the circle). A quantitative measure of this saddle height is 107% to 109% of the height of the symphysis pubis from the floor. The handlebars are placed in a position to enable the body to lean forward, placing the hip in flexion, which allows the use of the powerful gluteus maximus muscle during cycling. Research has shown that there is greater electrical activity in the hip extensors when the cyclist is in this low, crouching position, also known as the racing position, than when the cyclist is in the upright-trunk position. That the cyclist is able to exert more force in the racing position than in the upright position has also been substantiated by research in which strain gauges were utilized to measure the forces exerted on the pedals by the feet of the cyclist.

If the cyclist is not cycling in hilly terrain or is not attempting to achieve speed, the upright body position may be the preferred trunk posture. This might be especially true for older persons, persons with kyphosis, or persons who wish to isometrically contract the abdominal muscles while cycling, thereby improving strength in these muscles as a concomitant value. The upright position may also be advocated for persons who have excessive tension in the shoulder, neck, and upper back because of habitual work or sport postures. Conversely, the person with low back pain may prefer the flexed-trunk position to relieve stress to the lumbar region.

To increase the speed of cycling, competitors use toe clamps. These clamps help maintain the foot position on the pedal and allow the leg muscles to apply force during the upward movement of the pedal, as well as during the downward movement.

Thus it is evident that the muscle forces generated and required during cycling are dependent on many factors, and the kinesiologist must help the person attain efficiency in movement or speed or both. Fig. 16-1 depicts muscle forces used by a skilled recreational cyclist, as measured by electromyography.

Air resistance (drag). The amount of surface area encountered by the air can be decreased with a lowering of body position. The racing position decreases the frontal area exposed to the air, thus causing lowered frontal air resistance (drag). At least 20% greater drag exists in the upright position than in the racing position. In terms of power, the drag force multiplied by the velocity cubed is a reasonable estimation of the amount of power required for cycling. For example, if the velocity is 8 m/sec, the drag force in the upright position is 2 N, and the drag force in the racing position is 1.5 N, the power output needed to maintain this velocity would be 1024 Nm/sec in the upright position, compared with 768 Nm/sec in the racing position.

In team competitions the cyclists will travel

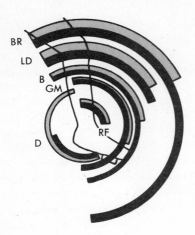

Fig. 16-1. Representation of muscle action during bicycling, based on electromyographic data. The solid arcs indicate high handlebar position, and the shaded arcs indicate low handlebar position. (*BR,* Brachioradialis; *LD,* latissimus dorsi; *B,* biceps brachii; *GM,* gluteus maximus; *RF,* rectus femoris; *D,* deltoids.)

closely behind each other so that only the lead cyclist encounters air resistance equal to the speed of cycling. The others travel in the "wake, or draft," of the others and may be thought of as traveling in a vacuum.

The bicycle. Since the circular sprocket design of the cycle is not efficient, but has two locations at which the cyclist has difficulty in maintain force and therefore momentum against the pedals, the beginning cyclist will have several problems. The feet will slip from the pedal, causing the pedals to stop and the cycle to decrease in speed. The result will be a problem in equilibrium if the cycle is one or two wheeled. The beginner must be taught to extend the leg through the down position, which is one of the two "problem spots." This action of one leg will help the other leg through the second site of inefficient force application. This site is the pedal-up position, at which spot the angles of the segments of the leg are such that leg extension is difficult to initiate.

The cycle environment itself, then, determines the level of efficiency of the cyclist, as well as the

adjustment the cyclist can make in body position as a result of saddle and handlebar positioning. The weight of the bicycle and the size and tread of the tires will determine how much effort is required to propel the cycle. The coefficient of friction between the tires, the supporting surface, and the weight of the cycle will determine how easily the cycle can be accelerated. Low friction and lightweight cycles are the goals for racing. At some point, however, and depending on the skill of the cyclist, lateral stability will become a consideration. If the cyclist has difficulty in balancing a bicycle, a wider-track tire may be required. The three-wheel cycle used for teaching children to ride cycles has also become popular with older persons who have problems in equilibrium or who wish to use the cycle as a vehicle to carry parcels. This type of vehicle is helpful for persons with neurologic problems or strength deficits or both.

As with walking and running, the speed of locomotion via cycles is influenced by the power capabilities and efficiency of the performer. Mechanical efficiency varies with speed. There is an optimal speed that will require minimal muscle force to keep the pedals rotating. This muscular force is assisted in the down phase by the weight of the leg. Speeds faster and slower than this optimal speed will require greater muscle force to propel the cycle. To allow for increased speed with minimal muscle force, a series of gear ratios have been built into bicycles. A change in gear ratio will cause the cyclist to pedal several revolutions while traversing only a short distance, thereby sacrificing movement efficiency for a gain in force efficiency. Using the tenth gear of a ten-speed bicycle increases the movement distance of pedaling to ten times that of the first gear to traverse the same distance on the ground. Thus improved efficiency for different types of terrain and different goals is possible with a ten-speed bicycle.

Unicycling

In unicycling the upright position is necessary for balance. Velocity is not as great a factor as with bicycling because unicycles are used primarily for stunts, changes of direction, and "cycle dances" rather than for competitive races.

SKATING

Although skating can be considered a form of stepping, its mechanics differ in several ways from those of walking. In ice-skating the differences are necessitated by two aspects of the situation: (1) the base of support is much smaller (the width of the skate blade compared to that of the shoe or foot) and (2) the supporting surface offers little resistance to a horizontal push (ice compared to ground or floor). In roller skating the base is wider, but the lack of friction between the rollers and the supporting surface affects the mechanics. Balance can be improved by using hip and knee flexion to lower the body's center of gravity; often the trunk is close to the horizontal plane. Since friction between skates and supporting surface is negligible, gravitational force cannot be used as a contributing factor in forward progress. The center of gravity must be kept over the supporting foot; it cannot be allowed to fall ahead. Otherwise, gravity encounters no resistance as it pushes backward, and balance is likely to be lost. In walking, running, and jumping there is resistance to the backward push, and the body can rotate about the motionless base.

In ice racing, while the skater is waiting at the starting line for the starting signal, one of two foot positions is commonly used. In one the skates are placed shoulder width apart, one ahead of the other and both at an angle of 40 degrees (more or less) with the starting line. In the other the front skate is pointed forward (at 90 degrees to the starting line), and the rear skate approaches a parallel with the starting line. Skaters who use the second position believe that it saves a fraction of a second in the start, since the foot need not be lifted and turned as the first step is taken.

At the starting signal the center of gravity is lowered by increasing knee and hip flexion; the weight is shifted to the rear foot so that the forward one can be lifted slightly for the first step. With this step the rear knee and hip extend. Here for a brief time the center of gravity falls ahead of the

supporting foot; this is possible because the angle of the skate resists the backward push of gravity and the extension of the rear hip and knee. This extension continues until the rear limb is straight and at an angle of about 45 degrees with the horizontal. After a short step the front foot has in the meantime been placed on the ice and angled, as was the rear foot. This type of stepping continues for three or four strides, each increasing in length over the previous one. During the beginning strides the arms move as they do in running, in opposition to the lower-limb movements.

After the starting strides the weight is carried over the front foot; now as the rear foot pushes, it does not affect the equilibrium. Here is seen the advantage of the low center of gravity; as the push from the ice is applied to the body, it is closer to the gravity plane than it would be if the body were erect. After the push, as the supporting foot glides, the rear foot is brought forward; as it passes the gliding foot, it takes the weight of the body. The push will have a sideward, as well as a backward, component. The former component should be minimized by placing the skate, as it takes the weight, in a forward direction and close to the other foot as it begins the glide.

After the starting strides the mechanics of action change somewhat with the length of the race. Filmstrips prepared in 1962 by Freisinger, 1964 Olympic team coach, show that in the 500-m race the trunk is slightly above the horizontal, whereas in the longer races it is horizontal. Also in the short-distance race, alternate flexion and extension of the spine are seen. At the end of the push one limb is well back of the gliding foot, and the trunk is fully extended; here trunk and limb balance each other over the supporting limb like two ends of a teeterboard. Marino investigated the factors that determine high acceleration rates obtained in the ice-skating start. Although their regression equation for the relationship between technique variables and acceleration showed a multiple correlation of only 0.78, the following factors were identified as forming the ideal skating start pattern: high stride rate, significant forward lean, low takeoff angle, and placement of the recovery foot directly under the body at the end of the single-support phase.

Roller skating

Although research does not exist concerning roller skating skills, the information given with respect to ice-skating can be used as a basic foundation for the analysis and improvement of roller skating skills. In fact, many of the principles described in this chapter are applicable to roller skating.

SKIING

Skiing is a form of locomotion within a relatively frictionless environment. In many ways, then, it is similar to roller skating, ice-skating, and water-skiing, in which the gear attached to the feet slides, or rolls, along the supporting surface. Therefore skiing becomes a sport in which it is paramount that the skier control the direction and magnitude of the sliding of the skis. This control (or regulation) of the slide is a matter of balance and steering.

The various mechanical and environmental considerations will be listed, and direct teaching applications will be described.

Effect of steepness of slope on movement. What is the optimal slope angle for executing skiing techniques? Is one slope best for all skill levels? Once again an understanding of the movement situation may be acquired by means of a free body diagram in which all the forces are identified. Before motion begins there are two major forces acting: body weight (gravity) and friction. Additionally there are the two forces that react to body weight and friction (termed reaction forces). Fig. 16-2 depicts these forces on zero slope (level ground). Notice that there is no propulsive force because gravity acts at right angles to the ground. Therefore the skier would have to exert an additional force—for example, pole plant and push—to initiate movement. Friction is equal to the coefficient of friction times the normal force. The normal force in this case of zero slope is equal to body weight.

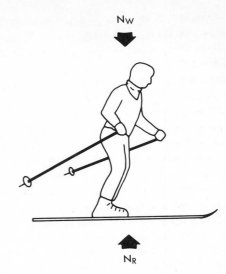

Fig. 16-2. Free body diagram depicting forces applied when slope is level and skier is stationary. (N_W, Normal force; N_R, normal reaction force.)

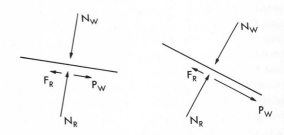

Fig. 16-3. Free body diagram representing magnitude and types of force acting on a skier under two different inclinations of the ski slope. (N_W, Normal force; F_R, friction force; F_W, propulsive force; N_R, reaction force.)

Definite alterations in force occur with the introduction of an incline, or slope (Fig. 16-3). As the slope increases, the normal force is now that component of the body weight which is perpendicular to the slope. Since the normal force decreases, the force of friction also decreases. Movement is therefore facilitated and will occur with less resistance or opposition than on a level surface. In addition, there is a component of body weight acting parallel to the slope. This component is termed the propulsive force because it causes the skier to be accelerated down the slope. This propulsive force increases in direct proportion to the increase in the slope. A skier, then, will have a speed of descent in direct relationship to the slope of the hill. The analysis of skiing is another example of the necessity for resolving one force vector into pertinent components, in this case with respect to the slope of the hill.

The optimal slope for skiing will vary with the individual and the techniques to be performed. There must be a propulsive force to cause motion, but this force must not be so great that the body accelerates so rapidly that the person panics or does not have time to react and execute desired techniques. A slope that is too low is less dangerous, although equally difficult in terms of performance, than a slope that is too steep.

Concomitantly one cannot disregard the type of snow and the surface of the skis. The interaction of these two materials produces a coefficient of friction that affects movement on a slope. An excellent treatise on this subject has been published as a result of the Winter Olympics in Sapporo, Japan, and the concern for maximizing the snow conditions for that event. The advent of indoor areas, artificial snow machines, and other advanced technology suggests that the near future will provide both the beginning and the competitive skier with ideal conditions for enhancing performance.

Too often the environment is ignored by the analyst of animal and human movement. Snow skiing, waterskiing, and surfboarding are excellent examples of activities in which the environment plays a dominant role in the success of the performer. Throughout this book an effort has been made to show the importance of the environment in mechanical and anatomic considerations. Truly the best performer is in harmony with the environment.

Balance. Persons are more stable on skis over packed snow than on shoes having the same type of surface as skis, since the base of support of skis is three to six times larger than that of shoes. This greater stability on skis is primarily in the postero-anterior direction, which is an asset when a skier is sliding down a steep slope. Keeping the skis apart, about hip width, will provide better lateral stability than placing the skis together. This wide position, called wide tracking, places the hips directly above the knees and the knees directly above the feet, thus ensuring that there will be equal weight on both skis and that the line of gravity of the skier will be midway between the skis when the skier is going down the fall line (line of slope that is the most direct). The weight of the body is distributed on the whole of both feet, the skis are flat, and the body is in a "natural position." This position (Fig. 16-2) places the center of gravity of the body lower than does the erect standing posture, thus increasing stability of the body. The term *natural position* means that the body segments are slightly flexed and thus able to respond easily to bumps and other changes in the terrain or to changes in the snow. This semiflexed position of the legs allows further flexion and also extension. The body faces squarely in the direction of travel, and it is in a state of differential relaxation; that is, only a minimal number of essential muscles are contracting, and these muscles are contracting minimally.

Turning on skis, walking on level ground, stepping around, and climbing the slope all necessitate transference of the line of gravity from between the skis to a position over one ski. The shift of body weight should involve as little modification as possible in the trunk, arm, or leg positions, since the shift is a lateral shift of the total body. Fundamental to being able to achieve skill in skiing is the ability to change the body weight line (line of gravity) from one ski to the other, and from one ski to both skis. The achievement of this ability, known as dynamic balance, can be fostered by placing the skier in situations that require combinations of single and double balance conditions. Thus dynamic balance may be practiced in such situations as stepping out (walking) at the end of a straight run (descent down the fall line), deliberately lifting one ski and then the other while in a straight run, and executing two steps to the side and back again during a straight run.

Steering. Steering refers to turning or changing direction of the slide of the skis. Since a turn requires greater movement of the tail of the ski than of the ski tip, the sliding action of a turn is also called skidding. Short skis, or the graduated ski length method (GLM), will provide greater success in learning the technique of skidding than will long skis. The reason is that longer skis will have the greater radius and greater arc of turn for the same angle of turn. There also is more time to commit errors, and greater centrifugal force is developed when long skis are used than when short skis are used.

Regardless of what length ski is used, the wedge, or V position, is recommended to facilitate turning. This position presets each ski at an angle to the fall line, thus creating a turning angle. Shifting the weight from the center of the V to one ski will cause the skier to execute a turn in the direction of the ski tip. A series of turns can be executed by alternately shifting body weight from a position above one ski to above the other ski. The speed and magnitude of the turn are dependent on the slope, snow, duration of single ski support, and edging, that is, tilting the ski so that one edge penetrates the snow while the other edge is elevated from the snow.

Edging and moments of force. When skis are in the traverse position (across the slope), they will tend to slide down the fall line if they are flat. The cause is the effect of gravity, which translates the skis as a unit. The speed of the slide will be directly related to the steepness of the slope and inversely related to the amount of friction between the ski and the snow. The friction is affected by such factors as the type and temperature of the snow and the type of wax used. In addition, the direction and speed of the slide can be regulated by the position of the line of gravity of the skier with respect to the ski length and to the amount of edging of the skis. If the skis are flat and the body weight is shifted forward, this places the line of gravity forward in relation to the balance point of the skis and creates

a moment of force, causing the tips to rotate downward. By the same reasoning, if the skis are flat and the skier leans backward, the tails will rotate downward. In both instances the results are caused by the creation of a moment of force. An analogy could be made to loading one end of a teeterboard with more weight than the other end. The weighted end rotates downward, and the lighter end goes upward.

The introduction of ski edging, however, creates a reactive force that can be greater than the moment of force produced by body weight. Thus edging the skis while leaning backward increases the friction on the tails, which prevents their rotation and causes the tips of the skis to rotate downward. Forward lean with ski edging causes the tails to rotate downward. Thus it is evident that the skilled skier has learned to create the precise moment of force required for a turn by regulating the amount of edging and shifting the line of gravity in the anteroposterior plane of the body.

Methods of initiating turns. The three major methods for initiating a turn, that is, shifting the weight and rotating the skis, are (1) rotation of body parts, (2) use of the external environment, and (3) unweighting. The anatomic, mechanical, and environmental considerations for each will be presented.

Rotation of body parts. Almost any body part can be used to initiate a turn. Rotations at the shoulder, spinal column, hip, knee, and ankle are executed in a direction counter to the turn and then in the direction of the desired turn. These actions are similar to the preparation, coiling, or backswing of many throwing movements. Each rotation can be forceful enough and can be in the correct direction. Knee steering (rotation at the knee) has two advantages over all the other rotations. The knee is at an equal distance between the center of gravity of the body and the ski. Thus the rotation at the knee is easy to control and does not displace the line of gravity excessively. Second, the knee is an important joint in the balance phases of walking. Therefore the use of the knee for locomotion is familiar. Likewise, rotation of the feet (heel thrust or foot steering) is an effective means of producing a turn because the feet are used in walking. Although closer to the ski than the knee, the foot has the disadvantage of being far from the center of gravity of the body. In addition, the range of motion is limited, as is the force. The heel thrust is used in deep powder snow and advanced turns and usually is combined with the method of unweighting.

Arm and trunk rotations, initiated by movements at the shoulder, hip, and spinal column, will cause the skis to turn if the action is forceful. This necessity for force, acceleration, and large motions is a source of "overturning" and loss of control. Usually the line of gravity is displaced a greater distance than necessary, thus causing the turn to be greater than 90 degrees and inhibiting the second turn or causing a straight run.

Use of external environment. A bump, or mogul, may be used to effectively initiate a turn. The ski tips or the area under the feet can be used as a pivot point as the terrain elevates tips, tails, or both from the snow. Change in body lean or the use of knee steering or heel thrusts can produce the pivot. Release of the edges of the skis may be the only action necessary to have an effective turn on a mogul.

The use of one or both poles may produce a turn. The friction between the ski and the snow may be decreased by transferring some of the body weight to the pole, or it may be eliminated altogether by transferring all of the body weight to two poles. The initial pole plant is nearly vertical but downhill from the position of the feet, so that the most effective reaction force can be attained.

Unweighting. There are two types of unweighting: up-unweighting and down-unweighting. Each has its use, although many beginning skiers find up-unweighting to be a more familiar or natural movement. In both cases the principle underlying the method is that the acceleration of the body mass can create a force that reduces the normal force, thus decreasing the reaction of the skis with the snow and decreasing the resistance to turning. If the acceleration is fast enough, the person can completely unweight, that is, have zero force between the snow and the skis, without leaving the ground. Acceleration of body mass is an outcome of rapid flexion or extension at the knee. The hips, trunk, and arms maintain their position and thus maintain the lateral position of the line of gravity. The unweighting method makes it possible to turn with the skis in the wide-tracking (parallel) position.

The up-unweighting technique consists of an acceleration of the body upward, which creates an overweighting followed by an unweighting when deceleration occurs as the legs reach the extended position (Fig. 16-4, *A*). The turn must be executed in the latter part of the upward movement of the body, when the friction is least. This fact, and the fact that, in general, upward movements are thought to be lifting, or unweighting, movements, probably are the reasons that beginners more easily learn to turn with this method than with the down-unweighting method.

The down-unweighting technique (Fig. 16-4, *B*) creates an unweighting in the initial part of the movement but an overweighting in the latter part of the movement. Therefore the turn must be executed in the early part of the downward movement. If the turn is attempted later, as in up-unweighting, the reaction force is greater than body weight and friction has increased proportionately, causing great difficulty and possibly producing no success in turning. Timing, or fast reaction time, is the key factor to success with this technique, since the down-unweighting technique utilizes gravity and has the potential for attaining greater acceleration than is possible with up-unweighting.

General concepts. Turns may be executed from the wedge, stem (one ski in partial wedge position), and parallel positions. The method of turn is dependent on the steepness of the slope, the type of snow, the radius of turn desired, and the speed of turn. Wedges and stems provide a slowing-down capability useful on steep slopes or difficult terrain. Edging, whether in parallel position or not, will reduce the skier's speed.

Human beings tend to be asymmetric; that is,

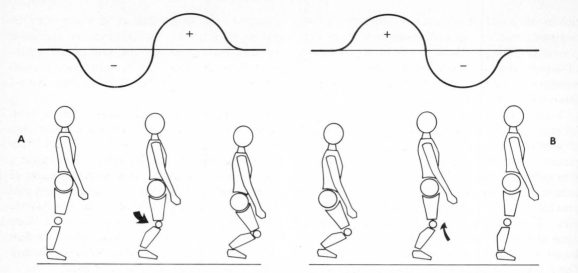

Fig. 16-4. Force-time histories obtained from force platform recording system. **A**, Negative and positive impulses during flexion at ankle, knee, and hip. In down-unweighting action, turn is initiated toward end of motion. **B**, Positive and negative impulses during extension at ankle, knee, and hip. Up-unweighting action initiates turn in snow skiing; illustration shows why turn must be executed early in motion.

they perform a turn more successfully in one direction than in the other. Leg dominance with respect to balance usually determines the preferred turning direction.

Turns are easier to perform when the skier is going fast and is close to the fall line. However, the acceleration rate and ultimate speed that can be tolerated by both the skier's leg muscles and the mind will determine the skier's need to check speed by stemming, edging, or deviating from the fall line. The larger the radius of rotation of the turn, the greater the speed and centrifugal force created—and therefore the more difficult it will be for the skier to remain in control of the turn. The major danger is that the skier will be unable to turn from the fall line to complete the turn started by a traverse. The reason is that centrifugal force causes the skier to "fly off at a tangent," that is, to continue in the tangential velocity at the midpoint of the turn, which is the fall line position (Fig. 16-5). Large-radius turns on steep slopes should not be

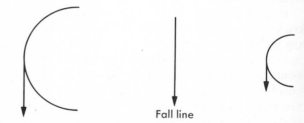

Fig. 16-5. Tangential velocity of skier for two radii of turns.

attempted by beginning skiers because they will not be able to adjust their speed appropriately and soon enough.

SURFBOARDING

Balance, or attaining a position or a series of positions of equilibrium on the surfboard, is the first skill in acquiring surfboarding expertise. Practice in still water and in a towing situation before beginning small-wave surfboarding will allow the person to realize similarities between the principles of equilibrium specified for walking, running, standing, and other land locomotion patterns and those utilized in surfboarding.

A low center of gravity produces greater equilibrium. A change in vertical position of the center of gravity should be made without horizontal displacement when moving from the kneeling position to the standing position. The line of gravity is kept near the midpoint of the base of support to provide the greatest distance for adjustments. The feet are positioned slightly more than hip width apart to provide control of the front and rear of the board without excess movement of the feet. The feet are set in a forward and backward stride position to provide control of the hydroplaning of the board. Lateral stability is achieved by a lateral spread of the feet approximately hip width apart. When riding the crest of a wave that elevates the surfboarder and the board, the surfboarder will lower the center of gravity by assuming a semi-squatting position.

Depending on the weight of the surfboarder and the length, width, weight, and design of the board, the position of the surfboarder will be forward or in back of an average position. This average position, the riding position, is closer to the rear of the board than to the front of the board. It is the position that allows the surfboarder to keep the "nose" of the board above water, which produces a hydroplaning effect comparable to that of the skis in powder snow. Any displacement of the tips of the skis or nose of the surfboard below the surface level causes the snow or water to act as additional drag and stops or decreases the motion of that part while the body and remainder of skis or board continue to move and are rotated upward. This action plunges the ski tips or board nose deeper and causes the person to capsize or fall.

Walking on the board is necessary as the velocity and height of the wave diminish. It is done to keep the correct degree of hydroplaning of the board. The board must be positioned to ride the wave and not be plunged under water with the leading edge (nose or side). Once the surfboard is positioned correctly, the surfboarder glides just as on snow skis. A turn is executed according to the basic principles of motion in a curved path.

The feet are placed with the rear foot at right angles to the line of the board, while the leading foot remains in the direction of the board. This stance resembles the fencing stance. To execute a turn, the person counterrotates toward the rear of the surfboard and then, using hip, knee, and foot steering as described in the section on snow skiing, rotates in the direction of the tip of the board. Once set, the surfboarder adjusts balance with body lean and rotation while maintaining contact with both feet, especially the ball of the rear foot.

Basic biomechanical principles may be more important to the surfboarder than to athletes on land, since the former must shift body weight in response to a moving environment that is also the base of support. The water and waves are a constantly changing medium that would be difficult to understand without formulating some general principles about motion and forces. The waves are not repetitive; each is different in height, direction, and place of occurrence. The surfboarder must "read" the waves and adjust the position of the surfboard by shifting the line of gravity right, left, forward, or backward, depending on the crest and direction of the wave with respect to the surfboard. In addition, the environment represents a four-surface frictional environment. The coefficient of friction between the feet and the surfboard and the coefficient of friction between the surfboard and the water may be two very different values. This difference, as well as the newness of the skill, often causes beginning surfboarders to experience muscle aches and "cramps" resulting from excessive tension in the muscles of the lower extremities, especially the feet.

SKATEBOARDING

Surfboarding and skateboarding appear to have several similarities, but there are also several ma-

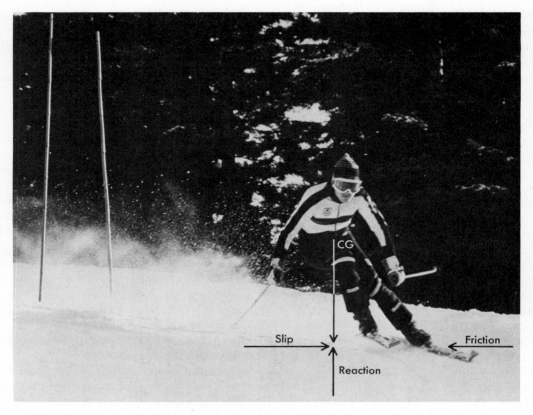

Fig. 16-6. Forces acting on skier during slalom turn. Frictional forces oppose slipping action of turn, and reaction of ground opposes weight of skier.

jor differences. The balancing techniques and shifting of weight front, back, right, and left are similar. When a performer is executing a turn, both activities utilize the same type of body position, the **C** shape. This position also is commonly used in snow skiing and waterskiing. The major differences between surfboarding and skateboarding are the greater speeds achieved by skateboarders and the static environment of the ground used for skateboarding. Speeds of 100 kmph have been recorded for skateboarding competitors. Such speeds allow a person to skate around the inside of a cylinder, becoming upside down during the midpoint of the loop. At such speeds the potential for

serious injury exists if the person loses control and falls. Elbow and knee pads, wrist and hand protection, and helmets are some of the devices necessary to the safety of skateboard competitors. Should the body weight shift quickly to one or two wheels, causing a proportionately greater friction on these wheels than on the other wheels, turns can occur. If the friction is too great, these wheels will be prevented from rotating and will "lock," thus causing the person to be catapulted from the skateboard at the velocity achieved before the wheels stopped. This is another instance in which the safety of the performer is dependent not only on performance but on equipment as well.

MINI LABORATORY EXERCISES

Using a bicycle, skis, skateboard, skates, or other gliding device, in an appropriate environment, perform the following:

1. Glide in a straight line and experiment with various body positions. Describe the balanced position of the body that appears to be best. State why.
2. a. Assume different amounts of lateral lean of the body when gliding in a curved path at three designated speeds: slow, moderate, and fast.
   b. Estimate the amount of lean possible for each of the speeds and discuss the basic principles involved in the determination of lean.
3. Take a small toy car or truck and attach a weight to the front.
   a. Push the weighted car down an incline.
   b. Describe the path of the car.
4. Repeat step 3, changing the weight from the front to (a) the rear, (b) the right, and (c) the left. Describe what happens to the path of the car for each situation and explain the reason or reasons.
5. Study Fig. 16-6 and explain the following:
   a. The forces acting on the skier
   b. The relationship of radius of the turn and the effect of these forces
   c. The magnitude of the displacement of the center of gravity outside the base of support with respect to speed and radius of turn

REFERENCES

Marino, G.W.: Kinematics of ice-skating at different velocities, Res. Q. **48**:93-97, 1977.

ADDITIONAL READINGS

Faria, I.E., and Cavanagh, P.R.: The physiology and biomechanics of cycling, New York, 1978, John Wiley & Sons, Inc.

Official American ski technique, Salt Lake City, 1966, Professional Ski Instructors of America, Inc.

Society of Ski Sciences: Scientific study of skiing in Japan, Tokyo, 1972, Hitachi, Ltd.

Terauds, J., and Gros, H.J., editors: Science in skiing, skating and hockey, Del Mar, Calif., 1979, Academic Publishers, Inc.

CHAPTER 17

Selected actions, concepts, and other forms of locomotion

This chapter discusses a number of movements and concepts not thought to be suitable for inclusion in other chapters. Many of the actions involve more than one motion; that is, they could not be classified as true jumping, running, throwing, and so on. In addition, it was thought appropriate to begin the discussion with children's early motor development in fundamental movements so that the reader can see how these movements relate to later adult patterns.

MOTOR DEVELOPMENT OF CHILDREN

Children's early motor development takes place in a sequential manner, from the reflex actions of the newborn to the more complex actions of the mature person.

The first actions of the fetus as well as of the newborn child are reflexive and are primitive and postural in nature. Their purpose is survival; that is, they are done for securing food (sucking) or for protection (attempt at righting from a falling action).

There are various ways to classify voluntary movement. Gallahue and colleagues list such movements as follows:

1. Rudimentary movements follow reflexes and, in the opinion of some, build on them. The reflexes begin 5 months before birth and continue for about 2 years.

2. Fundamental movements begin at 1 to 2 years of age and continue until 7 years of age. They involve walking, running, throwing, and jumping but are immature.

3. The complex sport skills begin at around age 7 to 10 years and are carried on into adulthood.

The reflexes are the first clues to later voluntary action. The stability patterns of creeping and crawling, followed by walking, and the manipulative patterns such as grasping, reaching, exploring, pulling, and twisting are the real basis for the later rudimentary and fundamental movements. The exact period for learning these skills varies considerably, but there is a range in age at which these movements are best learned. However, they are learned in an unvarying sequential manner, regardless of the age range.

Examples of the immature movements inherent in several actions include running, throwing, catching, kicking, and jumping.

Running. During the early learning period for running there is no observable flight phase, and the base of support is wide (the feet are spread apart; Fig. 17-1). The feet are rotated outwardly and laterally, and the stride is short. The center of gravity of the body is forward, and the action resembles tiptoeing rather than running. The arm swing is relatively rigid and is lateral and horizontal rather

Fig. 17-1. Child in running pattern. Note "tiptoe" style. There is no flight phase.

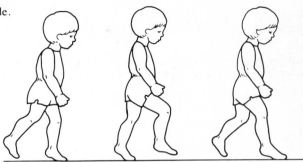

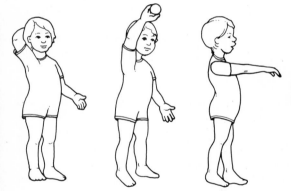

Fig. 17-2. Immature throwing pattern. There is no step with leg opposite from throwing arm.

than more vertical. As maturity is gained there is a definite flight phase with increased stride length and stride frequency. The support leg is more fully extended at takeoff, and the arms flex, extend, and move more vertically. (See also the discussion on mature running in Chapter 11.)

Throwing. In the early immature throwing action the movement at the elbow and part of the follow-through are similar to the mature action (Fig. 17-2). However, the center of motion is the elbow, with very little action elsewhere. The feet do not move, or at least there is no shifting of the feet into a step as the throw is executed. The axes at the

shoulder, opposite hip, and spine are lacking. The throw is accomplished from a fixed, almost rigid position. (See the discussion on mature throwing in Chapters 13 and 14.)

Catching. In the early stages of catching, the head remains stationary regardless of the angle and height of the incoming object (ball). The hands remain fixed and slightly flexed and are not adjusted to the height path of the ball. At the point of contact with the ball, the hands have very little "give"; the momentum is not attenuated. Mature individuals who catch in this manner are said to have "board hands." There is very little if any flexing at the knees to help absorb the shock of the ball's velocity. (See the discussion on mature catching in Chapter 21.)

Kicking. The young child initially makes very little movement of the upper body (arm and trunk) when kicking (Fig. 17-3). There is a very small amplitude of kicking of the leg in the backswing, and often there is very little or no follow-through. The arms are kept to the side for balance. The kicking leg contacts the ball while it is flexed. (See the discussion on mature kicking and striking patterns in Chapter 15.)

Jumping. The young child initially steps rather than jumps (Fig. 17-4). The pattern is a stride up or down as the situation dictates. Gradually the one- and two-foot takeoffs are learned. Frequently, in attempting to jump over a barrier, the young child merely jumps vertically rather than horizontally. The one-foot jump, after the step, is next in sequence, and then the two-foot takeoff is learned. A run and a step are combined in the leap. The ability to take off with one foot and land on two feet follows in the sequence. (See the discussion on mature jumping in Chapter 12.)

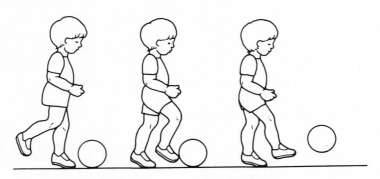

Fig. 17-3. Immature kicking pattern. Note small backswing of leg.

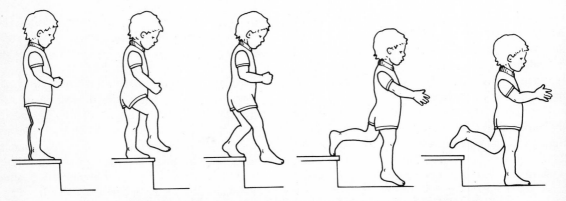

Fig. 17-4. Child jumping down is actually doing a step that is an immature jumping pattern.

DANCE

Dance involves types of movement that constitute a three-dimensional art form. Several factors play an important role in the performance of dance, namely, timing, rhythm, beat, and expression. These elements cause a dancer to have a different initial goal from that of a performer in a sport, artistic expression being an important consideration. Efficient movement is always given prominence, and fluidity and precision must be reckoned with in the execution of the actions.

The dancer is constantly shifting the body's center of gravity. This is not done at the expense of proper placement, which involves torso length and hip position. For example, the dancer often lifts one leg up and then brings it back to the original position without the disarrangement of the torso and head that usually accompanies the shifting of the center of gravity in one direction or another, depending on the objective. The dancer must know

and feel the location of the center of gravity as performance is accomplished. It might be said that the dancer executes a movement as would any sports performer but under artistic restrictions.

A brief analysis of one dance movement, the dance leap, is presented here.

Dance leap. In the leap the dancer strives for height or distance but also for an alignment of limbs that will give the illusion of floating in air even if in making these alignments the dancer sacrifices some height or distance. Fig. 17-5, *A,* shows the positions of segments of a skilled dancer at takeoff. The near arm is abducted to shoulder height toward the camera. As the body rises in flight, the front knee is extended, the rear limb is raised toward the back horizontal, and the arm is moved back to the position shown in the midair view (Fig. 17-5, *B*). This position is held during flight. It will be noted that when the dancer lands, the arms and rear limb have changed little; the

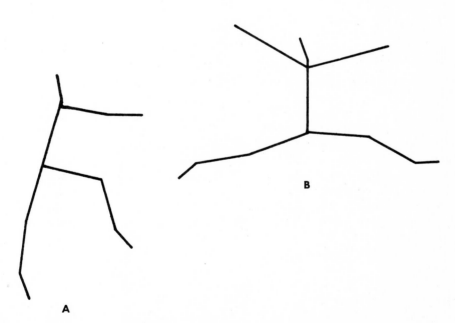

Fig. 17-5. Dance leap. **A,** Takeoff position. Center of gravity is well ahead of last contact point. **B,** Midair position. Horizontal alignment of limbs is held to give illusion of floating.

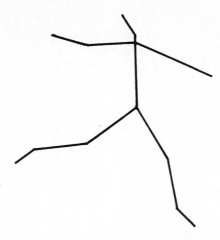

Fig. 17-6. Dance leap (landing position). Rear limb is still close to floating position shown in Fig. 17-5, *B*.

leading thigh and leg have been flexed to place the foot in contact position (Fig. 17-6).

LOCOMOTOR PATTERNS AND AGING

The stereotypic gait of the older person in American society consists of slow, short, shuffling strides in which there is decreased range of motion at all joints and a "slumping" of the head, shoulders, and upper trunk. That this pattern is not typical for ablebodied older persons has been shown by Murray in her extensive investigations of walking patterns of both ablebodied and physically impaired adults. Ablebodied males 60 to 65 years of age, for example, showed no differences in stance, stride width, swing, double-limb support, transverse or sagittal rotations of the pelvis, hips, knees, and ankles, or movements of the trunk when compared to younger men. Shorter steps (3.1 cm), shorter stride lengths, and increased out-toeing (2.7 degrees) were the only significant differences noted. Since this was a cross-sectional study rather than a longitudinal study, one cannot be sure that these differences were due to the age variable itself or to the sample within each age group.

Since individual differences in cadence, range, and speed of limb movements exist in every age group studied, the older person can be expected to be able to execute a walking pattern in the same manner as young and middle-aged persons. There are long striders and short striders, fast walkers and slow walkers, and persons with varying amounts of out-toeing and limb segment rotations among all age groups. Note the erect posture and "normal range and stride" of the 70-year-old woman depicted in Fig. 17-7.

If, however, parkinsonism or another pathological condition afflicts the older person, the gait pattern will be impaired. A "parkinsonism gait" can be described as one with short, unstable, shuffling strides, with the body flexed at the hips and throughout the spinal column. Another type of gait pattern seen among the older population afflicted with labyrinthine dysfunction is that of a widened lateral stance and lateral sway or lurching of the body during changing of the base of support. Persons with total hip replacement, however, appear to be able to establish a normal walking pattern, as noted by research conducted by Murray.

Investigations of vertical jumping patterns of older women who had not executed the pattern since high school years once again show no evidence of an age-related factor. The only difference

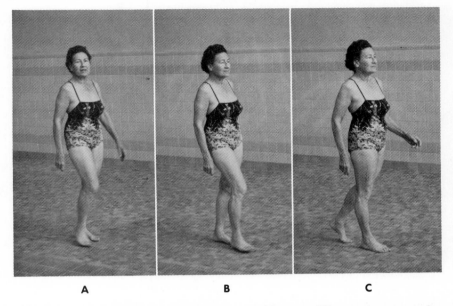

A   **B**   **C**

Fig. 17-7. Normal walking pattern of ablebodied 70-year-old woman. Note erect posture and normal opposition of arms and legs.

noted between data from college-age women and from an older population was in the lack of speed of extension of the leg at the knee joint. The sequencing of limb movements and the force-time histories were similar for both populations. The lack of extension speed may be due to aging, disuse, ratio of slow- to fast-twitch muscle fibers, or ratio of muscle cross section to body weight. More research is needed to better understand the capabilities of older persons.

GAIT PATTERNS OF PHYSICALLY IMPAIRED PERSONS

Locomotor patterns of physically impaired persons are unique to the type of impairment and to the general anatomic characteristics of all body parts. Modifications from normal locomotor patterns should be assessed from these perspectives, since adaptations in gait are made in response to a particular weakness or inability to move a particular body part. These adaptations are termed compensatory movements. Habitual execution of such compensatory movements enhances, by increase in muscle strength and development of neuronal patterning, the capabilities of physically impaired persons and establishes a locomotor pattern that is not easily changed.

The child shown in Fig. 17-8 is hemiplegic. Thus the movements of the right and left sides cannot be performed equally well or in the same fashion. The afflicted side will modify the "normal" side by the fact that its inability to perform will cause compensatory movements in the contralateral limbs. The trunk, also, will show compensatory movements to maintain dynamic equilibrium. Some of these compensations that "naturally" occur are beneficial, whereas others will interfere with attempts to achieve a gait pattern that is as nearly normal as possible. An assessment of capabilities, as well as limitations, in strength and range of motion must be made. Next, one must determine whether or not the limitations are permanent or can be changed. The movement analyst will then be able to determine the changes that will

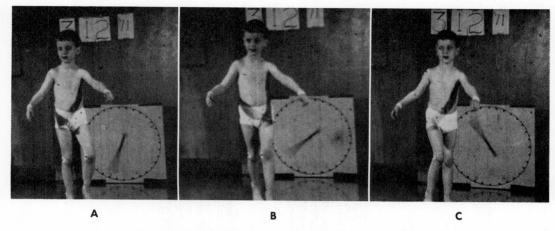

A   B   C

Fig. 17-8. Walking pattern of hemiplegic boy. (Actual film taken from testing situation.)

be beneficial and to predict the "biomechanically ideal" gait pattern for a given individual who is physically impaired.

Electrogoniometry has been used to identify normal and pathologic action at the joints of the limbs during walking, in both animals and human beings. A movement analyst can easily determine a decreased or increased range of motion, a change in angular velocity, and a difference in the timing of two or more joint motions in comparison with normal movements. Such records are useful not only in assessing locomotor patterns but in evaluating methods of treatment, such as exercise programs, surgery, and drugs.

MECHANICS OF PUSHING AND PULLING PATTERN

The pushing pattern is commonly used to project and to move objects while one keeps contact with them and the pulling pattern to move objects while one keeps contact with them. In the push and pull both hands are often used, and in some cases no joint action may occur in the upper limbs; in such cases these limbs serve as a connection between the body and the object, or they may not be used at all. For example, in a push the shoulder girdle may contact the object, and the force will be derived

from the action of the lower limbs. In general, one may say that in the preparatory phase of pushing the acting body segments are moved toward each other, and in the force-producing phase they are moved away from each other. In the pull the direction of the movements will be reversed in the two phases. For efficient action in both patterns the force developed by the body should be applied in a plane that is parallel to the desired direction of movement and that passes through the center of gravity of the object to be moved. Contact with the object will therefore be as close to that plane as possible.

Of the many patterns possible, only the push used to project an object will be described. This pattern is illustrated in Fig. 17-9, in which point *A* represents the shoulder joint and segment *AB* the upper arm, and point *B* represents the elbow joint and segment *BC* the forearm; the hand is not shown. In the preparatory position, *ABC*, the forearm has been drawn close to the upper arm; the shoulder is flexed 10 degrees and the elbow 170 degrees, bringing the distal end of the forearm to point *C*. To understand better the result of combined shoulder flexion and elbow extension, which will be used to develop projecting force, picture what would be the position of the distal end of the

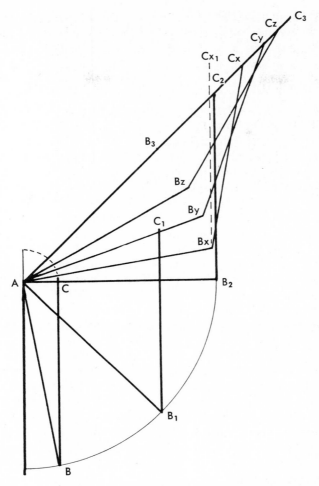

Fig. 17-9. Pushing pattern. AB, Upper arm; BC, forearm. As upper arm moves from B to B_2, equal angular velocity of forearm will move wrist through arc moving from B to B_1 to B_2. As upper arm moves from B_2 to B_3, angular movement of forearm must be twice as fast to move wrist along line C_2 to C_3.

forearm if either shoulder or elbow joint acted alone. If the shoulder were flexed 80 degrees and no elbow action took place, C would move along the small arc shown by the broken line and reach a position directly above A. The distal end of the forearm has moved a slight distance upward, which is the desired direction, but it has also moved a slight distance backward, which is an

undesired direction. Next, picture the position that C would reach if the elbow extended 80 degrees and no shoulder action occurred. The distal end of the forearm would be opposite the point B_1, and the forearm would be perpendicular to the line AB. Elbow extension moved C forward, a desired direction, but also downward, an undesired direction. When these joints act at the same time, the action in the undesired direction will be counter-balanced by the action of the other joint. After 80 degrees of movement in both joints, C will be at C_2, which is on the desired line of projection shown by the upper diagonal line AC_3.

After the first 80 degrees of movement, the upper arm has reached the horizontal (AB_2), and the forearm is perpendicular to the upper arm (B_2C_2). From this position, as both actions continue, the elbow must extend twice as fast as the shoulder flexes if C is to move along the desired line of flight (AC_3). This is shown in the illustration; from B_2 to Bx the shoulder has flexed 10 degrees, another 10 to By, another 10 to Bz, and 15 degrees from Bz to B_3. If the distal end of the forearm is to move along the line AC_3 during this time, the elbow must extend 20, 20, 20, and 30 degrees; the result of the combined actions is shown by Cx, Cy, and Cz. If the elbow had extended only 10 degrees from B_2 to Bx, the distal end of the forearm would be at point Cx_1. Surely one must marvel at the ability of the human mechanism to make the joint adjustments necessary to keep on the line of flight. One can be confident that the speed of joint action is not voluntarily controlled; only a mental picture of the line of flight is necessary, and the nervous system somehow produces the needed actions. This suggests the importance of developing in the performer a picture of the line of flight for a projection rather than a concentration on the target, which is the final goal of a projection.

The lever and its resistance arm, which is moved by shoulder joint action, will include the entire arm and hand to the center of gravity of the projectile; the lever moved by elbow joint action will be the same except for the upper arm. In projections the hand, which is not shown here, will be moved by wrist action; its lever and resistance arm will be the same as those for elbow action except for the fore-arm.

Determination of the contributions of shoulder and elbow action will be more complex in this action than in the underarm, overarm, and sidearm patterns. This is because of the undesired actions. At Cz each lever, moving diagonally, will have a vertical component—up for shoulder action and down for elbow action—and a horizontal component—backward for shoulder action and forward for elbow action. The moment arm for shoulder action will be almost twice the length of that for elbow action. Part of the force of each moment arm will be used in counteracting the force in the undesired direction of the other.

If the action is made with one arm, pelvic and spinal rotation can be added to the pattern; although the contributions of the pelvis and the spine will be similar to those described in Chapters 13 and 14, in the push the range of these actions is likely to be smaller than in other projection skills. In a two-arm push the trunk is often an additional lever, moving from a flexed position by extension at the hip. In both the one-arm and the two-arm push, extension of the lower limbs may add to the force developed.

In the following sections, specific patterns will be described. Obviously if opposing directions of movement, such as those described in the preceding paragraphs, occur, the force developed cannot equal that developed in other projection skills. Again, these specific patterns are not presented as best types of a general pattern; they are given to promote an understanding of mechanics.

MINI LABORATORY EXERCISES

1. Each class member should demonstrate both immature and mature patterns of movement in running, jumping, and throwing. Show where some of these movements might of necessity be used in gamelike situations.
2. Visit a dance class or performance and list the movement principles utilized.
3. Write a short paper on the differences between long jumping and triple jumping.
4. Calculate similar problems regarding projectiles, as listed in the body of this chapter.

REFERENCES

Gallahue, D.L.: Understanding motor development in children, New York, John Wiley & Sons, Inc. (In press.)

Gallahue, D.L., Werner, P.H., and Luedke, G.C.: A conceptual approach to moving and learning, New York, 1975, John Wiley & Sons, Inc.

Murray, M.P.: Gait as a total pattern of movement, Am. J. Phys. Med. **46:**290, 1967.

Murray, M.P., Drought, A.B., and Korg, R.C.: Walking patterns of normal men, J. Bone Joint Surg. **46A:**335, 1964.

ADDITIONAL READINGS

Broer, M.R., and Zernicke, R.F.: Efficiency of human movement, Philadelphia, 1979, W.B. Saunders Co.

MacGraw, R., and Foort, J.: Multi-joint electrogoniometric assessment of patients receiving knee implants, NHW Project 610-1128-Y, final report, Vancouver, B.C., 1979, Division of Orthopaedics, University of British Columbia.

McClenaghan, B.A., and Gallahue, D.L.: Fundamental movement: a developmental and remedial approach, Philadelphia, 1978, W.B. Saunders Co.

Wickstrom, R.L.: Fundamental motor patterns, ed. 2, Philadelphia, 1977, Lea & Febiger.

CHAPTER 18

Aquatic activities

Previous chapters have shown that movement of human beings and animals on land is made possible by the relatively rigid surfaces on which the living body exerts a force and by the coefficient of friction between the surfaces. This frictional element produces a resistance to movement. Friction is a result of the normal force's causing an equal and opposite reactive force, which results in deformation of the land surface. The air constitutes a nonrigid substance that normally produces a negligible resistance to movement of the body parts. Forces exerted by the human or animal against the air are virtually ineffective. The air moves away from the body part; it does not become deformed or compressed. The medium of water constitutes an environment that is less rigid (less compressible) than land, be it grass, asphalt, wood, or sand, but is more rigid (more compressible) than air. As with land surfaces and air at different altitudes and temperatures, not all water is alike. For example, saltwater, cold water, hot water, oil-saturated lake water, fast-flowing river water, and choppy, windswept water all change the aquatic environment slightly for the person attempting to use the water medium. These uses of a physical nature can be grouped into floating activities, therapeutic exercises, swimming, surfboarding, and all types of small-craft activities.

RELATIONSHIPS OF BODY AND WATER WEIGHTS

If the human body, either stationary or moving, is supported by water, the mechanical problems that it encounters differ from those encountered when it is supported by a more rigid surface and also when it is surrounded by air. When the body is supported by the ground or a floor, those surfaces are usually more than strong enough to resist the weight of the body and any additional force applied by moving body segments. When the supporting surface is water, this surface is unable to support the body; it gives way, and the body sinks, wholly or partially. It will sink until the weight of the displaced water equals the weight of the body. If the displaced water equals the weight of the body before the latter is completely immersed, the body will float. The first recognition of this weight relationship is attributed to Archimedes (287-212 B.C.), who said, "A body immersed in a fluid is buoyed up by a force equal to the weight of the displaced fluid." This concept is known as Archimedes' principle.

The weight of a body compared to that of an equal amount of water is known as the *specific gravity* of the body:

$$\text{Specific gravity} = \frac{\text{Weight of body}}{\text{Weight of equal amount of water}}$$

Human bodies differ in specifix gravity; those with greater proportions of bone and muscle will be heavier. However, all are close to a specific gravity of 1, some being slightly less than 1 and some slightly more.

The specific gravity of a given body can be determined by various methods. If the body is a regular geometric solid, its dimensions can be measured and its volume calculated. If the volume is known, the body weight can be compared to the weight of an equal volume of water.

If the body is irregular in shape, it can be submerged to determine the weight of the water that it displaces. If the body sinks, its weight can be determined while the body is completely submerged. The loss of weight when it is submerged is the weight of the displaced water.

$$\text{Specific gravity} = \frac{\text{Body weight}}{\text{Loss of weight in water}}$$

If the body does not sink or does not sink readily, additional weight may be attached to it to ensure complete submersion. The submerged weight of the attached mass should be determined. The loss of body weight in the water will be the total weight of the submerged body and attached mass minus the weight of the mass under water. The formula just given for bodies that sink readily can be applied to determine specific gravity.

In measuring 27 college women Rork and Hellebrandt found that after full inspiration the mean specific gravity was 0.9812, ranging from 0.9635 to 1.0614; when the lungs were deflated, the average was 1.0177. Only 5 subjects had a specific gravity of less than 1 on full expiration. According to these authors, their findings compare favorably with those reported by previous investigators. It is to be expected that in general the specific gravity of women will be less than that of men, and that of children will be less than that of adults, especially at ages when the trunk is a greater proportion of the total body mass.

Since the specific gravity of most nonpowered small craft (rowboats, canoes, kayaks, sailboats) is less than 1, these objects will float upright or when capsized. Because of the relative size of these objects, the volume of water displaced is high compared to their weights. Some small craft have air chambers, or float spaces, to provide or enhance their floating ability.

FLOATING POSITION IN WATER

Persons whose specific gravity is less than 1 will float with some part of the body above the surface of the water. The position of the body as it floats will depend on the relationship of the center of gravity of the body to the center of weight of the displaced water. In most individuals the lower limbs will sink because they are heavier than the water that they displace. However, the chest, which displaces water weighing more than this portion of the body, will float. The lungs assist in flotation by causing a balloonlike effect. The center of weight of the water displaced by the total body will therefore be nearer the head than is the center of gravity of the body. As the lower limbs sink, the spine will be arched, and the center of gravity will move toward a vertical line passing through the center of weight of the displaced water. When these two centers are in the same vertical line, the downward rotation of the lower limbs will cease.

Since in the adult the center of gravity is farther from the head than is the center of weight of the water, any changes in relative position of body segments that move the center of gravity closer to the head will bring the centers closer together. Raising the arms overhead in line with the trunk would do so, as would flexing the knees. For floating, the head, as well as all other body segments, should be resting in the water. The center of buoyancy of a body is also a factor in flotation.

Since muscle is heavier than fat, clearly a heavily muscled person will sink lower in the water than will a fatter person of the same size. This difference in body composition determines the extent of immersion in the water.

Knowledge of the relative position of the center

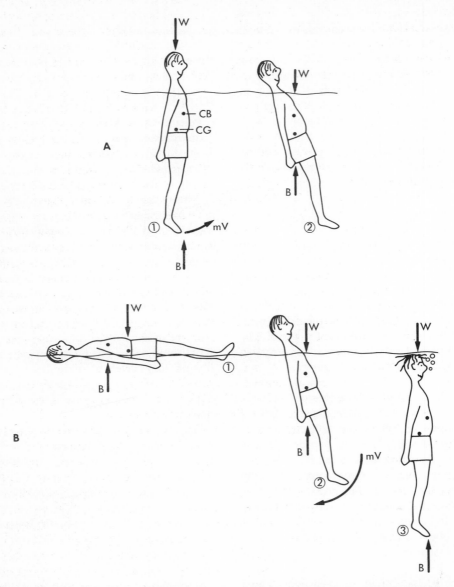

Fig. 18-1. Floating positions in relation to positions of center of gravity *(CG)* and center of bouyancy *(CB).* **A,** Buoyancy force *(B)* and weight force *(W)* create momentum *(mV)* to lift body to floating position. **B,** Momentum now submerges body.

of buoyancy in the body is helpful in teaching persons to float (Fig. 18-1). Since most persons float other than in a horizontal position, the legs and hips will descend into the water when a prone or supine floating position is assumed. Moreover, the descent of these body parts produces a rotation about the center of buoyancy, as well as a downward movement. Consequently the momentum created will cause the head of the individual to submerge, and any hopes of floating are soon dissipated.

A reverse momentum, creating a pleasant feeling rather than fear, occurs when a person begins the floating experience from a vertical position. The bouyancy force causes the legs to rise toward the horizontal position until the position of equilibrium occurs. Since the body motion is opposite the direction of gravity, the movement will stop at the point of equilibrium. This is not the case for the body descending from a horizontal position toward the diagonal floating position.

With respect to synchronized swimming, including stunts, the performer who floats horizontally has the advantage with respect to efficiency over the person who floats at a diagonal. Few or no sculling movements would be required to maintain the floating position. An action such as raising one leg above water, as in the ballet leg stunt in which the leg is perpendicular and completely above the water, requires a force only equal to the weight of the leg. The person who does not float horizontally is already using muscle effort to maintain the body position at the surface of the water. Additional force will be required to support the leg out of the water. Likewise, all the slow, propulsive strokes displaying exaggerated arm movements above the water level are more easily performed by the floaters.

FORCES ACTING DURING LOCOMOTION IN WATER

Resisting forces. As the body moves through water, its progress is resisted by this medium. Karpovich states that, as investigations on plane and ship models have shown, this resistance consists mainly of three factors: skin resistance, eddy resistance, and wave-making, or frontal, resistance. The opposing force of frontal resistance is the greatest of these. In addition, it has been found that a looser-fitting suit offers more resistance than does a tighter-fitting suit. In observing the drag, Karpovich found less resistance in the prone position than in gliding on the back. This finding has been disputed by some. Counsilman found that the prone position offers less resistance than does the side position and that, if the body is rolled by an external force, the resistance increases and is still greater with a self-rolling position. However, all top swimmers utilizing either of the crawl strokes roll their bodies to some extent. There evidently are advantages to the roll that are greater than those lost through resistance. Among them are the following: (1) The arm is closer to the line of the body rather than to the side, and consequently its pull is more effective; (2) the recovery of the arm is facilitated; and (3) the breathing position is improved. Because of the body roll, the legs often cross as the kick is executed. This allows the opposite arm and foot to work together. The feet kick "down and out" to counteract the effect of the one-arm recovery in a cycle.

Form, or frontal, resistance during swimming changes continuously as both the velocity and the body position change.

In observing the effect of the speed of the body on resistance, Alley found that when the body is in the prone position, resistance increases up to approximately 0.6 m/sec (2 ft/sec). At speeds between 0.6 and 1.5 m/sec (2 and 5 ft/sec), the lower limbs are lifted toward the body line. This action, of course, decreases the resistance. When the speed reaches 1.8 m/sec (6 ft/sec), a noticeable bow wave adds to the resistance. These observations were made while dragging the body through the water without changing limb positions. Resistance values during these towing conditions ranged from 1.0 N to 2.5 N at approximately 1 m/sec.

During the glide phase of swimming the resistance is termed passive and remains relatively constant. Active resistance, however, occurs during the remainder of the swimming cycle and varies as the position of the body changes with an application of force by the swimmer. Rennie and associates measured active resistance as 2.3 to 5.0 N at 0.9 m/sec for women swimmers. Thus twice as much resistance may be expected during the act of swimming than during gliding.

One of the more commonly investigated cross-sectional characteristics (and therefore an indirect measurement of form resistance) is the breast-stroke kick and its variations. For example, differences in the spread of the feet vary from about 30 cm in the preparation phase of the whip kick to 180 cm in the preparation phase of the breaststroke kick. The frontal area changes almost fourfold between glide and preparation in the latter kick. In addition, the duration of the preparation phase is longer for the breaststroke kick than for the whip kick (Fig. 18-3).

Alteveer recorded the minute changes in speed during swimming and found that the sidestroke, elementary backstroke, and breaststroke showed a loss in speed of greater than 50% during the recovery phase. This loss was attributed to the increase in frontal area during that phase. The crawl strokes and dolphin stroke showed less than 15% reduction.

Since active drag is one and one-half to two times that of passive drag, researchers have attempted to determine the effect of anthropometric characteristics on active drag. None of the correlations were greater than 0.46, an indication that anthropometric characteristics are not the primary factor in the production of active drag, but that swimming technique is more important.

Many practices have been utilized by swimmers and coaches to reduce frictional (surface) resistance, including shaving the body, oiling the body, and changing the material of the swimsuit. An exceptionally hairy man was able to reduce towing resistance by no more than 1% after having shaved. Woolen suits have been discarded because of their absorption of water and the consequent increase of resistance. Nylon and other artificial fibers have provided suits that prevent water absorption, but there are no other measurable differences among styles or materials.

Tethered swimming, swimming in a water treadmill, and swimming with hand paddles or other resistance devices all have been utilized by coaches to increase the work required of the swimmer. Since force characteristics change in these situations compared with free swimming, one may assume that the mechanical characteristics of the stroke itself may change. For example, when the swimmer is tethered, the water is churned up, and the same water is being engaged with each stroke, causing turbulence. This turbulence causes the water particles to move in a haphazard fashion, increasing the resistance but varying it in an unknown amount from one stroke to the next. Thus the application of force by the swimmer will not be the same for each stroke.

Nelson attached a resistance training device to the waist of women being towed in the prone position (Fig. 18-2). The average resistance during

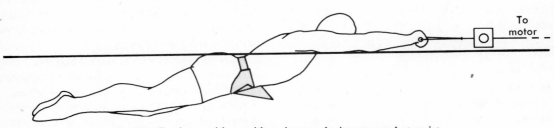

Fig. 18-2. Towing position, with resistance device strapped at waist.

towing with the device was 90% greater than during towing without the device, as recorded by strain gauges. One group of swimmers trained with the device and one group trained without the device. The following conclusions were drawn:

1. The resistance while a swimmer is wearing the device will vary among subjects because of the size of the sagittal-thorax area, which is the primary cause of turbulent flow into and around the device.
2. Wearing the device will drop the lower half of the body, thus causing a change in body orientation. This change could prevent the swimmer from practicing the specific movements of stroking needed to train effectively.
3. The evidence suggests that swimmers who continue to use the device believe that it is beneficial in spite of perceived problems with specificity of training.

Propelling forces. The aim of a good swimmer should be to push a larger amount of water a short distance because of Bernoulli's law, since water is a liquid and will move quickly away from the applied force. For this reason good swimmers are constantly pitching their hands to find "new" water and thus to apply a continual force against the water. This force is created by the velocity of the hand and by the path and pitch of the hand. Without the velocity, the forces will be small. It is an oversimplification to state that the water is pushed backward or that the hand searches for still water. Rather, one might state that the optimal combination of lift and drag forces (Chapter 5) is being sought by the movements of the arms, hands, legs, and feet. The hands and feet, which are at the end of the levers of the upper and lower limbs, should be oriented at angles that will provide the greatest push against the water. In arm strokes the hand position with reference to the arm can be changed as the arm moves, so that the hand is kept pushing with a sculling action, which helps the swimmer to apply a constant force against the water. Applications of the principles of lift and drag are seen in the sculling actions during treading of water, in performances of swimming stunts,

and in lifesaving courses. Lift forces have been identified recently in kicking as well as in the arm strokes of swiming. The eggbeater type of kick used in both synchronized swimming and in water polo is an example of such a kick.

The foot position with reference to the leg can also be varied, but this coordination is more difficult. A frequent observation is that many beginners, in executing the flutter kick without the arm stroke, will move backward instead of forward. The difference in direction of movement of the body in the water results from the position of the foot with reference to the leg. As Cureton has shown, the foot position can be such that it pushes backward on the downstroke as well as on the upstroke. As the hand and foot apply force, the resistance arm of the lever comprises the entire limb, and the fulcrum is at the shoulder or the hip joint. The distal segment, the foot in particular, can provide another lever, in this case acting at the ankle joint.

Because the hand can so readily be placed in a position to apply maximal force, it is to be expected that its contribution to forward movement will be greater than that of the foot. In fact, the feet exert little push in long-distance swimming. Karpovich found that in the crawl stroke good swimmers derived 70% of the push from the arms and 30% from the legs. Poor swimmers derived 77% from the arms. In the breaststroke, however, the legs are effective; it has been said that they contribute as much as 50% of the propelling force. In the crawl stroke the hand is more effective if the elbow is flexed. In this position the moment arm (distance between the shoulder and the hand) is shortened, and the shoulder muscles are more effective; in addition, the application of force is closer to the body and will have less sideward effect.

One of the more important factors in swimming performance is the continuous application of force by each of the segments in a sequence that will maintain the inertia of the moving body. Once the acceleration phase of swimming, much like that found in running, is terminated, the required muscle force is equal to the force necessary to overcome the types of resistance previously described. The dolphin and crawl strokes are best designed to propel the body efficiently, that is, with a minimal fluctuation of speed within a stroke cycle. From an anatomic point of view, the crawl strokes are more efficient than the other competitive strokes. Muscle effort to produce speed and power is more economical in terms of physiologic energy cost and mechanical power.

In a comparison between the arm stroke of the front crawl used alone and the leg stroke used alone, the arm stroke was found to be more efficient than the leg kick. There is a critical speed at which the arm stroke combined with the leg stroke is more efficient for crawl stroking than the arm stroke alone. This critical speed occurs at approximately 1 m/sec, which is slightly faster than the average competitive long-distance swimming speed. This is the reason that the leg kick of long-distance swimmers appears to be a balancing type of kick rather than a propulsive type of kick.

For the recreational swimmer the breaststroke and other gliding types of strokes may be used to increase long-term work efficiency at the sacrifice of power efficiency. For example, to initiate the next stroke, the recreational swimmer will prolong the glide phase and rest during this phase at the expense of reapplying force at near zero speed. As in walking, each individual can determine the optimal frequency of stroke execution for a given stroke used for long-term swimming without undue fatigue. Thus the recreational swimmer may be able to perform more work but will have decidedly less power.

The effectiveness of the whip kick in comparison to the wedge kick, or frog kick (or old-style breaststroke kick, as it has been termed), is unquestionable. Studies of the work and power used per stroke have shown that more force can be created in a shorter period of time when the whip kick rather than the wedge kick is used. Thus the efficiency as well as the effectiveness of the whip kick is superior to that of the wedge (Fig. 18-3). Several reasons can be listed for this superiority:

1. The preparation phase of the whip kick presents a smaller surface area, thus creating less form drag than the wedge kick.
2. The whip kick applies force in a relatively backward direction, whereas the wedge kick applies the majority of the force inward.
3. The stronger extensor muscles are utilized in

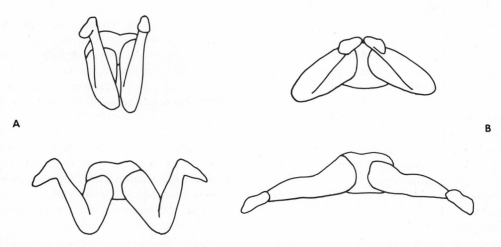

Fig. 18-3. **A,** Whip kick showing lesser drag. **B,** Breaststroke kick showing greater drag.

the propulsive phase of the whip kick, whereas the wedge kick depends primarily on the adductors.

Despite these mechanical attributes of the whip kick, concerns have been raised with respect to the possible risk of injury to the knee when the whip kick is executed. The force of the water acting on the lower leg (shank) produces a moment of force about the knee. Thus the equal and opposite reactive moment acts at the knee during the whip kick, but it acts at the less vulnerable hip during the wedge kick. If pain occurs in the knee during the whip kick, the swimmer should be advised to use another type of kick or to exercise the limb in such a way that all the muscles, tendons, and ligaments may be strengthened. Since the majority of daily living movements, as well as many sports, use sagittal plane movements, the knee of most humans is strong in the sagittal plane but not in the other two planes. Thus it is vulnerable to high-intensity twisting movements.

Scott attempted to isolate the factors necessary for proficiency in executing the whip kick. Numerous anatomic and physical characteristics were tested and correlated with performance. No single factor was found, nor was a cluster of factors shown to be a prerequisite to proficiency. She concluded that combinations of different factors may produce the same result, and that if a factor is desirable, more of that factor may not have any effect on performance.

Work and power are not easily measured during swimming, but swimming proficiency tests are common. These tests compare the frequency of stroke cycle with the distance traveled and the time for execution of the distance. Although the force is not known, the "power" improvement can be estimated with respect to a given individual, since a decrease in time of execution of the test indicates an improvement in power.

BASIC ANALYSIS OF SWIMMING STROKES

Those strokes which are anatomically feasible in the supine, prone, and side positions have been influenced, if not determined, by the anatomy of the body. The evolution of strokes as bilateral or alternating may be due to water conditions, purpose, and reflexes. For example, the crawl stroke resembles the reflex-based crawling pattern. The breaststroke is the best stroke for maneuvering in high waves such as are found in the ocean or a stormy lake. The dolphin stroke is an imitation of the propulsive movements of fish.

Refinement of strokes occurred as competitive swimmers desired to go faster, and lifesaving techniques were refined so that they would be more efficient. Synchronized swimmers developed hybrid strokes to produce certain aesthetic effects at the expense of maximal forward propulsion.

The purpose of all swimming strokes is to produce some propulsion so that the swimmer moves through the water. Propulsion can be accomplished by creating two forces, lift and drag, by means of muscular contractions. Although some mention of lift force occurred earlier than 1971, it was not until the publication of Bernoulli's theorem as it applies to swimming, by Counsilman that swimmers and researchers began to give serious attention to this force. Previously, persons had been taught to "push the water backward" to be able to move forward. This concept was identified as the application of Newton's third law, and drag force was used to cause the propulsion. Investigations of Olympic-caliber swimmers in the 1960s and 1970s showed no single, direct push backward in any of the competitive strokes. All the strokes included what Barthels has called an insweep and a medial and lateral fixed handle, that is, flexion at the elbow and adduction-abduction at the shoulder caused the hand to remain in the same relative position with respect to the forward-backward direction but to move medially or laterally. This action creates a lift force, as well as a drag force, that causes the body to move forward with respect to the hand, much the same as a canoe moves forward in relation to the blade of the paddle.

Schleihauf has shown this insweep to occur in the breaststroke, backstroke, and butterfly stroke, as well as in the crawl stroke. The amount of lift and drag is altered by both the path and pitch of the

Frame

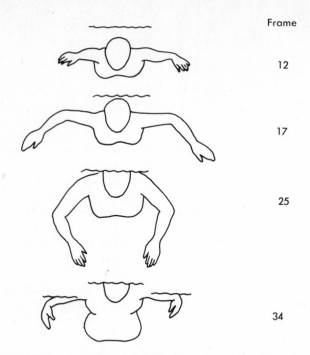

12

17

25

34

Fig. 18-4. Contourogram of arm stroke of dolphin butterfly stroke. (From Barthels, K.: Three-dimensional kinematic analysis of the hand and hip in the butterfly swimming stroke, doctoral dissertation, Washington State University, 1974.)

hand. Wood has shown that both these factors change as the swimmer tries to attain the most effective combination of lift and drag for each part of the underwater phase of each stroke. Barthels has shown that in the dolphin stroke the greatest body acceleration forward occurred during the insweep, at which time lift was the major contributor of the propulsion. Wood also calculated that the first part of the front crawl stroke had greater lift than drag in the production of a horizontal resultant. The second half of the stroke produced ten times the force forward, and the drag force was negligible at that time.

Researchers are applying the techniques of electromyography, electrogoniometry, dynamography, and cinematography separately and in combination, to better understand the role of lift

and drag in swimming. For example, Schleihauf noted three distinct hand patterns in the free style of world-class swimmers: (1) the classic sculling, more lift-dominated stroke, as used by Thomas, Spitz, Hall, Furniss, and Sintz; (2) the rapid-turnover, deep-pressing motion of Schwannhausser and Daum; and (3) the more drag-dominated stroke of Montgomery and Hershey, which had certain similarities to the classic style. The first style requires skillful manipulation of the pitch of the hand. Possibly a high-level kinesthesis is the governing factor for determination of its use. The second style relies on the latissimus dorsi muscle and a rapid turnover rather than on biceps-triceps action. Whether the strength and frequency of this stroke are inherent in the swimmers, or whether any swimmer can develop these factors, is not

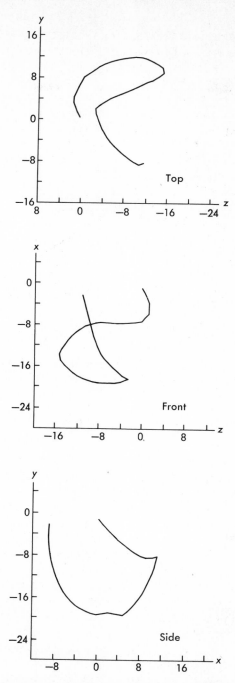

Fig. 18-5. Plots of path of hand during butterfly stroke. Front and side views were obtained from computerized analysis of movie film, whereas top view was extrapolated from two films. (Note *x, y,* and *z* axes.)

known. The last style might well be used because of the greater strength available than in the other two styles.

It is evident, then, that different styles occur, but one does not know cause and effect. Differences in morphology and acquisition of skilled use of a particular style may be dependent on many factors. Hand shapes and sizes influence types and amounts of forces generated by the hand, as well as influencing the amount of muscular force required at the elbow and shoulder to counteract these forces. The active drag during the different stages of the stroke and the various anthropometric measurements of the swimmer influence the nature and magnitude of both propulsive and resistive forces. Thus persons with large hands and feet produce large amounts of propulsive drag. If the musculature is sufficiently strong, or can be developed, to counteract the moment of force created by the drag on the hand, those persons with large hands and feet will be able to achieve greater velocity than persons with small hands and feet. Similarly, in fish with various sizes of fins and various breadths of the tail, size is related to ability. This is borne out by the fact that Scheuchenzuber found taller swimmers and swimmers with greater palmar area to be superior to those who were shorter and had smaller palmar areas.

PRINCIPLES OF PROPULSION

1. Continuous application of force by the hands produces the most effective and efficient stroke.
2. Body roll and shoulder elevation will increase the forward reach of the arm to increase the potential time and distance of force application.
3. A horizontal body position decreases the frontal resistance and therefore requires less muscle force to propel the body than if the body were in any other position.
4. During the recovery phases of arms and legs, the cross-sectional area of the limbs should be minimized with respect to frontal resistance so that the inertia of the moving body can be maintained.

5. The arm should continuously flex at the elbow until the shoulder is above the hand; then the arm should extend at the elbow. This action during propulsion utilizes strong shoulder muscles for application of force and reduces the moment of resistance.
6. The unilateral arm and leg movements should be near the midline of the body to prevent undesired rotations.

MINI LABORATORY EXERCISES

1. Experimentation with body and water weights and floating:
   a. Hold a diving brick or other heavy object and assume a back-float position.
   b. Adjust the position of the brick in the water and above the water; note the effect on the floating position or the sinking action.
2. Swim at a moderate pace, using a stroke of your choice. Assume a horizontal position on a table or bench and simulate the stroke. Can it be done? What are the noticeable differences? Observe others and discuss results.
3. Compare the swimming proficiency of three persons executing three different types of swimming strokes. Count the number of stroke cycles executed over a distance of 6 m (20 ft) and time the duration of this effort.

$$\text{Stroke proficiency} = \frac{6 \text{ m}}{\text{Number of strokes}}$$

$$\text{Stroke ``power''} = \frac{\text{Stroke proficiency}}{\text{Time}}$$

4. Measure drag force during towing. A spring scale can be used, or the devices reported in the literature can be constructed.

REFERENCES

Alley, L.E.: An analysis of water resistance and propulsion in swimming the crawl stroke, Res. Q. **23**:253, 1952.

Alteveer, M.: Minute changes in speed during execution of several strokes, master's thesis, Springfield College, 1976.

Barthels, K.: Re-evaluation of swimming movements based upon research. In Adrian, M., and Bramne, J., editors: Research: women in sport, vol. 3, Washington, D.C., 1976, American Association for Health, Physical Education, and Recreation.

Counsilman, J.E.: Forces in two types of crawl stroke, Res. Q. **26**:127-139, 1955.

Counsilman, J.E.: The application of Bernoulli's principle to human propulsion in water, Bloomington, n.d., Indiana University Publications.

Cureton, T.K.: Mechanics and kinesiology of the crawl flutter kick, Res. Q. **1**:87, 1930.

Karpovich, P.V.: Water resistance in swimming, Res. Q. **4**:21, 1933.

Nelson, L.J.: Drag and performance analysis of a resistance device in swimming, thesis, Washington State University, 1976.

Rennie, D.W., Pendergast, D.R., and DiPrampero, P.E.: Energetics of swimming in man. In Clarys, J.P., and Lewillie, L., editors: Swimming, vol. 2, Baltimore, 1975, University Park Press.

Rork, R., and Hellebrandt, F.A.: The floating ability of college women, Res. Q. **8**:19, 1937.

Scheuchenzuber, H.J., Jr.: Kinetic and kinematic characteristics in the performance of tethered and nontethered swimming of the front crawl arm stroke, doctoral dissertation, Indiana University, Aug., 1974.

Schliehauf, R.E.: A hydrodynamic analysis of swimming propulsion. In Terauds, J., and Bedingfield, E.W., editors: Swimming, vol. 3, Baltimore, 1979, University Park Press.

Scott, S.: Factors influencing whip-kick performance, thesis, Washington State University, 1969.

Wood, T.C.: A fluid dynamics analysis of the propulsive potential of the hand and forearm in swimming. In Terauds, J., and Bedingfield, E.W., editors: Swimming, vol. 3, Baltimore, 1979, University Park Press.

ADDITIONAL READINGS

Adrian, M.J., Singh, M., and Karpovich, P.M.: Energy cost of leg kick, armstroke, and whole crawl stroke, J. Appl. Physiol. **21**:1763-1766, 1966.

Clarys, J.P., and LeWillie, L.: Swimming. II. International Series on Sport Sciences, Baltimore, 1975, University Park Press.

Ringer, L.B., and Adrian, M.J.: An electrogoniometric study of the wrist and elbow in the crawl arm stroke, Res. Q. **40**:353, 1969.

CHAPTER 19

Airborne and arm-supported activities

Human beings are unique among terrestrial beings in their ability to execute complex stunts while airborne. Single, double, and triple somersaults, combined with twists of varying degrees, are performed primarily in the sports of Olympic gymnastics, tumbling, springboard and platform diving, acrobatics (including circus and ski acrobatics), and trampolining. These stunts can be initiated by applying force from a land surface, either by the feet or the hands, or from an arm-supported position involving swinging, mounting, and dismounting from gymnastics equipment. Success in the execution of these stunts is dependent on achieving adequate air time to complete the aerial stunts and on the ability to generate angular momentum and to regulate changes in angular velocity and changes in direction throughout the swinging and rotatory activities.

The planar arm-supported and aerial movements are relatively easy to analyze, as was noted in other airborne activities, but the activities that consist of movements in two or more planes are very difficult to analyze. These complex activities may be analyzed by separating each rotatory component and defining the basic mechanical principles and anatomic considerations involved in each component. The combination, however, must also be investigated, since a person who can perform one rotation

such as a twist, as well as another type of rotation such as a somersault, may not be able to perform a twisting somersault.

The head movement also will elicit a response from the body based on the tonic neck reflex. For example, an extension of the head, such as the act of "throwing the head backward" for initiation of a backward somersault, will elicit the tonic neck reflex, in which body parts respond reflexively to movement of the head as determined by tension in the muscles crossing the neck. Extension of the head causes both flexion of the legs and extension of the arms. These actions facilitate the backward somersault by decreasing the moment of inertia and the radius of rotation. This same reflex acts to flex the arms and extend the legs when the head is flexed. This time the reflex interferes with the execution of the movement pattern—the front somersault.

BASIC PRINCIPLES APPLIED TO AIRBORNE AND ARM-SUPPORTED ACTIVITIES

Some of the basic principles that can be applied to rotatory aerial stunts and arm-supported swinging activities are as follows:

1. Rotation can be produced only by an eccentric force; that is, the force must create a moment about the center of gravity of the

body and must not be directed through the center of gravity of the body.

2. The moment of force must be optimized. This requires that the person cope with the desired rotation and the speed of rotation without becoming disoriented.

3. Sufficient vertical height must be produced to facilitate the aerial skill. The required height can be mathematically calculated by using the equation of falling bodies:

$$s = \tfrac{1}{2}at^2$$

with t equal to rotary time of desired number of rotations.

4. While the person is airborne and during swinging, the principle of conservation of angular momentum will determine the speed of rotation with respect to changes in body position.

5. Movements while the performer is airborne will not change the flight of the center of gravity of the body, but they will create reaction forces within the body, causing movements of body segments that may or may not be desirable.

6. The time of execution of a movement will determine success or failure, or it may necessitate modification of the movement before it can be completed. For example, if the projection of the body is executed too early, the result will be insufficient height, greater horizontal velocity, and greater rotatory velocity than if the force for the body projection occurred at the biomechanically correct instant in time.

7. Movements of body parts, including hand positions, are easiest to perform at zero velocity during the swinging movements.

A twist requires a horizontal moment of force, whereas the somersault requires a vertical moment of force. Thus, when a person attempts to generate both moments of force, the result often is insufficient vertical force, since effort was required to produce the twist. Therefore the twist may occur, but the complete somersault might fail. In addition, the correct timing of each movement may be difficult to achieve. A simple one-rotation movement allows the person to concentrate on the time of initiation of that rotation. Initiating a second rotation approximately at the same instant as a rotation in another plane is a task of greater difficulty, although some persons have more difficulty than others. In addition, a movement requiring rotation in two planes changes the body's orientation in space compared with that of single rotation. Various reflex responses and possible disorientation may result.

REFLEX PATTERNS

Because the body is placed in upside-down positions and in other orientations to earth, and because the position of the head with respect to the trunk deviates from a straight line, many swinging, suspended, and airborne types of activities are often facilitated or inhibited by the labyrinthine righting reflexes and the tonic neck reflexes. The head will reflexively orient itself to the upright position in headstands, handstands, somersaults, cartwheels, and upward swings. This change in the position of the head for the purpose of righting the body often interferes with the maintenance of a stable support position, since the action of the head may move the line of gravity outside the base of support.

TRAMPOLINE AND DIVING SKILLS

Gaining height. Gaining height is essential in diving and trampoline skills to provide time for the desired movements of body segments while the body is airborne. The more complex the movements, the greater the height must be. Since the force of projection is derived mainly from the rebounding net or board, these surfaces must be depressed as much as possible when great height is desired. Depression is achieved by several means.

First, the performer approaches the net or board from a projection. In running dives this is the hurdle that precedes the final landing on the board. On the trampoline the performer uses repeated bounces. When the height of the bounce and the resulting depressions of the net were measured, the data shown in Table 19-1 were obtained from a film of a highly skilled performer.

These measures suggest that after a given height the resulting depression will be relatively less. The depression for any net will be affected by the tension in its springs.

Second, the center of gravity of the body should be directly over the feet as the contact is made, so that the direction of the landing force is kept directly downward.

Third, there is no "give" by the performer as the feet contact the net or board. Ordinarily the jar of landing is decreased by flexion of the ankles, knees, and hips. In dives and on the trampoline the depressing surface takes over the task of eliminating the jolt, and landing is made with full foot contact and with flexed ankles, knees, and hips held firmly as the feet land. The arms are extended downward and just back of the hips on landing. The relationship of these flexed positions should be such that the center of gravity is over the feet.

Fourth, as the surface depresses, the flexed joints extend, pushing the net or board downward, beyond the depth that it would reach were the landing the only force acting on it. On the trampoline the ankle reaches an angle of 90 degrees; the hips and knees extend to bring the legs, thighs, and trunk into a straight line. The arms, at the same time, are swung forward and upward and add to the downward force. In dives the knees are not fully extended; they reserve some of their power for the projection.

Table 19-1. Bounce and depression in trampolining

	Height	Resulting net depression
First bounce	0.53 m (21 in)	0.51 m (20 in)
Second bounce	1.14 m (45 in)	0.76 m (30 in)
Third bounce	1.50 m (60 in)	0.78 m (31 in)

When great height is desired, the trampoline performer takes repeated bounces; the diver can use only one landing, and for those dives which require longer time in the air a high diving board is used.

Projectional direction. From the low point of depression the performer rides upward on the rebounding surface. During this time the center of gravity develops a velocity equal to that of the canvas or board, and at the departure point this velocity is increased by ankle extension and some further shoulder flexion and in dives by the remaining amount of possible knee extension. The direction of the center of gravity during flight is determined by the position of the center of gravity in relation to the feet at the final thrust. The diver must have some forward lean to enter the water a short distance from the board. The position of the entry will depend on the lean. Beginning divers are likely to lean too far forward as they attempt a straight front dive; they concentrate on clearing the board rather than on gaining height, and, consequently, as they enter the water their bodies approach a horizontal, rather than a vertical, line. Since the center of gravity follows a parabolic curve, the time of flight from takeoff until the hips enter the water is a measure of the height attained. Block has suggested that in working with women the beginner be given a distance goal of 1.5 to 2.4 m (5 to 8 ft) from the board as the desirable entry and that the diver attempt to develop a projection that would have a minimal time of 1.1 seconds. Such projections would mean that the center of gravity would have an inclination of 22 to 30 degrees beyond the perpendicular at takeoff and a velocity of 3.9 to 4.2 m/sec (13 to 14 ft/sec). These goals were found, experimentally, to be

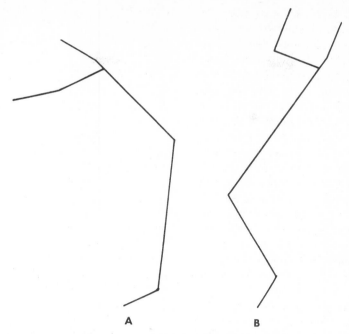

A   B

Fig. 19-1. A, Takeoff position, from trampoline, of highly skilled college man for forward somersault. **B,** Takeoff position from trampoline for backward somersault. Position of center of gravity determines direction of total body rotation.

within the capacity of beginning college women divers. Groves found that with an expert male diver the lean for various dives ranged from 20 to 34 degrees at takeoff and that the height reached by the center of gravity ranged from 0.73 to 1.4 m (2.4 to 4.6 ft).

On the trampoline no forward component of velocity is needed, and the center of gravity can be in a line that is perpendicular to the final thrust. In bounces to gain height this will be done to convert the rebounding force as much as possible into an upward projection.

Rotations and twists in flight. As the performer leaves the canvas or board, the position of the center of gravity also starts the body rotations in the sagittal or transverse planes or both. The amount of lean depends on the amount of rotation desired during flight. The performer riding upward on the rebounding surface has the desired body rotations in mind and makes adjustments to place the center of gravity in the needed relationship to the final thrust. In Fig. 19-1 are shown line tracings at takeoff of an expert performer planning to execute forward and backward somersaults during flight. In the forward movement the center of gravity has been carried ahead of the toes by hip and shoulder flexion. The thrust will start the rotation in a counterclockwise direction. For the backward movement knee flexion has carried the center of gravity back of the toes, and rotation in a clockwise direction will be started. Once the body is in flight, joint actions will add to the speed of rotation of the segments.

Reuschlein measured on film the rotation of body parts of an expert performer executing a forward somersault in the pike position. The degrees of rotation in space of the trunk and the lower limbs and the changes in the hip angle were measured. Rotation was produced by creating a moment of force before becoming airborne. The trunk, slightly above the horizontal at the beginning of flight, rotated counterclockwise until it reached the 12-o'clock position—more than 270 degrees—whereas the lower limbs, starting near the 6-o'clock position, rotated more than 360 degrees counterclockwise. In the first 0.284 second the trunk rotated 110 degrees and the limbs 61 degrees. Trunk movement was facilitated by gravitational force, while the lower limbs opposed gravity. In the next 0.521 second the limbs rotated faster than the trunk. Thus to speak of an angular velocity of the total body may not always be valid, since positioning of the limbs and changes in the angles at the joints mask the total body rotation.

If greater speed of rotation is desired, the body will assume a tuck position to shorten the length of the moment arms. While the body is in midair, the speed of rotation will be decreased by extending the limbs and the trunk, as is done in preparation for landing or entering a body of water.

A diver does not assume as much trunk flexion as the trampolinist, because the diver's flight will always have some horizontal velocity. The diver can use full body lean to displace the center of gravity of the body in front of or behind the base of support. For the reverse and inward dives the body position appears similar to that of the trampolinist. Swain studied dives performed at an Association for Intercollegiate Athletics for Women (AIAW) national diving championship and discovered a relationship between type of dive (number of rotations) and body position at takeoff. The more rotations, the greater the lean. The lean was unique to each classification. Fig. 19-2 depicts film tracings of these findings.

ROTATORY CAPABILITIES OF HUMAN BODY

The human body can rotate about the three principle axes: vertical, frontal-horizontal, and saggital-horizontal. These rotations are termed (1)

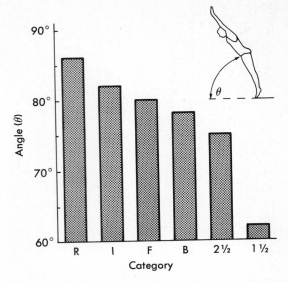

Fig. 19-2. Relationship of body lean to type of dive. *R,* Reverse layout; *I,* inward layout; *F,* front layout; *B,* back layout; 2½, somersault back layout; 1½, somersault front pike.

pitch, which is about the frontal-horizontal axis as in a front somersault; (2) yaw, which is about the saggital-horizontal axis as in a cartwheel; and (3) roll, which is about the vertical axis as in twists. In addition, the body may rotate about any diagonal axis or about more than one axis. In certain movements it is possible for a person who is rotating about one of the horizontal axes to lean the body to one side and be able to twist about the vertical axis. By redistributing the body mass the performer may change the direction of the main axis, which may give rise to a conical motion about the axis of momentum and cause the performer to rotate about more than one axis at the same time.

Usually, angular momentum is produced while the performer is on a supporting surface, whether a foot support or arm support. Thus rotations are begun before the person terminates contact with the supporting surface. Even in twisting movements the body shifts the line of gravity from be-

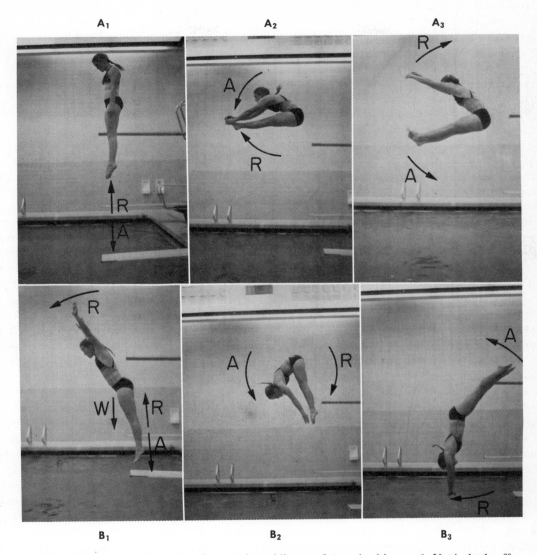

Fig. 19-3. Effects of rotation and action-reaction while a performer is airborne. **A,** Vertical takeoff results in foot first entry with no total body rotation despite efforts of the diver to execute a pike somersault. **B,** Total body rotation in sagittal plane is produced by eccentric action. (*A,* Action; *R,* reaction shown as vector and moment; *W,* weight.)

tween the feet or hands and toward one of the supports before the instant of takeoff. When the performer is in the air, the arms or lower limbs or both are moved to accentuate the twist.

Ramey and others have shown that the human body cannot execute even one complete rotation of the body in the pitch or yaw planes if no angular momentum exists at the time of takeoff. The reason is the principle of the conservation of momentum, which states that momentum cannot be created or destroyed once the body is airborne and no external forces or couples are acting on the body. Stated another way, the law of interaction functions in airborne situations to produce a counterrotation of one body part whenever a rotation is produced with another body part. For example, the front pike dive will result in a leg entry, as shown in Fig. 19-3, *A,* if the upper body flexes after the diver becomes airborne and the total body has no angular momentum. The lower body will rise to meet the upper body because of the law of interaction. Contrast this with Fig. 19-3, *B,* in which angular momentum exists before the upper body flexes. The lower body reaction still causes the upper and lower body parts to approach each other, but the pitch rotation places the body in a more favorable angle for entry into the water.

The "biomechanically ideal" method of assuming the extended inverted position from this jackknife position is to use minimal acceleration of the legs as extension at the hip is executed. The equal and opposite reaction, therefore, will also be small and can be counteracted by muscle force at the hip joint. Should the leg extension be one of moderate to great acceleration, thus creating a high velocity, the upper body reaction will be pronounced. The back will most likely arch, and the head and arms will rise. Persons with weak abdominal muscles will experience pain in the lumbar region of the spine and have an uncontrolled landing.

Although pitch, and the rarely used yaw, rotations cannot be initiated successfully while the diver is airborne, twisting movements can be and are initiated at that time. This is possible because the rotation is about the longitudinal axis of the body. The body parts may be redistributed about this axis to produce favorable moment-of-inertia ratios with respect to the law of interaction. The easiest way to understand this concept is to visualize the twist as it is initiated from a pike position, with the upper body inverted and the legs horizontal, as shown in Fig. 19-4. As the arms are moved to cause the upper body to twist, the opposite reaction in the legs will be one of low velocity, and therefore low displacement and counter twist, because of the high moment-of-inertia ratio. The legs have a long moment arm and a small twist in the horizontal plane, in contrast to the short moment arm of the horizontal twist by the upper body. The arms and trunk will move at a greater velocity and have a large angular displacement because their moment of inertia is small compared to that of the legs. This example not only provides an understanding of the biomechanical principles but illustrates how important it is for the performer to execute movements at precisely the most optimal point in time within a movement pattern.

Twisting movements can be executed in a variety of ways. Individual differences may account for one performer's method in comparison with another, or the particular stunt may influence selection of the method of initiating the twist. Many gymnasts use what is termed a high arm throw, whereas the low arm throw is more common to divers. Thayer studied these two types of arm actions used in diving. Although her data are not conclusive, the results suggest that the high arm action is biomechanically better because the velocity is in the direction of the twist, and in addition, the line of direction of the possible muscles involved and the moments of inertia appear to be better during that action than during the low arm action. More research should be conducted with different populations and with respect to twisting movements in general.

MINI LABORATORY EXERCISES

One of the best examples of conservation of angular momentum is achieved by standing on a freely rotating board (such as a twister board) or a chair (swivel type)

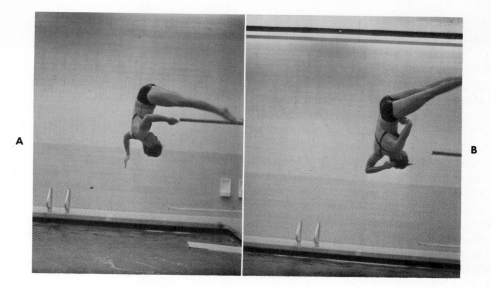

Fig. 19-4. Twist executed from pike position creates only a small amount of movement reaction since the moment of inertia of legs is great compared to rest of body.

and changing the moment arms of the upper extremities while spinning.

1. Spin a person who is standing on a freely rotating surface.
2. Have the person begin with the hands at the sides (anatomic position).
3. After the spin has started, ask the person to abduct the arms to the horizontal position. Note the decrease in angular speed.
4. Now spin the person, beginning with arms in the abducted position and adduct the arms during the spin. Note the increase in angular speed.
5. Add weights to the hands and repeat steps 1 to 4.
6. Other examples of the conservation of angular momentum can be observed in sports. One of the easiest and safest ways to experience the increase in angular speed is with the forward roll. Since the person is not airborne, there is little danger if the person fails to achieve high angular speeds. In fact, failure to do so is safer than developing too much speed. Thus one can experience the trade-off that occurs between the moment of inertia and angular speed (velocity). Estimates of differences in moments of inertia of body parts among persons and between one person's body

parts may be made by estimating differences in angular velocities by means of time or radian measurements.

ARM-SUPPORTED SKILLS
Mechanics of arm-supported skills

In many gymnastic skills the body is supported by the hands as it is rotated in a vertical or horizontal plane around the support. In the vertical plane as the body rotates downward, gravitational force aids; as the body rotates upward, gravity resists the movement. Therefore on the downswing the skilled performer will move the body's center of gravity as far as possible from the center of rotation; this is done by full hip extension and shoulder girdle depression. On the upswing the center of gravity will be moved toward the center of rotation by hip flexion and shoulder girdle elevation. In skills in which the body is rotated in the horizontal plane, the joint actions will be those that tend to keep the center of gravity directly over the supporting base.

Simple underswing

The simple underswing (swinging back and forth) is a preliminary movement that is used in preparation for the execution of more advanced moves. The hands provide the point of support and the center of rotation. To develop a simple underswing the hips should flex on the upswing (forward or backward), thereby shortening the radius of rotation (with the result that the center of rotation moves closer to the center of support). The performer, by elevating the shoulder girdle when the body is directly under the point of support, may also help increase the angular velocity. In gymnastic terms this is known as *hollowing* the chest. As the body starts downward at the end of the swing, the velocity can be increased by hip extension and shoulder girdle elevation.

Giant swing

The giant swing may be done both backward and forward. On the upward swing the radius of rotation is shortened by flexion of hips and also by shoulder girdle elevation. Actually the hollowing of the chest has the effect of causing a slight flexion as well as depression of the shoulders to take place. (If the arms were flexed, the radius of movement would be shortened much more; however, in topflight gymnastic competition the flexing of the arms is considered poor form.) This brings the center of gravity closer to the center of support (shortening the radius) and in turn accelerates the upward angular velocity. As the center of gravity moves over the center of support (the hands), the grip has been moved upward, and the performer momentarily pushes the body up to a handstand position. On the downswing the body is fully extended. The extension is made just before the body reaches the high vertical position to gain the full effect of gravity and to develop the greatest possible velocity in preparation for the next upward swing. (See Figs. 19-5 and 19-6.)

Following are kinetic findings reported by Vallière on performers executing the backward giant swing on the still rings.

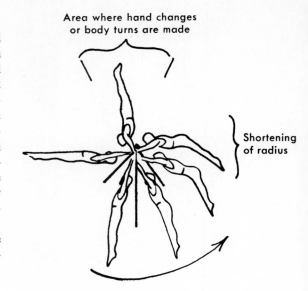

Area where hand changes or body turns are made

Shortening of radius

Fig. 19-5. Reverse-grip giant swing on high bar.

1. A decline in force was exerted during the descent phase.
2. A sudden increase of force coincided with the greatest shoulder joint velocity.
3. A drop in force coincided with the whiplike action of the legs, occurring at the bottom of the swing.
4. A sharp increase in force moving to a maximum coincided with the upward lift of the body in the ascent phase. (See Fig. 19-7 for a view of this special apparatus; see also Fig. 19-8 for the force-time curve.)

Stunts on parallel bars

In the swing from the supine position (Fig. 19-9) on the parallel bars, much of the skill depends on adjustments made to keep the body's center of gravity over (or near) the supporting hands. Note that in the supine position the arms are tilted to the left and the hips are flexed; both adjustments move the body mass toward the vertical plane of the hands. In the prone position the el-

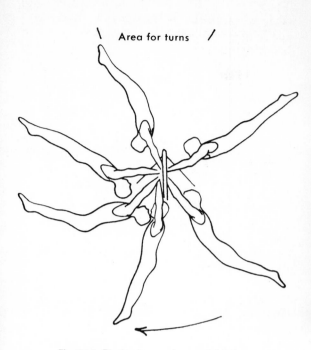

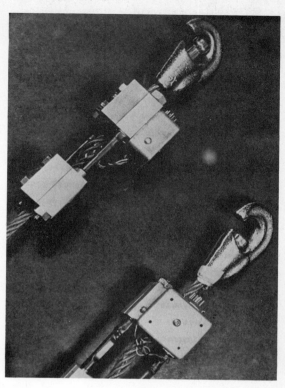

Fig. 19-6. Back giant swing on high bar.

Fig. 19-7. Special strain gauge transducers used by André Vallière in his study of backward giant swing.

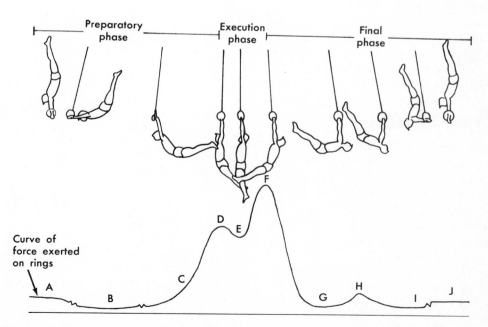

Fig. 19-8. Kinetic and kinematic diagram of backward giant swing executed on still rings. Selected points on strain gauge recording were synchronized with corresponding body positions taken from film sequence. (From Vallière, A.: Kinetic and kinematic analysis of the backward giant swing on the still rings in gymnastics, doctoral dissertation, Indiana University, Aug., 1973.)

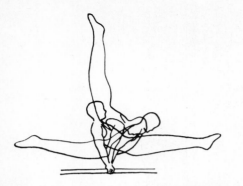

Fig. 19-9. Swing in support position on parallel bars. A deduction would be made for bent arms shown in prone position; thus this competitor would lose points.

bows are flexed; this is a reversed muscle action that moves the upper arm and with it the upper portion of the trunk to the right to balance the lower limbs. In the final position, extension of the spine and backward rotation of the pelvis have moved the lower limbs close to the support to balance the head and shoulder girdle. As the arms moved to the right on the downswing, the effect of gravitational force was increased by increasing the distance between the hands and the center of gravity; as the elbows flexed on the first part of the upward swing, that distance was shortened to make better use of the momentum developed on the downward swing.

Stunts on uneven parallel bars

The same principles involved in swinging activities on the high bar and on parallel bars apply to swinging on the uneven parallel bars. In addition, however, the transfer of a swing on one bar to the other bar increases both the complexity and the possibilities of stunts that can be performed. The lower bar also may be an obstacle to the execution of stunts that normally are routine on a high bar. For example, women are performing the giant swing of the high bar on the top bar of the uneven parallel bars. The downswing essentially is the same as in the high bar performance, but the up-

swing necessitates a piking and an upward extension of the body, which is by far more difficult than the upswing on the high bar.

One of the most important mechanical principles is that of continuity of angular momentum, that is, the maintenance of the rotatory momentum for the execution of a series of stunts, especially those which involve transference from one bar to the other.

The cast-off from the high bar to a back hip circle on the low bar is one of the more common stunts, and it is one that shows the applications of swing and moment of inertia. The swing is begun by a clockwise rotation of the lower body to overcome inertia, produce a forceful counterclockwise rotation, and thus acquire the greatest height for the starting point of the swing (Fig. 19-10). The body is extended, with chest hollowed to provide the longest lever possible for the downswing. As the center of gravity reaches a point below the bar, the body arches slightly and causes the legs to move behind the trunk. As the trunk leads, the lever length is decreased somewhat, and angular velocity increases. This facilitates the piking action necessary to execute the back hip circle around the low bar. The piking action increases the angular velocity considerably and, when perfectly timed, will cause the axis of rotation of the body to coincide with that of the lower bar axis. The body will rotate around the lower bar with a minimum of pressure between the bar and the body. In essence, this back hip circle is similar to the back pike somersault dismount from a high bar. The only difference is that the bar contains the horizontal velocity and maintains a fixed axis of rotation about the bar. The performer then grasps the lower bar with her hands and increases the moment of inertia by extending into the front support position.

The amount of muscular activity in selected shoulder muscles during four stunts on the uneven parallel bars has been studied by Landa. She used surface electrodes to record the action potentials from the pectoralis major, three heads of the deltoids, the biceps brachii, the superior and inferior heads of the trapezius, and the latissimus dorsi.

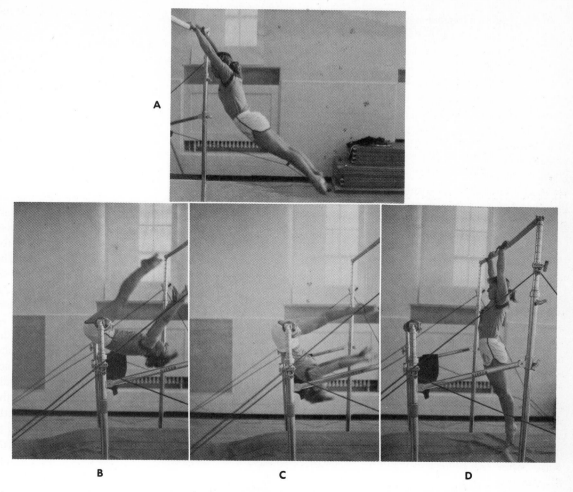

Fig. 19-10. Cast-off from high bar to back circle on low bar of uneven parallel bars. Note periods of long radii and short radii, and movements with gravity and opposing gravity.

Muscle activity was positively related to increase in swing amplitude, which also meant that it was related to swing velocity. Both the stationary hang into a squat on the low bar and the jump-catch swing into a squat on the low bar showed less activity than did the cast-off into a pike around the low bar and the cast-off into a back hip circle on the low bar. The latissimus dorsi contributed a greater amount of electrical activity with respect to potential than any of the other muscles. Landa

concluded that strength improvement exercises in the shoulder and upper back, especially for the latissimus dorsi, are vital for performers on the uneven parallel bars.

Oglesby also investigated muscle activity in women gymnasts. She studied the upper, middle, and lower portions of the rectus abdominus muscle to determine their magnitude and time of activity in the kip and single-leg shoot-through on the uneven parallel bars, as well as in three floor exercise stunts and two balance beam stunts. She found that the muscle, especially the lower portion, performed a major function in the execution of five of the seven stunts. Each stunt showed a unique pattern of electrical activity, which suggests that exercises which simulate the stunts should be used in abdominal strength training.

Another anatomic consideration of importance to successful performance on the uneven parallel bars is the length of the body. It is essential that the levels of the two bars and the distance between the two bars be adjusted precisely to the length, and therefore the swinging distance, of the body of each performer. Beginners, who strike the bar and possess little thigh mass, may find padding useful and necessary during the learning stages of movements such as back hip circles after swinging movements from the high bar. Improper timing will cause impact trauma to the body rather than a ''wrapping of the body around the bar.''

Flyaway

The flyaway is a type of dismount that usually follows a giant swing. The performer first does a giant swing and then prepares for the flyaway by increasing speed. The radius of rotation is short-

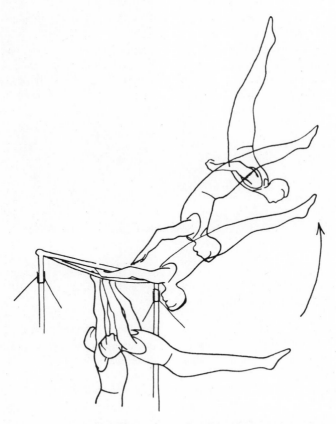

Fig. 19-11. Flyaway (layout) from back giant swing on high bar. Head appears to extend too early. Although some gymnasts still do extend head in this manner, it would generally be considered too early to obtain maximum lift. In final drawing, arms should be extended to lift center of mass of body upward.

ened as the body passes over the bar. This is done by flexing the hips and depressing the shoulder girdle. (The arms could be flexed, but this is considered poor form.) The back is then arched (by extension) just before coming directly under the bar on the downswing. This arching helps shorten the radius as the body rises in the upswing and aids in accelerating the angular velocity. As the body rises above the horizontal, the arch is continued with the head held well backward (upper back and head extension) and the hips and arms (slightly) flexed (Fig. 19-11). The reaction from the bent bar gives added upward velocity to the performer. Centrifugal force pulls the body away from the bar.

Action on still (stationary) rings

The performer on the still rings demonstrates the principles of good balance by shortening the lever arm (radius) and also shows the value of continuous movement throughout the exercise.

Back uprise to a handstand on rings. To execute the back uprise to a handstand on the still rings (Fig. 19-12), the performer swings the body to and fro by alternate trunk flexion and extension to gain momentum, and on the downswing the radius (the distance from the hands to the toes) is lengthened. The center of gravity is kept under the point of suspension of the cables. On the upswing the radius is shortened by arching the back and in-locating the shoulders, that is, internally rotating the humeral head in the glenoid fossa. (This helps overcome the force of gravity and gives the performer accelerated upward angular velocity.) The body is moved forward, placing the center of rotation nearer to the point of support (hands), which is kept behind an extended line from the shoulders. The center of gravity is still kept under the point of suspension of the cables and rings. As the point of support moves under the point of suspension of the rings, the center of gravity moves upward and inward at the same rate. The performer pulls the

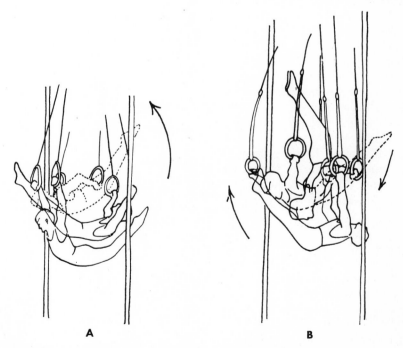

Fig. 19-12. A, Back uprise to handstand on rings. **B**, Shoot to handstand on rings.

body up by forceful scapular abduction and shoulder extension and then pushes upward to a handstand in continuous motion as the rotary swing diminishes. This is accomplished by flexing the hips and abducting the scapulae. (See Fig. 19-12).

Since the rings should be as stationary as possible while the exercises are being performed, the performer should attempt to stop or prevent movement of the cables. Usually swing occurs when the performer fails to keep the center of gravity under the point of support and along the rope suspension line. When the swinging begins, it is difficult to stop, and thereafter all movements on the rings are difficult to execute. Developing a certain amount of swing is inevitable during the course of a competitive routine, and the accomplished gymnast learns to ''kill,'' or stop, the swing in some movements and use it to advantage in others. Usually one of two things happens: the swing continues to increase (most commonly) or may be controlled or partially dissipated. Movement of the center of gravity of the body against the direction of the swing may help control or stop it.

Cross-hang position on the rings. The cross-hang position is an exercise of simple joint action requiring tremendous strength because the supports (the hands) are not directly above the body's center of gravity but rather at arm's distance from it horizontally (Fig. 19-13). To maintain the arm position the shoulder adductors must contract forcefully. The elbow and wrist joints must be stabilized; however, the muscular effort for maintaining the positions of these joints is not great if the shoulder position is held. From this position upper trunk rotation takes place to either the right or the left.

Side horse activities

The movements on the side horse are normally those of pendulum-like swinging, rotary movements, and variations of these two.

A type of pendulum-like swinging is observed in the execution of simple leg cuts and scissor actions (Fig. 19-14). The points of suspension of the pendulum are the shoulder joints. The radius is shortened as the performer moves the center of

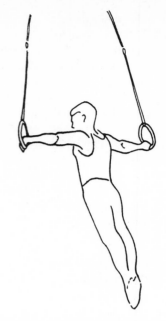

Fig. 19-13. Cross-hang position on rings.

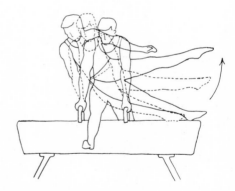

Fig. 19-14. Pendulum swing in scissors action on side horse.

gravity nearer to the base of support on the upswing and is lengthened on the downswing to increase angular velocity. This is accomplished by flexing the hip, accompanied by flexion and lateral rotation of the trunk. On the upswing the top thigh

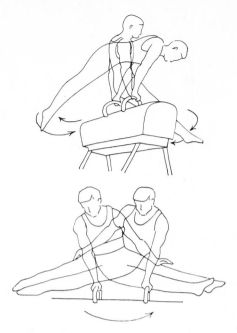

Fig. 19-15. High double-leg circle on side horse.

while the action takes place, or the performer will fall off the apparatus.

Balance beam

The gymnastic event executed on the balance beam is one in which the woman performer is called on to do many acrobatic stunts while maintaining balance. The duration of the movements on the beam is restricted to not less than 1 minute 15 seconds and not more than 1 minute 35 seconds.

To counteract toppling in one direction, the gymnast rotates her arms and sometimes the non-supporting leg in the direction of unbalance to cause the rest of the body to move in the opposite direction, thus abating the overbalance.

It is evident that this event, in which a mounted beam of narrow width constitutes a performance area where dance steps, turns, jumps, leaps, and gymnastic twists are executed, calls for great skill involving principles of equilibrium. The placement of the body's center of gravity must be directly over the feet so that the performer is able to stay on the beam after executing a move. During the execution of the stunt the center of gravity must move in the direction of movement so that the movement flows as progress is made back and forth on the beam (Wilkerson).

Vaulting

Vaulting may be thought of as consisting of two jumps, one from the feet and one from the hands. Therefore many of the principles described in the chapter on jumping can be applied to the skill of vaulting. Since the goals of vaulting and jumping differ, however, some differences are evident. Since the distance allowed for the approach in vaulting is less than 8 m, vaulters do not attain maximal running speeds before takeoff. Average speeds of skilled vaulters immediately before contact with the takeoff board have been reported as being 6.09 to 7.31 m/sec (20 to 24 ft/sec). Little or no speed is lost during board contact, because of the rebound capabilities of the board as well as the vaulter's ability to apply force during the contact phase. Less skilled vaulters are not able to main-

is abducted. The resistance arm of the level (distance from the point of support to the center of gravity of the combined mass of the trunk and lower limbs) is also shortened on the upswing and lengthened on the downswing. As the upswing diminishes until the velocity is zero (with the upward velocity and the pull of gravity nullifying one another), the performer flexes the hip, flexes and laterally rotates the trunk, and executes leg crosses and scissorlike actions.

When high double-leg circles are executed, the center of gravity must be kept over the center of rotation and base of support during most of the move. The body rotates about the center of support by means of lateral trunk flexion, with the shoulders held more or less at the same elevation (Fig. 19-15). The shortening of the radius and raising of the center of gravity during the movement allow the return swing to be made more easily. Takemoto and Hamaido liken this action to the spinning of a top. No pause (or slowing down) may occur tain their speed and show decreases of 1 or 2 m/sec during this phase.

The speed of the approach is a major determinant of flight speed. The faster the approach speed, the greater the possibility for a more skilled performance. Dynamic control of the approach speed is the next determinant of skilled performance, since the takeoff determines the angle and speed of the preflight (airborne phase between takeoff from the board and contact with the horse), just as the direction of the initial contact with the horse will influence the effectiveness of the postflight (from leaving the horse to landing on the mat). The preflight velocity of skilled vaulters is greater than that of less skilled vaulters.

Research on the handspring vault shows that vaulters contact the takeoff board at an angle producing 75% horizontal force and 25% vertical force to the board. Their takeoff velocity shows approximately equal horizontal and vertical components.

As with other forms of jumping a compromise must be made between magnitude of force and magnitude of time during the takeoff phase. Skilled vaulters have a relatively short contact time, both on the board and on the horse. Contact times on the takeoff board are about 0.1 second (100 msec) but will vary with respect to type of vault, type of board, and vaulter. Contact times on the horse for handspring vaults of 10 advanced female gymnasts ranged from 130 msec to 295 msec. The best vaulter had a contact time of 17 msec. This vault was characterized by a takeoff from the horse before the body passed the vertical. Less skilled vaults were characterized by takeoffs after the body passed the vertical position on the horse (Daniels).

As the equipment changes, vaulting styles may change, and the types of vaults will become more complex. The following basic principles may aid the teacher and performer in attaining vaulting achievements:

1. Attain an approach speed that is as fast as possible without loss of dynamic equilibrium.

2. Learn to obtain maximal mechanical energy from the takeoff board. Penney has shown that skilled vaulters adapt to the rebounding surface, but some vaulters exceeded the limits of the Reuter board, formerly used extensively for vaulting competitions.

3. Determine the angle of that preflight which will result in the best body position and the least amount of inhibiting or detrimental reaction force at contact with the horse.

4. Apply force during contact with the horse to attain adequate velocity of the postflight.

MINI LABORATORY EXERCISES

1. a. Observe a dive foreward roll.
   b. Describe the angular velocity during different phases of the roll.
   c. Estimate the radius of rotation (length of lever).
2. Ask the performer to execute the roll in the following ways:
   a. Tuck as soon as possible and maintain the tuck throughout the roll.
   b. Extend the legs and maintain this extension until upside down and then tuck rapidly.
   c. Extend legs and assume a pike position as soon as possible; assume the tuck position when upside down.
3. a. Observe the rolls performed in steps 2.
   b. Evaluate whether or not the performer executed the task.
   c. Assess the performances as in step 1.

REFERENCES

Block, J.: Teaching the running front dive through progressive goals, thesis, University of Wisconsin, 1952.

Daniels, A.: Cinematographic analysis of the handspring vault, Res. Q. **50:**(3), 1979.

Groves, W.H.: Mechanical analysis of diving, Res. Q. **21:**132, 1950.

Landa, J.: Shoulder muscle activity during selected skills on the uneven parallel bars, thesis, Washington State University, 1973.

Oglesby, B.F.: An electromyographic study of the rectus abdominis muscle during selected gymnastic student, thesis, Washington State University, 1969.

Penney, J.B.: A cinematographic analysis of the effect of vaulting board pads on the takeoff velocities during vaulting, thesis, Washington State University, 1975.

Ramey, M.R.: The use of angular momentum in the study of

long-jump take-offs. In Nelson, R.C., and Morehouse, C.A., editors: Biomechanics, IV, Baltimore, 1974, University Park Press.

Reuschlein, P.: An analysis of the forward somersault in the pike position, unpublished paper, University of Wisconsin, 1962.

Swain, R.: A comparison between coaching cues and the execution of that dive, unpublished paper, Washington State University, 1979.

Takemoto, M., and Hamaido, S.: Gymnastics illustrated, Tokyo, 1961, Ban-Yu Shuppan Co., Ltd.

Thayer, A.: A mechanical analysis of two methods of twisting in a forward somersault with one twist, master's project, Washington State University, 1980.

Vallière, A.: Kinetic and kinematic analysis of the backward giant swing on the still rings in gymnastics, doctoral dissertation, Indiana University, Aug., 1973.

Wilkerson, J.: Kinematic and kinetic analysis of the back handspring in gymnastics as performed on the balance beam, doctoral dissertation, Indiana University, 1978.

ADDITIONAL READINGS

George, G.S.: Biomechanics on women's gymnastics, Englewood Cliffs, N.J., 1980, Prentice-Hall, Inc.

Kreighbaum, E.F.: The mechanics of the use of the Reuter board during side horse vaulting, doctoral dissertation, Washington State University, 1973.

CHAPTER 20

Fencing, martial arts, and self-defense

Since fencing, judo, karate, and self-defense are combative activities, each of them consists of attacking movements such as striking, kicking, pushing, or pulling and of defensive movements for blocking the attacks. Thus the application of the basic principles of stability, $\Sigma F = ma$, impulse-momentum, and work (kinetic energy) are often easily recognized.

FENCING

In fencing, an implement (foil, saber, or épée) is used to deliver the "blow" to the opponent. Speed is therefore important, as is the direct line of action of locomotion of the body and manipulation of the hand. Deception, however, is a major concern. Therefore movements need to be made with the fine muscles of thumb and index fingers. As in judo, too firm a hold on the weapon usually will cause arm and shoulder muscles to produce large movements when only the fingers should apply force and will thus prevent adaptability to the opponent's movements. Ultimately the major problem of the fencer, as with all performers of movement, is the inability to eliminate all extraneous movements and muscle tension. To paraphrase Basmajian, high-level skill is not recognized so much by what one does as by what one avoids doing.

The basic stance is one in which the feet are at right angles to each other, with the lead foot facing the opponent. This provides both lateral and sagittal stability. The width of the feet is such that the center of gravity may be lowered for stability and for increased distance of flexion at the knee from which to execute a forceful lunge. In addition, the knees should be above the feet to reduce the movements of force and therefore stress at the knee joints. The feet should also be spread a distance that provides optimal mobility.

Fig. 20-1 shows electromyographic and electrogoniometric data on lunging, both correctly and incorrectly. Note the differences in muscle action potentials with respect to position of the knee. Such data not only can assist a fencer in determining performance faults but can be used to determine which muscles are vulnerable when performance is incorrect.

High-speed photography will also assist the movement analyst in noting the movement of the muscle itself. Fig. 20-2 shows the movement of the triceps surae (the gastrocnemius and soleus considered together) during a fencing lunge.

The fencing lunge is the attack of the fencer. The force is obtained through extension of the rear leg and movement of the lead leg and rear arm. The more directly horizontal this force can be directed, the faster and more effective will be the lunge. Note in Fig. 20-3 the differences in peak

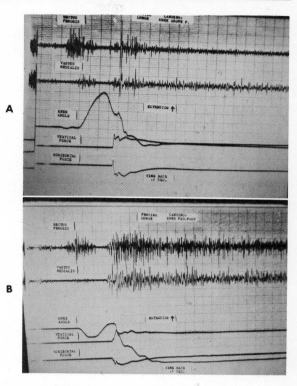

Fig. 20-1. Electromyographic and electrogoniometric recordings of the fencing lunge. **A,** Knee is above base of support at end of lunge. **B,** Knee is outside base of support at end of lunge.

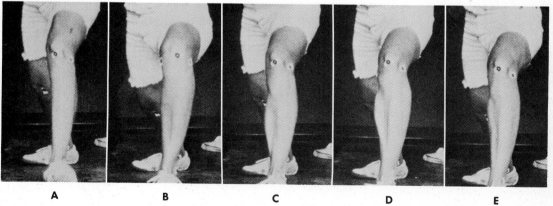

Fig. 20-2. Deformation of triceps surae muscle at instant of contact during fencing lunge. (Filming speed was 200 frames/sec.)

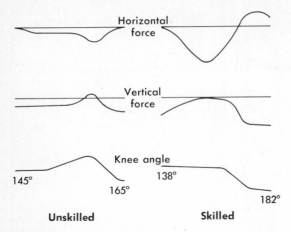

Fig. 20-3. Force-time histories (rear leg) of unskilled and skilled performers during fencing lunge.

forces of the rear leg during the lunge of a skilled performer and that of an unskilled performer. The unskilled performer did not extend the rear leg completely until after landing, and vertical forces were greater than horizontal ones. In addition, the vertical impulses were greater than the horizontal impulses. The skilled performer developed 355 N of peak force and five times more impulse in the horizontal direction than did the unskilled fencer. The skilled fencer showed no vertical force greater than body weight.

JUDO

Judo may be thought of as the art of throwing an opponent. To do so one must cause the opponent to become unbalanced and must time the execution of the throwing action when the opponent is in this unbalanced position. Timing is more important than strength, since the use of the opponent's actions and momentum necessitates less strength on the part of the thrower.

Balance may be upset in eight conventional directions: forward, backward, right, left, and in the four corners. Force application patterns used to produce this loss in equilibrium consists of (1) push, (2) pull, (3) push followed by a release, (4) pull followed by a release, (5) push-pull (force couple from the use of both hands), (6) pull-push (force couple), and (7) combinations of all the above. Combinations of push-pull and pull-push always produce rotations of the opponent's body about its longitudinal axis.

The defensive position is taken with the center of gravity lowered by flexion at the knees. The feet are more than hip width apart, and they are at right angles to each other to provide both lateral and anteroposterior stability. This stance is similar to the fencer's stance, but in judo the torso is facing the opponent.

As the judoists face each other in this defensive stance, they grasp one another's lapel and sleeve. The material is held with the third and fourth fingers while the other fingers and thumb exert little pressure. This grip can be changed easily to achieve better leverage. Grasping the lapel causes any force by fingers or hand to control the midline of the opponent's body, whereas the grasping of the sleeve causes a moment of force to be applied to the torso.

Since the judoist must always be prepared for an attack, locomotion is made with short, quick steps of a sliding nature, with a lowered center of gravity. These movements provide maximal stability and promote maintenance of balance during the locomotion itself. The weight is often maintained over the leading foot so that the rear foot can be quickly used for sweeping and other attacks.

Basic principles applied to seoinage (hip throw). Fig. 20-4 depicts the throw, termed seoinage, in which the thrower (tori) rotates in front of the one to be thrown (uke). The circle begins low and moves diagonally upward as the uke is pulled into the circle of the hip. As contact is made, the uke has become off balance, and the throw is executed. The following principles are applied:

1. Maintain a low center of gravity.
2. Take short preparation steps to maintain equilibrium.
3. Place the center of gravity below the level of the opponent's center of gravity.
4. Move continuously and in a circular fashion.
5. Unbalance the opponent.

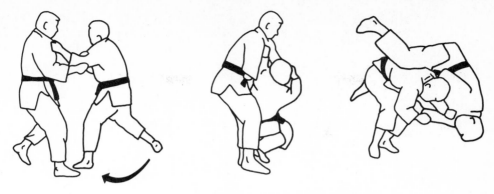

Fig. 20-4. Contourograms of judo throw (seoinage).

6. Draw the opponent forward, rather than moving toward the opponent.
7. Throw in the direction of the opponent's movement, which is the unbalancing movement.

Preparation before action will consist of an interplay between the opponents in which they search for the precise time in which unbalancing can be created. For example, after some pushing and pulling and sliding of the feet, the opponent may push. A counteraction may be pulling against this opponent with greater forcer than of the push. This action will offset the opponent.

The seoinage is typically done toward one side. Thus a judoist may become overdeveloped on one side of the body. Since judo is basically a unilateral sport, except for highly skilled participation, scoliosis, which is due to shortening of muscles on one side of spinal column, may result unless there is concomitant development of general body strength.

Another sports medicine problem caused by the force production and by the timing of the throw to coincide with the ideal position of the opponent's gravitational line is that of elbow injury. This injury is similar to "baseball pitcher's elbow," "tennis elbow," and other conditions caused by stress on the elbow.

Taiotoshi. Anatomic considerations affect the nature of the throwing technique. A stronger, larger or taller person will use a technique modified to fit his or her anatomy as well as that of the opponent. Seoinage will be preferred, so that the uke is thrown with a rotatory method. A shorter tori will prefer to use taiotoshi (Fig. 20-5); the uke is pulled forward, shoulders square, and thrown over the body. Force-time curves for taiotoshi will show the effects of these differences. The sequence of positive and negative impulses will allow a coach to determine whether or not the movements were executed precisely at the correct time.

Taiotoshi uses a sweeping action of the leg (Fig. 3-8). The sweep is executed in balance, that is, with the body rotating about its center of gravity rather than displacing the center of gravity. Other throws involving the foot sweep require large distances so that the sweeping action develops kinetic energy. The foot sweep will be similar to that of a soccer kick in that the leg is extended through the object (opponent) and the hips are rotated to the "open" position.

Breaking the fall. Since all throws involve a landing, the basic techniques described in Chapter 21 are applicable. The hand slap is unique to judo. Although the slap does not absorb a great deal of force, it is useful in placing the rest of the body, especially the trunk, in the most advantageous position of landing. The large surface area is the goal. Muscle force is used to position the body for such a landing.

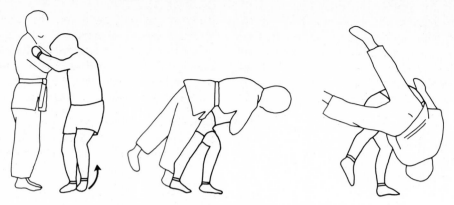

Fig. 20-5. Contourograms of judo throw (taiotoshi).

If the landing will be a rolling type, the back is curved and the head is flexed to produce a low resistance to rolling.

KARATE

Karate is the art of hand and foot fighting, also known as unarmed self-defense. Attacks are commonly made with hand or fist (punches) and foot (kicks). Again, both the defensive and attack positions require a lowered center of gravity and a stable base. Except for a lateral position, the other stances resemble the semilunge position of fencing. Since the goal is to deliver the punch or kick with as much force as possible, the body parts must be moved as rapidly as possible; thus muscle shortening must be achieved as rapidly as possible. The application of the following two principles is therefore paramount to success:

1. Apply the force through a great distance to achieve great kinetic energy.
2. Apply the force over a period that is a compromise, that is, long enough to develop adequate momentum but short enough to prevent the opponent from blocking the attack.

To apply these principles, the karateka (person performing karate) sequentially times the forces much the same as for other maximal efforts. The strong muscles begin first, and then the weakest or smallest ones complete the sequence. The optimal

time for each succeeding force to start is at the greatest velocity (zero acceleration) of the preceding force.

If locomotion is necessary to the attack, the center of gravity of the body should move in a straight line, ideally with no vertical motion. Likewise, all limb movements should be in a straight line and in the direction of the described application of force. Thus this martial art is very different from judo, in which rotatory movements are predominant. Karate primarily consists of linear movements, since the shortest distance to an object is a straight line.

The principles of collision and of receiving impact forces can be applied to the impact of the punch and kick. To increase the time of impact, the person thinks of "going through the person" and is thus able to maintain velocity and prevent early deceleration. In addition, the muscles are tensed at contact, which produces less deformation of the striking limb, less recoil from the joints, and therefore less absorption of the force by the striker. Additionally, the wrist and ankle are firm and in alignment with the limb, making a rigid bar at impact. The entire body is rigid, with the rear foot and leg extended to act as a brace against which to counteract the collision.

To intensify the effect of the impact, the performer must apply the greatest pressure (force per square centimeter) to the opponent. This can be done in two ways: by decreasing the contact area of the striking part, and by decreasing the contact area of the body part struck. For example, the hand strike is made with the side of the hand proximal to the fifth finger, rather than being made with the palm. The two knuckles of the fist are used, rather than all four. The lateral edge of the foot is used, rather than the sole of the foot. Furthermore, the target should be a vulnerable area of the body, such as the bridge of the nose.

In reality, the hand and foot are not rigid bars, but they do deform. The skin and then the muscles or tendons deform to absorb some of the force of impact, thereby protecting the body part from injury. The impact force has been measured as high as 3000 N for breaking concrete blocks and almost 700 N for breaking wood. The velocity of the hand was 14 m/sec to develop such a force. The front kick, side kick, and both downward strikes developed these velocities. Thus a mistimed or misplaced action on the part of the karateka could be dangerous. In addition, the trauma to the part of the body used in striking and kicking causes either injury or anatomic changes resulting from adaptation to trauma. Hypertrophy of two knuckles occurs as one of these adaptations.

SELF-DEFENSE

Self-defense may be considered an application of the principles of both judo and karate, as well as an avoidance of the need for self-defense. The use of devices such as canes and keys is also included in the art of self-defense. However, whereas judo and karate are a combination of arts and competitive sports, self-defense is not. The visual alertness needed in karate and the use of vulnerable areas as the sites of blows are also applied in self-defense. Likewise the tactile and kinesthetic awareness of judo (and wrestling) and the application of leverage are also utilized in self-defense.

MINI LABORATORY EXERCISES

1. Explore the use of leverage in the following ways:
   a. Grasp a person's arm in the following three positions and then attempt to turn the person:
      (1) Near the shoulder
      (2) Below the elbow
      (3) At the wrist
   b. Name the levers involved and the relative success of each; explain why success differs for the three situations.
2. Observe a judo class practicing throws. Describe the positioning of the center of gravity of the two bodies and discuss the relationship of success to failure with respect to the positions of the centers of gravity.

REFERENCES

Basmajian, J.V.: New views of muscular tone and relaxation, Can. Med. Assoc. J. **77:**293, 1957.
Basmajian, J.V.: Muscles alive: their functions as revealed by electromyography, ed. 2, Baltimore, 1967, The Williams & Wilkins Co.

ADDITIONAL READINGS

Adrian, M., and Klinger, A.: A biomechanical analysis of the fencing lunge. I. Fencing Coaches Magazine, p. 14, 1979.
Feld, M.S., McNair, R.E., and Wilk, S.R.: The physics of karate, Sci. Am. **240:**150-158, 1979.
Klinger, A.K.: Teaching mechanical principles through self-defense. In Dillman, C.J., and Sears, R.G., editors: Proceedings, Kinesiology: a national conference on teaching, Urbana, 1977, University of Illinois.
Kodokan, Kodokan Judo, Kodansha, Tokyo, 1968.

CHAPTER 21

Catching, falling, and landing

MECHANICS OF STOPPING MOVING OBJECTS

Among the variety of motor skills that human beings perform is the ability to stop a moving object. The object may be external, such as a ball, or it may be the performer's own body, as in landing from a height. The pattern of joint actions varies with the situation, but in all situations the mechanical principles are the same. If the stop is skillfully made, the momentum of the moving object is decreased gradually by joint actions. These actions are such that the object is permitted to continue its motion as its velocity is gradually decreased. If the object is contacted with the hands and the arms are out to meet it, the joint actions are those of a pulling pattern, usually extension of the upper arm and flexion of the forearm. Although the joint actions in pulling and stopping are the same, the source of energy differs. The momentum of the oncoming object moves the segments in the direction in which the object was moving; at the same time muscular effort resists that motion. As the upper arm is extended by the force of the object the shoulder flexors resist; as the forearm is flexed, the elbow extensors resist. In pulling, the object to be moved resists while shoulder extensors and elbow flexors contract. Likewise, when the body lands from a height, the momentum of the center of gravity tends to cause flexion at the ankle, knee, and hip joints. These actions are resisted by the extensor muscles at the joints.

Catching, falling, and landing are specialized cases of impact, or collision. They represent the impacting of a living body with another living body or with an external object. Each impact creates a situation that might cause injury to the performer. Chapters 15 and 20 were also concerned with collisions between external objects. Although many of the principles described in those chapters are apropos here, their emphasis was on maximal or optimal transference of force (impulse) to the external object without concern for injury.

The basic mechanics involved in stopping a moving object or one's own moving body in action are based on the effective and efficient manner of dissipating the kinetic energy of the moving body without injury to the performer. The kinetic energy ($\frac{1}{2}mV^2$) of an object can be reduced to zero or to other safe limits by the following methods:

1. Using as great a surface area as possible in the catching or landing.
2. Using as great a distance as possible. This may be accomplished through movement of body parts, deformation of body parts, or moving the entire body.
3. Using as great a mass as possible in the catching or landing.
4. Regulating the position of one's center of gravity for dynamic control. For example, in falling, the person is able to continue movement of the body into a controlled rolling action that terminates in a stance, rather than lose equilibrium, which causes the body to

tumble several revolutions and in uncontrolled directions, terminating in an upside-down position.

5. Using materials other than the human body to perform steps 1 to 4.

CATCHING

Catching is the act of reducing the momentum of an object in flight to the point of zero or near zero velocity and retaining possession of it at least momentarily. This is accomplished by using the hands, body, feet, and auxiliary pieces of equipment. The momentum of the object is transferred to the receiving mechanism. When an object is light in weight and traveling slowly, a human being can easily stop it. However, if the object is heavy or is traveling at great speed or both, the transfer of momentum must be gradual to prevent injury to the hands or other parts of the body and to allow the receiver to control the object once in possession of it.

When one part or parts of the body, such as the hands, are held rigid at the moment that a fast-moving object comes in contact with it, the part must absorb the full force of the impact. In sports the momentum of an object being caught is decreased by increasing the distance at which it is caught; this process is known as *giving,* or *recoiling,* with the object until it is traveling slowly enough to be controlled accurately.

If the object to be caught is heavy, such as a large medicine ball, or is traveling unusually fast, such as a fastball thrown by a baseball pitcher, to dissipate its momentum over a long distance may be difficult and will take more time than can be allowed during the process of playing a particular game. The more practical procedure is to increase the mass (inertia) of the stopping mechanism and decrease the distance over which it travels. For example, the baseball catcher dissipates the momentum of the ball thrown by the pitcher by placing the body directly in front of the path of the oncoming ball. He assumes a stance whereby the feet are placed in a stride position with the knees bent and the center of gravity low; this is the best posture in which to recoil from the force (momentum of the ball), and at the same time it offers as much of the body to absorb the momentum of the ball as possible.

The receiver must be careful not to make unnecessary body motions when running to receive an object. Unnecessary up-and-down movements (raising and lowering the center of gravity and thereby moving the head and eyes up and down through a vertical plane) may cause the receiver to lose track of the path of flight of the object. Outstretching the arms (shoulder flexion and elbow extension) while running may cause the receiver to slow down because he is not using the arms properly in the run and also is projecting the center of gravity too far forward. It also may tense the arms and cause him to drop the ball.

A ball is not caught with the fingers; rather it is received first against the middle of the palm of the hand (made into the form of a cup), and then the fingers close around it, preventing it from escaping. If it is caught against the rigid heel of the hand, it is likely to rebound too quickly from the hand and may also cause injury to the hand.

The effective catcher (receiver in any sport or endeavor) has loose, flexible hands to catch the object and to dissipate its momentum gradually. Correct body posture is also essential. Placing the hands in the best possible position is another requirement for success. For example, a ball traveling in flight at a height below the waist is caught with the fingers pointing downward. In all instances the hands are placed so that they have a basketlike quality. Seldom does a good performer not make use of two hands, even though the actual catch is made with one hand. The object (such as a ball) may rebound out of one hand if the momentum is not properly dissipated. The use of both hands aids in trapping the object.

Large objects thrown with great speed, such as a football (which is also thrown with a spin), are caught and then quickly cradled; that is, the receiver pins the football against the body as soon as possible to prevent its escape because of the reaction. If the arms do not have to be extended fully for the catch, the receiver, in this instance, should not do so. In the flexed position the arm muscles can withstand the force of the impact with no chance for injury, since the impact will elicit flexion.

When gloves are used to catch fast-moving objects, two principles can be considered. The first principle is to allow some part other than the human body to absorb the force of impact, which can be considered as having a certain amount of either kinetic energy or momentum. The second principle is that of dissipating the force through a distance. The use of catcher's, fielder's, and first-base gloves is based on these principles (Fig. 21-1).

The catcher's glove usually provides for the material itself to deform; thus the ball embeds in the glove and dissipates its force through a large surface area. The material deforms and provides the increased distance through which to dissipate the force (energy). The first-base glove functions more on the principle of increasing the distance through which the glove moves, thus dissipating the kinetic energy of the ball. The distal end of the glove, and thus the ball, will move approximately 15 cm after initial contact and then, because of its moment of force, cause the hand to move. Then the elbow, shoulder, and other joint angles of the body will change. The fielder's glove incorporates certain features of each of the previously mentioned gloves.

The quantification of what actually happens during catching may be described, with the skill of cradling a lacrosse ball in a lacrosse stick being used as the catching example (Fig. 21-2). When the ball strikes the lacrosse basket, the materials of ball and basket deform, but only the deformation of the basket can be seen. These deformations are not sufficient to prevent rebounding of the ball. Thus the movement of the stick and arms must be performed in the direction of ball flight.

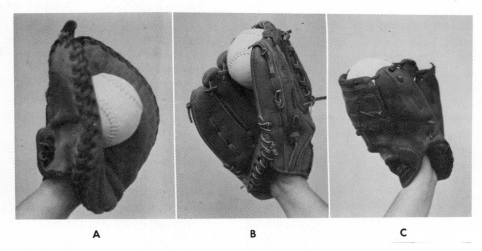

| A | B | C |

Fig. 21-1. Catching a softball with three different mitts. Note the differences in moment arms (ball to wrist) and possible arcs of movement after ball contacts glove (views **A** and **B** as the catching action).

If the flight velocity of the ball had been 20 m/sec before impact, its kinetic energy would be ½mV², or 480 Nm, or joules (based on a ball weight of 2.4 N, which is 0.5 lb). Both deformation of the basket and the reactive forces caused by the lengthening and narrowing of the basket opening reduce the kinetic energy of the ball as much as 90%. Thus the ball velocity for rebounding may be no more than 5 m/sec. Movement of the arms and stick adds mass to the moving ball system and reduces the ball velocity to 0.2 m/sec, based on the conservation-of-momentum principle. Observation of the performance indicates that a distance of 0.6 m is required to reduce the velocity of the ball and arms to zero.

During the game of lacrosse a catching distance of 0.6 m requires too much time and places the ball and stick in an unsatisfactory position. An alternate method of catching involves the cradling, or rotation, of the stick about its longitudinal axis, which causes the ball to rebound from one side of the basket to the other. Thus linear displacement is replaced by rotational displacement for the dissipation of kinetic energy of the ball.

In most sports situations the momentum gained during the catch may be used in starting the next movement. If the next action is to be a throw, the ball is drawn back during the catch in preparation for throwing. Whenever possible the receiver should move the body into position for the next action as the catch is made, to reduce still further the time required for the complete movement. In addition, the momentum of the body and the reconverted momentum of the ball (since it seldom

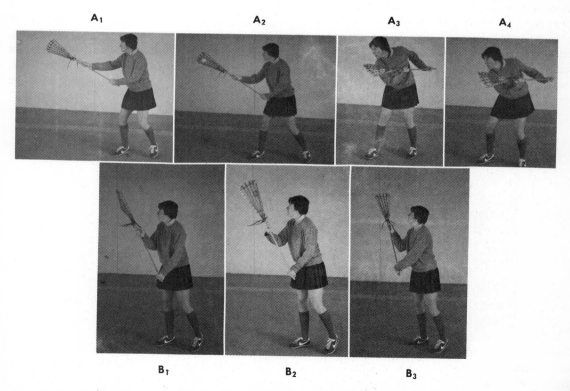

Fig. 21-2. Catching, **A**, and cradling, **B**, techniques used in lacrosse to dissipate kinetic energy of ball.

comes to a complete rest but usually continues in a small angular path as the arm is moved to throw) may be used in moving the ball in the new direction.

FALLING

Correctly performed falling involves a gradual reduction in the momentum of the body when it comes in contact with the floor, ground, or other surface. Four general principles and techniques of protection in falling may be listed:

1. In the sit-down-and-roll technique the center of gravity is lowered, and the action in falling is such that the weight of the body is distributed over a large area. If the fall is vertical, the momentum should be transferred from vertical to horizontal as soon as possible to reduce the force of the fall.
2. The bony projections of the body must be protected by using the fleshy parts as striking surfaces.
3. Extended levers offer a greater potential range of motion than do flexed ones. Therefore when the legs or arms strike the surface in falling, they should be prepared for the contact by being placed in extension or near extension. Care must be taken to avoid hyperextension, which causes the joint to be rigid and to resist flexion of the limb. With the joint at an angle slightly less than 180 degrees, the force of the fall can then be taken by a gradual flexion of the legs or arms.
4. During a fall the landing is made on the feet to maneuver to bring the center of body weight near a position above the feet, thus utilizing the shock-absorbing action of the ankles, knees, and hips.

The recovery from a stumble is mainly reflexive. Both the righting reflex and equilibrium reactions (which are instinctive) are activated. As the ___ trips over an obstacle and the body starts to fall ___ equilibrium reactions are initi- ___ head and trunk are extended to ___ ard momentum. The shoulders ___ to assist in regaining balance. ___ arts to fall to the right side, for

example, usually elevates and abducts the shoulder and extends the elbows (with arms out to the sides). The body is shifted to the left to help check the momentum to the right. The side of the buttocks is offered as the landing surface. The legs are flexed to decrease the force of the blow and to lower the center of gravity so that the distance of the fall is reduced. A rotation of the trunk may take place so that the momentum of the fall is dissipated in two directions—opposite and to the rear. Protective extension of the arms is often used to help dissipate the momentum of the fall. This action, however, has proved dangerous when the elbow has gone into hyperextension. Gymnasts, dancers, and others must be cautioned not to use the rigidly extended arm to attempt to stop the fall.

LANDING

Landing is a type of fall that is both controlled and expected and that enables the performer to strike a surface without incurring injury to the body parts if possible. Landings occur in many activities of life, from the mild ones of foot landings during walking to the landings of ski jumpers, sky divers, and pole vaulters. When a body falls, its vertical force, kinetic energy, and momentum are directly related to the distance through which it falls. Since the rate of falling is 9.8 m/sec^2, the velocity of the body increases exponentially, not linearly, as the height of fall increases. Therefore landing on a rigid, rather nondeformable material is dangerous from heights of 3 m or more. If the landing is headfirst, the result is often death, except for the very young. In the sports arena specialized landing surfaces are required for high jumping, pole vaulting, long jumping, and certain gymnastics events. When a landing cannot be made with the feet, the fleshy parts of the thighs, hips, and shoulders are preferred landing areas. These parts are the primary landing sites in judo. For ectomorphic persons, however, no area of the body may have sufficient ''padding'' for a safe landing, even with landing mats. In such instances the landing should be with the feet unless protective equipment is worn.

Kneepads are common in the sports of volleyball, basketball, football, skateboarding, and soccer. Shin guards are recommended for field hockey and soccer. Thigh pads are used in softball, baseball, and football. It is recommended that hip or thigh protection be used for gymnasts performing on the uneven parallel bars. Padding of the bars may be an alternative to padding the human body. The higher the skill level, the greater the forces are apt to be; however, the lower the skill level, the more it is likely that there will be uncontrolled landings.

In activities in which the landing is the terminal point of the movement pattern, such as in high jumping and pole vaulting, the landing surface is padded, rather than the performer. Both the pole vaulting and landing pits are above ground to decrease the falling height, and therefore the final velocity, of the performer at landing. The pits are made so that the penetration by the performer into the landing pit is approximately half the depth of the landing pit at the time the performer reaches zero vertical velocity. This distance allows a safe rebound from the pit.

Since the vertical drop in long jumping is much less than in pole vaulting or high jumping, and since the landing is on the feet, an elevated landing pit is not needed. A sand pit in which the body can penetrate from 10 to 30 cm into the sand is adequate for safety.

During recent years the public has shown a concern for reducing the injury rate in sports. Manufacturers have produced more and better protective devices to be worn by the performer or on which the performance takes place. Sometimes there are conflicting problems in the manufacturing of a product that must be designed not only to improve safety but also to improve performance. Often an improvement in safety alters the performance capabilities or prevents the attainment of a satisfactory performance. For example, shoulder pads restrict the ability of football line players to raise the arms above shoulder height. Original tumbling mat design and construction allowed the impact forces to be absorbed at landing but prevented a second tumbling movement to be executed directly from that landing. As new materials were developed,

mats with an elastic component were constructed. These mats not only attenuated the energy of landing but gave a "spring" to the performer. As skill levels in tumbling improve and more complex stunts at greater heights are executed, the mats may no longer be safe, or the safe mats of today may limit the acquisition of skill, especially for Olympic-caliber performers.

A similar inadequacy of sports equipment has been noted with respect to jogging. Many persons, estimated in the millions, are jogging several miles on concrete sidewalks and paved streets, and competing in long-distance races on similar terrain. Jogging shoes were not originally designed with the shock attenuation qualities necessary for such conditions. Research that identifies the impact forces and the sites of impact is now helping manufacturers to design safe shoes for jogging.

The Committee on Sports Facilities and Equipment of the American Society for Testing Materials is the standards-setting body in the United States that studies the safety and performance of the equipment and facilities used in sports. Teachers and coaches can help the committee to identify problems and can provide the following information:

1. What types of injuries occur in a specific activity?
2. What landing surfaces and protective devices are used when injuries occur?
3. Which products are unsatisfactory?
4. What is the nature of the performance in which injuries occur—for example, falling from a height, rotary movements, or absorbing forces.

RECEIVING A SPIKE OR SERVICE IN VOLLEYBALL

Served balls and spiked balls usually are received by means of an underarm hit termed a forearm bounce pass, bump, or dig. In these situations the volleyball possesses greater speeds, and therefore more kinetic energy and momentum, than in any other situation occurring in the volleyball game. Thus the volleyball player uses the wrists and forearms as rebounding surfaces, rather than the active flexion of the fingers seen in passing situations. The speed and angle of the incoming spike and serve will determine whether the receiver will attenuate (absorb) the force or will apply force to the ball, and they will also determine the manner in which the force will be directed.

The first goal of the performer receiving a spiked or served ball is to establish a stable base of support. This base is best taken in a parallel stance so that the arms can descend between the legs and the person can achieve the deep squat position necessary for receiving certain spiked balls. Many players modify this stance by placing one foot slightly ahead of the other. This modification may be a compensation for eye and hand dominance. Care must be taken to maintain a stance that is as nearly parallel as possible, for ease in maneuvering and lowering the body. If a one-arm hit is used, a lunge type of stance will replace the parallel stance. Since spiked balls have a primarily downward flight, there is no need to widen the base of support in the anteroposterior direction. Even in the case of served balls, the trajectory is apt to be 30 to 60 degrees with the horizontal. Thus the horizontal momentum will be less than one third that of a fast-pitched softball traveling 257.44 kmph (160 mph) and can be received without loss of balance.

The type of contact and the surfaces of contact will determine the amount of rebound velocity of the ball. Any forward motion of the arms will apply a force to the ball and thus impart additional velocity to it. If the arms are stationary at contact, the amount of tension and the amount of fleshy tissue will determine the amount of attenuation of the force of the ball. For example, a ball dropped from a height of approximately 7 m will rebound almost 2 m after impact on a wooden floor, whereas the ball will rebound only half that distance if the impact is made on a maximally tensed, bony, tendinous surface such as the forearms. If, however, little effort is made to tense the arms, the rebound will be greatly reduced, to less than 20 cm. Thus it is important both to develop kinesthetic awareness of the amount of tension in the arms,

including the shoulder stabilization tension, and to be able to estimate the speed and angle of the incoming ball.

Learning can be facilitated by holding certain environmental considerations constant. Players should be able to use uniformly inflated balls with the same elasticity characteristics and the same material from one day to the next. Any change in ball material, clothing of players, or ball covering may alter the coefficients of friction and of elasticity during contact. Thus an understanding of these mechanical considerations will enable the learner to progress more rapidly than is possible with blind trial and error.

Contour and size of contact area will influence both the consistency of execution of the skill and the likelihood of injury to the body. "The greater the surface area, the less force per square centimeter" is a principle that can be applied to this skill. Injury is not likely to occur to hands; however, forearms do become bruised because the ball impacts against the flesh surrounding the radius and ulna. If there is insufficient adipose tissue or muscle, the deformation caused by the impact will force the small blood vessels against these bones, causing hematoma. Clothing is often worn to protect the forearms from bruises.

The flatness of the contact area is paramount for consistency in directing the ball. Theoretically the anterior surface of the wrist and heel of the hand are best because of their flatness and large surface area. There is the problem of stabilizing the two hands so that the forearms act as one unit. Normally it is not recommended that the hands or the heels of the hands be used for contact on the bump. The contact should be above the wrist and below the elbow, on the fleshy portion of the forearm, although some persons do clasp the hands together and use the radial surfaces of the hands as the contact site.

The positioning of the rebounding surfaces for the desired angle of rebound is done primarily by means of shoulder flexion. The angle of the arms with respect to the trajectory of the ball determines, in part, the angle of rebound. For example, if the ball enters at a 90-degree angle to the arms, it will rebound at a nearly 90-degree angle. These angles of rebound and incidence are nearly alike in volleyball except for balls with spin and for impacts in which the arms are moving. This statement is based on Newton's third law and the coefficients of friction and elasticity. As the ball rebounds, the speed can be vectorally added to show the influence of spin, elasticity, and friction. Knowing the incoming speed of the ball, a person could predict the speed and angle of the rebound. Fig. 24-1 shows two volleyball spiking patterns.

MINI LABORATORY EXERCISES

1. Rank the kinetic energy (KE) of the following falling bodies (vertical direction) and the approaching objects (horizontal direction), using the formula $KE = \frac{1}{2}mV^2$.
   a. Adult, 588 N, jumping from a bus step, 1 m above ground
   b. Diver, 490 N, diving from a 3-m board
   c. Ball, 19.6 N, traveling 10 m/sec
   d. Long jumper, 588 N, with center of gravity 2 m above ground
   e. Ball, 9.8 N, traveling 30 m/sec
   f. Pole vaulter, 534 N, clearing a 5-m bar with a 1.5-m landing pit

List one or more factors or methods useful in dissipating the kinetic energy of these moving objects.
2. Observe persons catching two medicine balls of different weights. Describe the effectiveness of the action in response to both a moderate speed of flight and a fast speed of flight.
3. Catch a softball in the following manner:
   a. With "board hands," remaining stiff and letting the ball rebound
   b. With hands
   c. With forearms and abdomen
   d. With hands and under conditions of increasing speed of flight until the ball "stings" at impact
   e. With a mitt and at increasing speeds (greater than those used in step d)

ADDITIONAL READINGS

Broer, M.R., and Zernicke, R.F.: Efficiency of human movement, Philadelphia, 1979, W.B. Saunders Co.

Doherty, J.K.: Modern track and field, Englewood Cliffs, N.J., 1964, Prentice-Hall, Inc.

Hodgson, V.R., and Thomas, L.M.: Biomechanical study of football head impacts using a human head model, final report, Detroit, 1973, National Operating Committee on Standards for Athletic Equipment.

Hay, J.A.: The biomechanics of sports techniques, ed. 2, Englewood Cliffs, N.J., 1978, Prentice-Hall, Inc.

CHAPTER 22

Activities of daily living

Probably the most important area of concern to the expert in analysis of movement is the area of movement patterns that have been identified as activities of daily living (ADL). Herein lie the foundation for survival and the basis for many work and leisure activities, including sports and dance. A large number of an adult's waking hours are spent in ADL or activities of work. Data from the 1970s show that persons over 60 years of age spend almost all their time with ADL and engage in few, if any, other types of activities. As one becomes older, the ADL become more difficult to perform, especially if these activities have been performed inefficiently—that is, in less than a biomechanically sound manner—in one's youth. The research in this area has been conducted mainly to identify problems of physically disabled persons, dysfunctioning, and unsafe conditions. In addition, ADL research is important to the construction of prostheses, braces, and other orthotic devices. Limited research exists concerning normal ADL analysis. This chapter will describe and analyze ADL for which research has been conducted. Although some reference will be made to the need for adequate strength, range of motion, balance, and other anatomic attributes, Chapter 23 will describe exercises for improvement of these attributes. The reader then can use the principles identified in that chapter to improve specific ADL for persons showing weaknesses in one or more areas.

The six major classifications of ADL are as follows:

1. Locomotion: walking, ascending and descending stairs, stepping into buses
2. Changing levels: moving from chair to standing, moving from bed to standing, stooping, reaching
3. Lifting and carrying groceries, suitcases, and other objects
4. Pushing and pulling: using a wheelbarrow, manual lawn mower, rolling pin, typewriter
5. Working with long-handled implements: axe, hoe, broom
6. Working with small implements: pencil, saw, hammer, knitting needles, eating utensils, hatchet

In general, ADL consist primarily of movements performed at slow to moderate speeds, the majority of movements requiring little muscle effort. When the task could be strenuous, persons (especially older persons) will rest frequently or avoid performing the task.

LOCOMOTION
Walking

Since walking patterns were discussed in Chapter 10, the reader is referred to that chapter for a general analysis of walking. A checklist is provided here to enumerate the basic considerations for the analysis and improvement of walking patterns of older persons in their homes and life spaces and of persons with physical disabilities.

1. Is the coefficient of friction optimal for prevention of slipping and for generation of

force? If not, which surfaces can be changed?

2. Have the anatomic characteristics of the person changed since successful walking occurred and present walking dysfunction was noted? Assess the weight, specific muscle strength of "walking muscles," postural deviations, and neuromuscular functioning (such as balance) to determine which factors are probable causes of walking dysfunction. Determine a means for modifying the walking pattern or correcting the factor.

3. Do imposed environmental conditions, such as carrying packages, interfere with an otherwise skilled walking pattern? If so, use the principles of moments and the assistance of devices to alleviate the problem.

Ascending stairs

Ascending stairs poses a problem to many persons who have weak leg extensors. The leg is lifted by the contraction of quadriceps and flexors at the hip, and the foot is placed on the next step, which is usually 23 cm higher than the preceding one. The body weight, then, must be lifted 23 cm, which has been selected as the optimal height for the average adult. One can easily see from Fig. 22-1 that stairs are not easily executed by children. The amount of leg lift and the optimal angles at the hip and knee joints will differ for individuals who have varying leg lengths. However, all persons show a greater range of motion at the knee, hip, and ankle during stair locomotion than during walking on level ground. Thus muscle weakness will affect the stair climbing pattern of obese and short persons to a greater extent than that of tall and lightweight persons.

Lifting the body requires that the center of gravity of the body be shifted from the rear foot to the

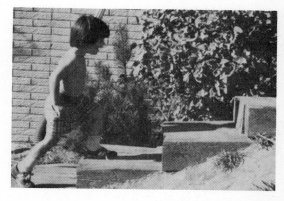

Fig. 22-1. Stair climbing by young child. Note angle at hip and at knee during initial contact, with lead leg on ground.

new supporting foot and that the rear foot initiate plantar flexion. This plantar flexion will raise the center of gravity of an adult male with a size 7 foot approximately 8 cm. Thus one third of the total distance through which the body weight must be lifted may be achieved by this action. This action is not as effective for persons with smaller feet, notably children. The ideal sequential timing of extension at the hip and knee of the lead leg with respect to plantar flexion of the rear foot produces a series of acceleration forces caused by these muscle contractions. Thus the summation of these forces facilitates the raising of the center of gravity of the body the necessary 23 cm to the next step. In this manner a person can compensate for weak quadriceps muscles, which are the primary muscles used by many healthy young persons in stair locomotion.

Correct placement of the total foot on each stair tread is important for individuals who have balance problems. Unfortunately, some stairs do not have sufficiently wide treads to allow large persons, who often weigh more than average, to place the total foot on the tread. One must be careful not to place the foot so far forward that the toe catches on the lip of the step as the foot is lifted.

Placement of the total foot on the tread allows the muscles crossing the ankle joint to relax and places the foot in a neutral position. From this position the foot dorsiflexes as the other leg enters the swing phase of ascent. This dorsiflexed position allows the person to generate greater force because of the greater distance through which plantar flexion can be accelerated, compared to the person who uses the ball of the foot during the support phase of ascending stairs.

Another advantage of the neutral position of the foot is that it releases tension in the gastrocnemius and thereby facilitates extension at the knee. This facilitation occurs because the gastrocnemius crosses the knee, as well as the ankle. With the absence of tension in the gastrocnemius, the quadriceps can move the leg with less force than if cocontraction between agonists and antagonists existed.

There is, however, a critical speed of ascent at which most persons will prefer to use only the ball of the foot rather than the whole foot. Although this critical speed will vary with individuals, it represents the speed at which the person rapidly passes through each single-support phase; that is, there is no sensing of a static single-support position. The faster the speed of ascent, the more pronounced will be the absence of full foot contact. With speed, however, the likelihood of the person's ascending two steps at a time is great. A person may again use the full foot contact, since the height to which the leg must be lifted is lowest with a full-foot landing than with any other type of landing. In addition, passive plantar flexion of the foot can take place, thus shifting the center of gravity of the body forward and upward with little muscle effort.

Physical disabilities and ascending stairs. Common modifications made by persons with physical disabilities when they are ascending stairs are of two types: (1) a handrail is used, and (2) the person

marks time, that is, places both feet on each tread. The use of a handrail not only compensates for balance dysfunction but provides a reactive surface for the hand. Arm extension thus produces another force for raising the body and compensating for weak quadriceps.

Persons who have had a stroke or other trauma that has resulted in the failure of one leg to function as well as the other should lead with the non-traumatized leg when ascending stairs. For these persons total foot placement, strengthening of extensor muscle groups, strengthening of lateral and medial stabilizing muscles, and exact control of the center of gravity with respect to the base of support are important requirements for success in ascending stairs.

Descending stairs

The problems imposed by the act of descending stairs are opposite those of ascending stairs. Whereas ascending stairs results in positive work (the product of body weight and height), descending stairs is negative work, since the muscles eccentrically contract to regulate the speed of descent caused by gravity. Once again, the line of gravity is shifted from one tread to the next via each foot, and greater stability is achieved with contact of the total foot than with the ball of the foot. The ball of the foot, however, usually makes the initial contact with the tread; thus the body weight may gradually be lowered the final centimeters of the total distance of descent.

Persons may turn the foot for a diagonal placement if the foot is too long for the tread width. This pattern is noted frequently in persons running downstairs. However, in this case the ball of the foot may be the only part of the foot contacting the stairs. A person using a fast descent allows gravity to accelerate the descent of the body, thereby minimizing the amount of eccentric muscle contraction. The person has confidence that the end of the stairway will be reached before the acceleration causes lack of body control.

Physical disabilities and descending stairs. Persons with physical disabilities should lead with the disabled leg when descending stairs, since maximal stability is required on the upper tread during the lowering of the lead leg. The nondisabled leg can be lowered quickly as soon as the lead leg is supported. This action minimizes the amount of time during which the impaired leg is the sole support of body weight.

The same principles are applicable for both descending and ascending stairs. The person maintains dynamic stability, utilizes forward and upward momentum to maintain dynamic inertia, and involves a sequencing of muscle contractions to create acceleration of the body in the desired path. Modifications are made in the pattern according to anatomic characteristics of the performer and environmental conditions. When the coefficient of friction is less than optimal, horizontal forces are reduced and vertical forces increased.

MINI LABORATORY EXERCISES

1. Measure the angles at the knee and hip for persons of different heights as each assumes a stair-ascending position with each foot on a different tread. Rank the persons with respect to ease of ascent, based solely on the collected data. Give reasons for your choice of ranking.
2. Calculate the work done by four individuals of different body weight when they are ascending one set of stairs, using the following formula:

$$\text{Body weight} \times \text{Total height of stairs} = \text{Work done}$$

3. Calculate the maximal power achieved by these same individuals when they ascend this same set of stairs as fast as possible, using the following formula:

$$\text{Work} \div \text{Time of ascent} = \text{Power}$$

4. Ask one person performing in steps 2 and 3 to perform with a packsack, heavy coat, heavy boots, or other weight attached or carried. Calculate work and power. (NOTE: Body weight now includes addition of clothing or load.)
5. Discuss the results of steps 2 to 4.

CHANGING LEVELS

Rising from a bed and chair and lowering oneself to these pieces of furniture involve the same general principles as described in locomotion on stairs. Weak quadriceps muscles usually are the limiting factor in the ability to rise from furniture. The lower the furniture, the more difficulty will be encountered by the person, since the person must perform more work (raise the center of gravity a greater distance) and will begin the movement at an unfavorable angle of muscle pull. In addition, the type of material and the construction of the furniture seat influence the method of rising. Mattresses and cushions do not provide a sufficiently rigid surface for the generation of reactive forces and therefore pose a greater problem than do rigid chairs.

The following general principles and movement analysis are useful for the improvement of the act of rising from furniture. The first action by the person desiring to rise from a chair is to move the center of gravity near the edge of the chair seat. Next, the person places one foot under the chair and one foot slightly in front of the chair legs. The person shifts the center of gravity over the new base of support, the feet, and stands by means of leg extension. If the muscles of the leg are not strong enough to raise the body weight at the initial angle of execution, the person may accelerate the trunk by alternating actions in the sagittal plane and may use the acceleration (which might be redefined as energy or momentum) of that body part to assist the muscles of the legs to create the necessary force to lift the weight of the body. In addition, the arms can be used to add a counterforce to the body weight, by pushing against the chair or against the thighs. The latter action directly aids in extension at the knee joint.

Another example of the use of momentum of a body part to facilitate the performance of a movement pattern is found in the act of rising from a bed. Since the full length of the body may be distributed on the bed, the legs can be raised from the bed and then allowed to swing toward the floor with the help of gravity. This leg swing then raises the trunk to a sitting position. If the leg swing is facilitated by muscle contraction, the momentum of the leg swing may produce enough trunk motion to propel the person into a standing position with the help of a hand push against the bed. This technique utilizes both the strong muscles that cross the hip joint and the momentum of approximately one third of the body mass to compensate for weak muscles crossing the knee.

Stooping, squatting, and sitting on the floor or ground are patterns common to scrubbing floors, placing items in drawers and cabinets, dusting furniture, picking up shoes and other items from the floor, and doing certain gardening tasks. With the advent of many laborsaving devices, some of these tasks have been eliminated from daily activity patterns, and others have even been eliminated altogether. There are instances, however, when stooping or sitting on the floor may be necessary and desirable. Laborsaving tools do not find items that are dropped on the floor, do not clean the corners of the room, and are not worth the cost or effort for such tasks as putting one potted plant into the ground. These activities require greater ranges of motion at the hip and knee joints than walking and stair locomotion. Greater strength is needed to initiate the upward movement from the squat or sitting position on the floor than is required to rise from a chair or bed.

There are numerous ways to descend to and rise from the floor-sitting position. Persons over 70 years of age and young children select methods on an individual basis. Three patterns of young children are shown in Fig. 22-2. Older persons use all these patterns. The strength of the quadriceps with respect to body weight, the distribution of body weight, balancing capabilities, and previous experiences with success at the initial learning age are some reasons that may be cited for the particular method selected by a person. Several patterns are nevertheless possible because none requires maximal contraction of muscles. Therefore persons can be inefficient until the task becomes one of maximal, or nearly maximal, effort because of a physical disability. Then efficiency is sought in the pattern. For example, efficiency is a necessary requirement in teaching a stroke patient to rise from the floor.

Since one side of the body usually is disabled after a stroke, the stroke patient should place the foot of the disabled leg close to the hips when attempting to rise from a seated position on the floor. The other leg is raised to a position supported by the knee and shank. The center of gravity is shifted to the foot, and the hands exert a push against the floor. If the leg is not strong enough to extend to the standing position, the person should grasp a piece of furniture to assist the extension of the leg, much the same as the handrail is used in stair locomotion.

A major concern of kinesiologists is the incidence of injury to the knee as a result of squatting, kneeling, and stooping. As the squat position is achieved, the knee is placed in an open position, or what is sometimes termed a loosely packed position. This makes the knee vulnerable to dislocation and rupturing of ligaments or muscles crossing the joint. If these tissues are strong, it is unlikely that an injury will occur. There is, however, a danger of injury because of loss of balance or a deliberate twisting motion that would place excessive stress on the knee. The knee would then be injured because of the torsion, not the separation in the sagittal plane. Obese persons, persons who discover that they cannot rise from the squat position, and persons who attempt to perform movements requiring greater balance and strength capabilities than they possess are the most vulnerable to injury during squatting activities.

Persons desiring to perform the squat after not having attempted a squat for some length of time should test their ability to do so as follows:

1. If possible, perform the movement in water.
2. Assume the squat position while horizontal to check the range of motion and to eliminate the effect of gravity.
3. Assume a semisquat position.
4. With the assistance of a person, chair, or some other aid, assume the squat position.

At the first sign of pain the movement should be discontinued until strengthening exercises can increase the stability of the knee joint.

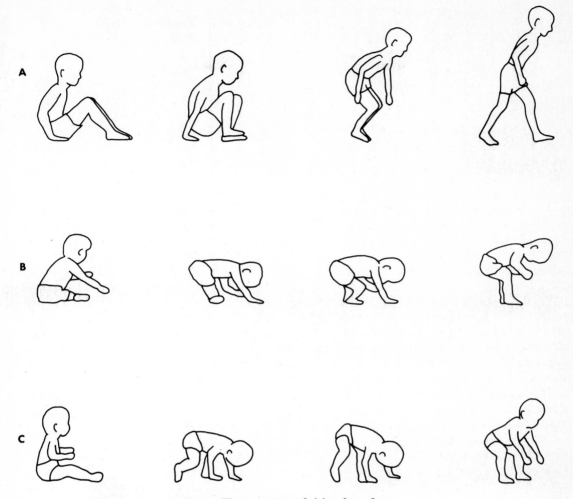

Fig. 22-2. Three patterns of rising from floor.

LIFTING

The proper way to lift objects from the floor or other low position has been a topic in most kinesiology textbooks and industrial safety pamphlets because of the vulnerability of the human body to low back injury. Fig. 22-3 shows three methods of picking up an object. The weight vector for the object and its moment arm from the principal axis of lifting motion can be drawn. Based on these facts, position A would have the least moment of resistance force and would have the least stress on the trunk, more specifically the lumbar region. Position B would primarily need lumbar extensor muscles to counteract the object being lifted. Depending on the weight of the object, however, either one or the other or both may be acceptable methods of lifting the object. Position C is never acceptable because it places stress on the posterior of the knee and stiffens the legs in a position of genu recurvatum.

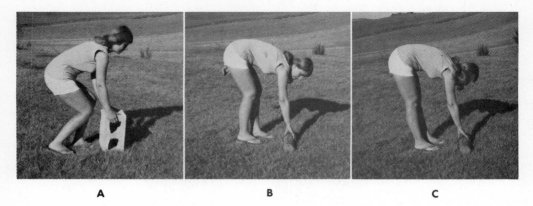

Fig. 22-3. Three methods of lifting an object from the ground. **A**, Least stress on spinal column. **B**, Acceptable stress on spinal column. **C**, Undesirable stress on knee and spinal column.

If the weight of the object is light, either position *A* or *B* is acceptable, providing the person is not so heavy that the musculature cannot control the action of stooping and returning to a stand. The obese person is more apt to stoop rather than squat because the leg strength would probably be insufficient for rising from a squat. If the object is heavy, an obese person might not be able to achieve success with position *A* but could swing the object toward the legs, using position *B* in much the same way a weight lifter does. The moment arm for the resistance is decreased, and then the object can be lifted with the back. There is danger in such a pattern because the swing may not remain in one plane and could therefore cause a twisting of the trunk and vertebral damage. Probably a combination of slight knee flexion and trunk flexion is the most effective and safest method of lifting heavy objects.

Chaffin has shown that there is a direct relationship between the amount of stress in the lumbar region on one hand and the horizontal distance of the object from the person's base of support and the vertical distance the object is moved on the other. Therefore the safest position is one in which the object is near the center of gravity of the body. This position minimizes the moment arm of the resistance.

USE OF IMPLEMENTS

Long-handled implements. When human beings use long-handled implements such as rakes, hoes, brooms, axes, and shovels, the interfacing of the body size to the implement is an important consideration. For taller-than-average individuals, the commercially available long-handled implements may be too short for efficient use. The person must then assume a stooped posture that promotes excessive tension in the neck and upper back muscles, as well as possible tension in the lumbar region. Taller persons should thus adapt to the implement by performing the task with an increased flexion at the knees and hips to maintain a more efficient trunk position. Shorter-than-average persons must adapt to the average-length implements by adjusting the placement of the hands.

Long-handled implements require the user to establish the most efficient lever system possible, sacrificing movement distance for force improvement in many cases. For example, when using a long-handled shovel to lift a load of dirt, the person will separate the hands to produce a first-class lever system. The hand nearer the load will act as the fulcrum (axis of rotation), and the more distant hand will exert a force downward through a long distance (Fig. 22-4). Thus the hand supporting the weight of the shovel and dirt is at or near the bal-

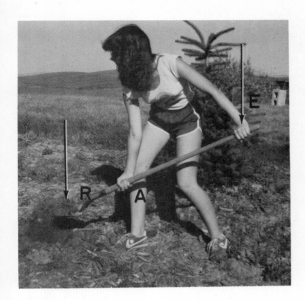

Fig. 22-4. Lifting dirt with long-handled shovel. This is a first-class lever system. (*R*, Resistance; *A*, axis; *E*, effort.)

ance point of the system. The long moment arm of the handle of the shovel allows movement with a significant mechanical force advantage. Use of the large muscle groups—the leg muscles and the oblique muscles of the trunk—to lift and even to support the implement is also a means of utilizing the implement more efficiently.

In some instances the person will push, slide, or pull the implement to move a resisting material, rather than lift it. These other actions, such as sweeping and raking, require less muscle effort and produce less work (and therefore less energy) than does lifting. The exception is the type of action in which there is an unusually high coefficient of friction for the materials involved, such as shoveling wet, heavy snow.

The act of chopping wood with an ax resembles many of the actions described in tennis serves and in other overarm patterns used in sports. The use of the implement necessitates holding the handle near the ax head on the upswing to decrease the resistance moment arm and to increase control over the implement. The other hand is placed at the end of the handle. The body counterrotates, and the ax is lifted in a curved path above the head. The back hyperextends and the legs flex. On the forward swing of the ax the body rotates, the trunk flexes, and the legs extend as one hand slides to meet the other hand at the end of the handle. This latter action increases the moment arm and thus the arc and velocity of the ax head as the ax swings forward and downward. Trunk flexion carries the force of the ax through the wood as the muscle force and gravity combine to accelerate the weight of the ax head.

As with sports skills, the greatest acceleration occurs at the instant of contact, and the best performer accelerates the fastest or through the greatest distance. The taller and longer-limbed person has the potential for creating the greatest force. However, since multiple levers are acting, the coordinated timing of these levers and the body's neuromuscular speed determine the effectiveness of the act. Thus shorter persons might outperform taller persons even when using a less coordinated pattern. Note the path of the ax head for a tall person and for a short person chopping wood, as depicted in Fig. 22-5.

MINI LABORATORY EXERCISES

1. Describe the pattern of hoeing.
2. Given the following conditions, explain how the basic pattern just described would be modified. Use the theoretical model presented in Chapter 2.
3. List the key concepts and principles that necessitated the modifications you indicate.
   a. Condition A: hoe blade decreased in size by 50%
   b. Condition B: ground made up of hard clay
   c. Condition C: handle reduced by 0.66 m

Small implements. Most ADL skills involve the use of small implements. One of the best approaches to the study of these movements has been developed by the time-motion analysts (human engineers). These persons have analyzed movements required in industrial tasks and have set guidelines and made modifications in the human-machine task or in the environment to improve the

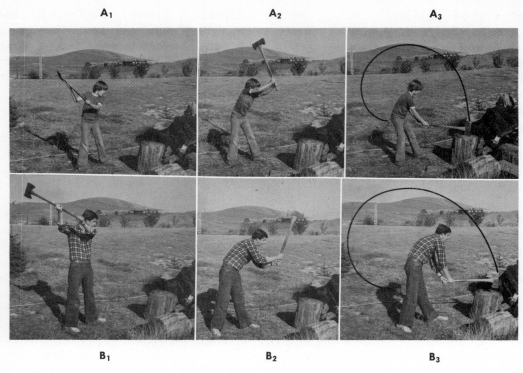

Fig. 22-5. Movement pattern of ax during wood chopping by two persons of different stature.

efficiency of the human-machine operation. Because of the financial need to obtain maximal production for minimal cost, including minimal cost in human years of productivity, the analysis of industrial tasks has a solid scientific basis. Scientific analyses of ADL involving small implements are needed if we are to accrue these same benefits of human productivity in daily life. Persons who are older, the weak, or physically disabled need efficiency in their daily tasks. The young and strong need to learn this efficiency to help others or help themselves, especially in later life.

The three basic components to be considered, once again, are time, space, and force. The direction, range, speed, and rate of sequencing of each directional part (thurblig) of a movement task are studied to determine whether or not the values of each allow the person to perform the task with a minimum of force and a minimum of nonessential movements. In addition, the required posture for the task is evaluated by the same criteria. The last step in the analysis is to identify variations and inefficiency caused by anatomic differences.

For tasks in the home that will be repeated or performed for several minutes' duration, the following guidelines may be considered as biomechanical principles for efficiency:

1. Keep the distance of travel of the arms and hands in an area that allows the trunk to remain stable and without excess tension. The shoulders should be in a relaxed position, not elevated, retracted, or protracted. The arc of a horizontal plane depicting this travel would be approximately 120 degrees, with mid position being at the midline of the body and a radius of the length of the person's arm. The vertical space to be used is approxi-

mately from shoulder to elbow. This vertical distance provides the optimal working position for the trunk and causes minimal lifting of the upper arms, thus maintaining a low energy level.

2. Whenever possible, use curved movements rather than linear movements requiring changes in direction. An increase or a decrease in the curvature of motion requires less force than stopping movement in one line and initiating movement in another line. The inertia of a moving body increases the efficiency in the former action but decreases efficiency in the latter action.

3. Horizontal movements have an advantage over vertical movements. The work against gravity is virtually zero in movements in the horizontal plane. One need only counteract the mass of the limbs, since there are no vertical accelerations. Most movements that are slow to moderate in speed and that require little force are performed more efficiently with horizontal movements than with vertical ones.

4. When gravity can be used to facilitate the movement, vertical movements have an advantage over horizontal ones. The upward lifting of the arms is performed close to the body to decrease the moments of force. On the downward movements the arms are moved away from the body and allowed to accelerate without muscle effort. Thus gravity-assisted movements are very efficient. An example of such a movement is the act of hammering a nail into wood.

5. Allow the large (strong) muscles to perform the work task. Pulling motions are usually done best in the anteroposterior plane, and pushing motions are done in the horizontal plane (lateral movements). Women, especially, tend to have weak forearm extensors and thus are ineffective in pushing with the arms solely in the anteroposterior plane.

6. Perform essential movements only.

7. Establishing a rhythm tends to eliminate nonessential movements and to utilize the momentum of one thurblig in the next thurblig. (See Chapter 9 for details concerning the use of rhythm in movements.)

Fatigue becomes a factor to consider with many ADL, hobby, and work tasks. The rate at which work can be done decreases with time unless the optimal pace is set for the individual. This pace may have to be determined by trial and error, but the number of trials necessary to find the optimal pace may be decreased by following these steps.

1. Ask the person to select a pace and rhythm.
2. Observe the person's performance, noting signs of excessive tension such as shoulder bracing and head movements.
3. If tension is noted, ask the person to decrease the pace. If tension is not noted, ask the person to increase the pace.
4. Observe the performance again.
5. Make further corrections in pace if necessary.

POSTURES

Standing posture for ADL. It has been suggested that the commonly used standing position for work tasks is a potentially harmful one, and it is one that has been reinforced in many school and work situations. This deleterious position is one in which the feet are together, the lower limbs are stiffened, and the upper body is in a flexed position. This posture produces sustained tension that may lead to loss of normal elasticity of the tissue, reduced circulatory efficiency, progressive reduction in the range of movement, and chronic general fatigue.

If persons work with their hands while in a standing position, the tendency is to hyperextend the legs and to create excessive tension in the chest and cervical regions. Persons should be taught to actively relax the muscles in the chest and neck and to flex the legs while performing work and ADL tasks. The feet should be separated into a forward and backward position for balance and reduced tension.

To avoid pooling of blood in the legs, excessive pressure on the blood vessels, which may cause partial occlusion of flow, and increased muscular

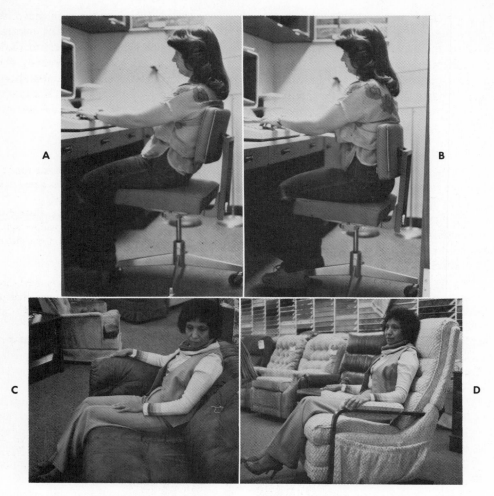

Fig. 22-6. Effects of chair design on sitting posture. **A**, Lordosis. **B**, Erect trunk. **C**, No support for head. **D**, Feet do not reach floor.

tension, a person should move about frequently, at least every 10 minutes. A 10-minute rest during each hour of physical labor is recommended for more productive work.

Sitting postures. Just as persons may assume, out of habit, a standing posture for long periods of time that is not efficient and may in fact cause postural deviations, they may also assume undesirable sitting postures (Fig. 22-6). In some instances the sitting posture is assumed incorrectly because of preference; in other instances the furniture evokes a particular posture. For many years, the design of seats in commercial airplanes produced a forward tilt of the head and discomfort in certain passengers with respect to upper trunk position and sitting height. Fortunately, these seats have been redesigned by some of the airline companies to eliminate the problem.

The soft-cushioned chair produces a different type of problem: pressure on thighs and lumbar

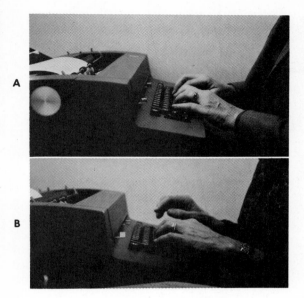

Fig. 22-7. Two styles of typewriting. **A,** Hands and forearms are relatively stable, with muscles in continual state of contraction. **B,** Hands lift intermittently, providing periods of muscle relaxation but also causing muscle effort to raise hands.

curve. The straight-backed chair provides the best support of buttocks, thighs, and back. However, the height of a chair also affects the comfort of the sitter. The feet should reach the floor, with a leeway of no more than a few centimeters. If the feet-to-floor distance is not optimal, persons may assume a slouch position (Fig. 22-6, *D*) that is inefficient and places the body trunk in a potentially dangerous position. The abdominal muscles and the erector spinae muscles or both may contract to form a rigid bridge of the lower trunk, or there may be excessive pressure on the trunk in the lumbar region. Increased lumbar curvature (lordosis) may result from prolonged sitting in this manner.

What, then, is the best furniture design for persons with back problems? The furniture must provide support for the lower back, forcing the lumbar curve to flatten. Any number of designs can be used to achieve this goal, but the straight-backed, rigid chair designed centuries ago still remains one of the best designs, along with the newer reclining chair.

MINI LABORATORY EXERCISES

1. Compare the two styles of typewriting shown in Fig. 22-7. Apply the principles of efficiency and determine which style is more efficient.
2. Attach a pedometer or estimate the amount of walking or running performed by the following:
   a. Airline cabin crew members on one flight
   b. Players in a basketball game
   c. Yourself on a typical weekday
3. Discuss the adjustments in equipment and technique that would be made by a carpenter having a choice of four hammers with two different head weights and two different shaft lengths. The carpenter would hammer nails for 2 hours each under the following conditions:
   a. Into a floor
   b. Into a ceiling
   c. Into a wall

REFERENCE

Chaffin, D.B., Herrin, G.D., Keyserling, M., and Garg, A.: A method for evaluating the biomechanical stresses resulting from manual materials handling jobs, Am. Indust. Hyg. Assoc. J. **38,** Dec., 1977.

ADDITIONAL READINGS

Carlsöö, S.: How man moves: kinesiological studies and methods, London, 1972, William Heinemann, Ltd.

Hilleboe, H.E., and Larimore, G.W.: Preventive medicine, ed. 2, Philadelphia, 1965, W.B. Saunders Co.

Metheny, E.: Body dynamics, New York, 1951, McGraw-Hill Book Co.

Williams, M., and Lissner, H.R.: Biomechanics of human motion, Philadelphia, 1962, W.B. Saunders Co.

CHAPTER 23

Biomechanics of exercises

Exercises should be based on biomechanical and physiologic principles. The goals of the exercises should be clearly defined, and the exercise pattern must ensure that the goals are met and that no deleterious "side effects" result. From the biomechanical perspective, exercises may be classified in four general groups: (1) exercises to improve strength of muscles, ligaments, or bones, (2) exercises to improve power of muscles, (3) exercises to increase range of motion, and (4) exercises to increase neuromuscular functioning. Most exercise programs center on the first and third groups and, from a physiologic perspective, on the improvement of the cardiovascular and respiratory systems. This latter category, however, can be considered from the biomechanical perspective as well. For example, improvement of the strength of the heart and respiratory muscles occurs as the cardiovascular and respiratory systems improve.

MUSCLE STRENGTH AND POWER

Improvement of strength. Since improvement of strength in bones and ligaments cannot be measured directly in living beings, this section will describe the biomechanics of improvement of strength in muscles. The assumption must be made, then, that the ligaments of the joints crossed by the contracting muscles, and the bones to which these muscles are attached, will be strengthened concurrently with the strengthening of the muscles.

Exercises to improve strength may have as their goal an increase in strength for a particular sport competition, activity of daily living, or job-related skill; the rehabilitation of an injured limb; or the modification of upright posture. The muscle or other body part to be strengthened should be identified so that the type of exercise that will produce maximal benefits can be selected. The movement plane and the angle of the limb should be specifically defined and adhered to throughout the exercise, since changes in position may negate the original purpose and muscle function. Finally, the resistance and the resistance moment of force should be quantified to determine relative difficulty of the exercise and probable degree of improvement.

The importance of these guidelines is illustrated by observing the two positions of a person performing a leg press on a machine such as the Universal Gym. Note the undesirable position in Fig. 23-1, A and B, which necessitates a lighter load for success as compared to the position in Fig. 23-1, C and D, in which it is possible to move a heavier load. The persons in A and B have an unsatisfactory mechanical advantage for the hip extensors and an undesirable force vector against the foot plates. Knowledge of moment arms and muscle angles of pull and an ability to estimate them will allow the exercise directors and participants to determine the relative difficulty of each selected exercise. They will also be able to determine the

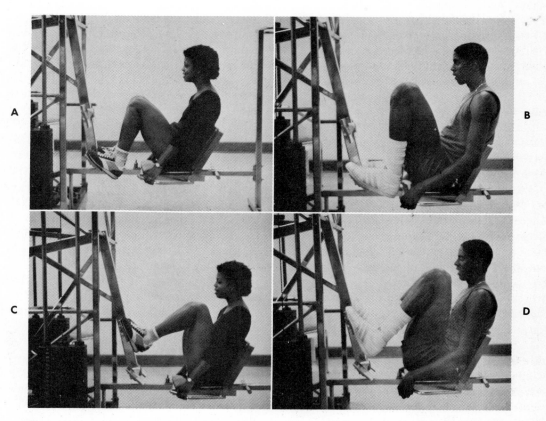

Fig. 23-1. Two persons performing leg press on weight machine. Differences in body segment angles, muscle angles of push, and direction of application of force are depicted for both foot plates.

most scientifically sound initial load and to progressively increase the load according to the individual's increase in strength. In this way the optimal regimen for improvement of strength may be formulated.

Since the human being walks on two feet in an upright position, the anterior muscles of the trunk tend to be underdeveloped and weak. The abdominal muscles in particular are usually inadequate for protection of the lumbar curve of the spine during both heavy lifting and the carrying of a fetus. To understand the role of the abdominal muscles, ask a person to lie down in the supine position. When a person is lying supine, the lumbar curve increases, and persons usually can place their hands under the curvature and encounter no resistance. This increased curvature causes an increase in compression at the posterior edges of the disks of the vertebrae. The rectus abdominis muscle can contract to tilt the pelvis and thereby decrease the curve and reduce the stress to the spine. If the abdominal muscle is not strong enough to reduce this stress, there is potential danger of damaging the disks.

One of the most common abdominal strengthening exercises is the sit-up, with its many variations. As the sit-up is initiated, the iliopsoas muscle contracts, tilting the pelvis into an increased lumbar curve and preventing trunk flexion. This lack of trunk flexion prevents the shortening of the moment arm of the part of the body being lifted from the floor, thereby creating a large moment of force about the vertebrae as the person lifts the upper body from the floor. Only the anterior ligaments and muscles can oppose this resistance moment. Thus the rectus abdominis contracts to decrease the lumbar curve, thereby facilitating trunk flexion during the sit-up and reducing the stress to the lumbar vertebrae.

Based on the equation of moments of force, a selection of gradated exercises may be made. Fig. 23-2 illustrates the differences in resistance moments for various sit-ups. The resistance is equal to the weight of the upper body, that is, from the hip joint to the top of the head, including the arms.

The moment arm is measured by the distance from the hip joint to the center of gravity of the upper body according to the distribution of the body parts. When an external weight is added to the upper body, the total resistance is the sum of this external weight and the weight of the upper body. Note the variation in moment arms and the effects of the weight of the legs on the resultant resistance moments of force that are illustrated in Fig. 23-2.

One must understand the anatomy of the body to know precisely what roles the muscles are likely to perform. In the example of the sit-up, the rectus abdominis does not create flexion at the hip joint or cause the sit-up action. It stabilizes the pelvis in the desired position to prevent injury to the spine, and it facilitates the flexed trunk position. The action of the iliopsoas and other flexors at the hip can be more nearly equalized with that of the rectus abdominis by performing sit-ups with flexed legs in the hook lying position.

If a sit-up is too difficult, the deleterious effects may outweigh the beneficial effects. An increased lumbar curve resulting in pain in the lumbar region may result despite the fact that the rectus abdominis has increased in strength. The reason is that the iliopsoas also gains in strength during sit-ups, and quite often this gain in strength is several times greater than the strength gain in the abdominal muscles. If the back is not flexed during sit-ups, little gain in abdominal strength results. Thus, rather than the complete sit-up, persons with weak abdominal muscles might well do head and shoulder raises, static V sitting positions, or sit-downs.

Strength exercises may be subdivided into isotonic (same tension), isometric (same length), and isokinetic (same velocity) exercises. Isotonic exercises, though misnamed, are the most common because the exercised body part moves through an angular displacement, as when weights are used and in everyday tasks. Quite often, however, the starting position is a weak position when weights are being lifted. Thus the capability of the muscle at all positions other than the starting position is

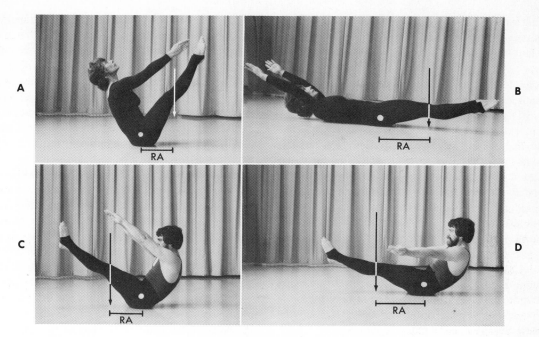

Fig. 23-2. Differences in moment arms during V types of sit-ups. (Arrows represent gravitational force acting on legs [weight of legs]; *RA*, moment arm of resistance [weight of legs].)

not even approached during the exercise. Furthermore, the person exercising in this manner is likely to accelerate the weight rapidly after the initial inertia is overcome, causing momentum to be the primary force throughout the remainder of the movement. Since muscle action is necessary merely to begin movement, strength is not developed in other segments of the range of motion to the same degree as at the start of the movement. To ensure maximal benefits from isotonic exercises, the performer should move at a nearly constant velocity rather than allow momentum to vary and facilitate the movement.

The use of free weights such as barbells in weightlifting competition is a classic example of the use of acceleration to enable the lifter to succeed. If the timing is exactly correct—that is, if the barbell has begun to accelerate upward—the lifter can change from a position in which the shoulders are above the bar to one in which the shoulders are below the bar. Full arm extension can then be used to lift the weight above the head. In other lifts the bar may be swung toward the thighs to reduce the moment arm and to utilize the inward swing to overcome the inertia of the stationary bar.

When weights are lifted from a semisquat or full-squat position, there is a danger of injuring the joints (ankle, knee, hip, lumbar spine) because of the increased moments of force (torques) acting at these joints. One might suppose that the moments of force would increase proportionately with the increase in weight lifted. This linear relationship does not always exist with human beings. As the weight changes, the person changes the kinematics of the lift. Furthermore, all persons do not change their kinematics in the same fashion. Hay found that one lifter, in changing from a weight 60% of maximum to one 80% of maximum, increased the moment of force at the knee twofold, whereas another individual showed a decrease in the moment of force at the knee.

Thus the most important factor for safety and for improvement is the manner in which the weight is lifted. Increasing the resistance may produce different benefits or may pose different dangers than are found with the lighter resistance. For example, arm extensions with free weights or attached weights may not increase the strength of the triceps brachii because persons may rotate the arms outward and thus utilize the strong shoulder girdle muscles (rhomboids) to change the angle at the shoulder. This change in angle may cause the arm to accelerate so that the weaker triceps brachii can be aided in producing extension at the elbow. Other compensations may include rotation of the body along its longitudinal axis and the use of the momentum of the body and the stronger arm to begin the arm extension. The weaker arm is therefore bypassed or allowed to extend only after upward acceleration has occurred.

Although isometric exercises produce no actual work, they may be useful in strengthening muscle groups. In particular, persons who have broken or sprained a body part will find that isometric exercises are the only possible exercises to prevent atrophy of certain muscles enclosed in a cast. This type of exercise is convenient to perform and appeals to persons who do not wish to exert themselves unduly or to perspire while exercising. Since occlusion of the blood supply to the muscle occurs, and since persons reflexively tend to hold their breath during isometric exercises, the duration of each muscle contraction should be short, preferably less than 6 seconds. Counting is a useful means of achieving normal breathing during isometric exercises.

Isometric contractions can be combined with yoga exercises and tension control programs, which will be described in later sections of this chapter. Isometric exercises have the following limitations: (1) Muscle strength improves primarily at the angle at which isometrics are performed, and (2) only slow-twitch muscle fibers are activated. Thus it is unlikely that a muscle will be strengthened throughout the range of motion solely by isometrics. Neither will all the muscle fibers be activated by isometrics; that is, fast-twitch fibers will not be contracting.

The concept of zero acceleration and graphic output of force applied during exercise was incorporated into strength-conditioning programs in the 1960s. This system of exercising was termed isokinetics. Since the limb is not allowed to accelerate, muscle force must be initiated to cause movement throughout the exercise. The addition of graphic displays of the force-time curve or force-angle curve ensured that the performer would attempt to apply muscle force throughout the exercise, rather than "cheat through the move."

Isokinetic machines can be set to move at various specified rates for improvement of strength or power. Both the resistance and the speed can be varied, thereby providing a variety of work outputs. Since the same work output may be produced by using either a high resistance (force) with low velocity or a low resistance with high velocity, the product of force × distance × repetitions will be identical for a given time period.

Strength improvement can be measured by the resistance (load) overcome (lifted) or by the work done. During isometric exercise one can pull against a dynamometer and record the total force produced. No work can be calculated, since the load is not moved. According to the definition of work, the work was equal to zero (Force × Distance = Zero). The degree of muscle tension involved for the particular isometric contraction can be measured and compared to other persons' scores or to one's own chart of progress.

During isotonic and isokinetic exercise, positive work accomplished is equal to the distance the weight is lifted, multiplied by the weight. No credit is given for lifting the body part itself in most calculations, although this does require muscle force. Likewise, no credit is given for lowering the weight, but this work is negative and is caused by eccentric contraction of the same muscle used in the production of positive work. The total work performed is equal to the work done for one lift, multiplied by the number of repetitions of the lift.

Thus in a strength exercise program the total work output should increase gradually. For example, swimmers swim more laps, joggers run more kilometers, and persons walk longer distances to increase their work output.

Improvement of muscle power. Strength alone is not sufficient; the improvement of power also is desirable. Power is the rate of doing work:

$$\text{Power} = \frac{\text{Work}}{\text{Time}}$$

As exercises are performed at gradually increasing speeds, the amount of resistance that can be overcome decreases. This is evident if one remembers that power also is equal to force multiplied by velocity. Power exercises are designed to improve the velocity at which loads of varying weights can be moved. Fast-twitch muscle fibers are activated during high-velocity movements, and all muscle fibers become involved as fatigue causes the velocity of the movement to decrease. Isokinetic devices have made it possible to quantitatively assess power and to exercise in a more scientific manner than was possible previously. However, these devices have limitations in speed; their maximal speeds do not approach those used in sports. Since so many of the sports movements require power, it is important to construct exercises to improve muscle power and consequently improve performances of individuals. Mastropaolo suggests that the person exercise at the level of power overload, that is, that load which is greater than the load for which maximal power was achieved.

Instrumentation for development of muscle strength and power. Computerized variable-resistance exercisers have been described as a means of facilitating maximal muscular involvement and of optimizing exercise productivity. A computer or microprocessor is connected to an exercise machine, and a person is tested on the machine for the purpose of diagnosing strength at various angles and of various body parts. Baseline data are stored in the computer, and initial loads are selected by the computer. Force curves can be displayed and com-

pared with other curves, and a new exercise program can be selected by the computer. The computer can assign resistance values for various angles and degrees of strength. Work output and power output can be recorded and displayed. Programmable treadmills and strength devices are being used for rehabilitation programs, athletic conditioning programs, and physical fitness assessment in general. The growth potential of commercial equipment using computers or microprocessors or both to record, program, and modify programs of exercise appears to be rapid and profitable.

RANGE OF MOTION

Range of motion (ROM) exercises are designed to increase the motility of all joints of the body in all the planes possible for each joint. For maintenance of ROM one may exercise faster and less often than if specific movements are to be enhanced. As with strength exercises, care must be taken to prevent an increase in performance in one plane or direction at the expense of performance in another plane or direction. For example, exercises to increase plantar flexion of the foot without concomitant exercises of dorsiflexion are likely to cause a foreshortening of the Achilles tendon or triceps surae muscles or both and thus severely limit the amount of dorsiflexion possible. Such a condition causes pain in walking barefoot or uphill.

Most ROM exercises are designed to improve posture and symmetry of body. These exercises lengthen certain muscles, thereby increasing ROM at a joint, and attempt to equalize the respective roles of agonist and antagonist muscles. Since the shortened muscle is usually stronger than the lengthened muscle, strength exercises should complement ROM exercises.

ROM exercises may be performed alone, with the aid of others who produce a force (passive exercise for the exerciser), or with the use of walls, towels, or other devices. In each condition the movement may be conducted at various speeds and with or without the influence of gravity. Yoga exercises and other slow exercises are safe and combine an isometric strength advantage with the ROM benefits. With practice and continual exercising, persons beyond the age of 40 years can achieve ROM values not possible for them for the previous 20 years.

As Wells and Luttgens have stated, there is a potential danger when ROM exercises are performed with high velocities or accelerations. In these situations either the muscle force or the force of gravity causes a momentum that may override the myotatic reflex, which normally protects the body from injury. In other instances the myotatic reflex is elicited, causing a contraction in muscles that should have been lengthened. Thus the purpose of the exercise is defeated, muscle shortening having been promoted rather than muscle lengthening.

Muscle strain or complete separation can result when one attempts to increase the length of the muscle beyond its strain limit. Older persons, who have a decrease in the elastic component, and persons who have fibrous tissue or calcium deposits are particularly susceptible to injury if ROM exercises are performed rapidly. Exercises performed while the body part is under water are especially safe for these persons. Moderate speeds of movement and the use of gravity, under control, sometimes provide a means of attaining ROM goals not possible in slow movements.

The importance of ROM exercises with respect to biomechanics cannot be underestimated. As with strength, the inability to perform normal ROM exercises at a specific joint may indicate severe restrictions on normal functioning and may prevent performance of some common necessary movements. For example, ROM limitations have prevented many persons from putting on and taking off shoes and stockings. Lowman has described numerous postural deviations and shown how each has a deleterious effect on athletic performance. Cardiorespiratory function and endurance, as well as movement efficiency of limbs, have been hampered. There is evidence that athletic performance may produce postural deviations

that must be corrected through appropriate ROM and strength exercises.

Most ADL and job-related patterns of movement tend to promote kyphosis (contracted pectoralis major muscles) and elevated shoulders. These characteristics also are noted in weightlifters and persons involved in other sports. Through an assessment of ROM restrictions, individualized ROM exercises can be constructed to correct unique anatomic characteristics.

NEUROMUSCULAR FUNCTIONING

The exercise category of neuromuscular facilitation, or perceptual-motor exercises, involves the development or maintenance of balance, speed, agility, coordination, and other eye-hand or eye-foot exercises. During the early years of life these exercises are necessary to assist the child in learning to move effectively. Late in life, disuse, pathologic conditions, or the aging process may create a need for persons to relearn these basics. Research with rats has shown that exercise increases the size of neurons and facilitates neuronal pathways of the central nervous system, including enhancement of the brain. Therefore one might speculate that continued practice of coordinated movements might improve or at least maintain neuromuscular functioning during the latter years of life.

Eye-hand coordination skills, reaction time skills, movement time in all planes of movement possible, eye-foot coordination skills, and bilateral, contralateral, ipsilateral, and other combinations of upper and lower extremity patterns can be selected and made part of a daily exercise program. Additional benefits of strength and ROM will also occur with many of these perceptual-motor exercises.

One other type of neuromuscular facilitation exercise is that of tension control. Basmajian states that skilled persons know how to effectively reduce the tension levels in muscles that are not necessary to a movement. The unskilled person cannot do so, and excessive tension from undesirable muscles interferes with the success of the movement. Woods has shown that the Jacobson method of tension control is effective in learning to regulate tension levels. Again, the biomechanical principles center on the perception of a moment of force, a quantity of work, or a postural deviation. The ability to recognize and regulate tension in one muscle is the basis for achieving efficiency in all movement patterns.

ANATOMIC CONSIDERATIONS

The selection of exercises should be based on scientific principles. As Flint has said, "Just be-

cause an exercise is commonly found in exercise programs does not assure its quality or qualify it for future use."* There are kinetic hazards that may cause injury if they are not recognized. For example, when exercises are conducted in large groups on command or on count, the taller persons tend to move faster than the shorter persons. Either the taller persons do not execute the exercises completely and therefore receive little benefit, or

---

*Flint, M.M.: Selecting exercises, JOHPER **35**:19, 1965.

A   B   C   D

E   F

G   H

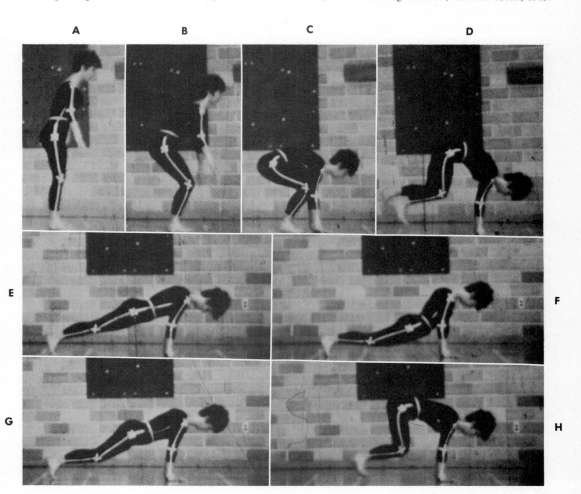

Fig. 23-3. Position of trunk when squat thrusts are done as fast as possible. Note extreme curvature of lumbar region.

the taller persons generate momentum during certain phases of the exercise that may cause injury. Fig. 23-3, *F*, shows a typical dangerous position when squat thrusts are executed on a count of 4. The stress on the lumbar curve may be excessive and could cause serious damage. This is not to say that group and cadence exercises are never to be used, but the biomechanics of each exercise should be analyzed fully to guard against common problems.

Individualized exercises provide a means of regulating the duration, intensity, and frequency of the exercise program. These three components make the difference in whether or not the program maintains, improves, overloads, or has little beneficial effect. The force, time, work, and power can be calculated for each exercise, and progression can be determined on an individual basis. For example, two persons, one weighing 801 N (180 lb) and the other weighing 1080 N (240 lb), each of whom is more obese than muscular, would be doing different amounts of work when performing stair climbing, pushups, chin-ups, jumping jacks, and so on.

MINI LABORATORY EXERCISES

1. Select various arm positions and weights for a person performing sit-ups. Estimate the magnitude of muscle effort for each position.
2. What is the relative difference in work done by persons with long trunks compared to persons with short trunks?
3. Is there any advantage in performing a sit-down compared with a sit-up? Explain why you chose your answer.
4. Calculate work done during pushups for persons of different body weights. (Hint for understanding the work done: Place hands on a scale to record the reaction force. Have the person perform the pushups slowly, and observe the changes in the scale recording.)
5. Develop a rationale for individualized exercise programs as opposed to programs in which all persons perform the same exercises the same number of times and with a standardized number for each level of achievement based solely on age or sex.

REFERENCES

Basmajian, J.V.: Muscles alive: their functions revealed by electromyography, ed. 4, Baltimore, 1979, The Williams & Wilkins Co.

Hay, J.G.: The biomechanics of sports techniques, Englewood Cliffs, N.J., 1973, Prentice-Hall, Inc.

Lowman, C.L.: Faulty posture in relation to performance, JOHPER **29:**14, 1958.

Mastropaolo, J.A.: Personal communication, 1979.

Wells, K.F., and Luttgens, K.: Kinesiology, ed. 6, Philadelphia, 1976, W.B. Saunders Co.

Woods, M.: Tension control, unpublished report, Seattle, 1980, Tension Control Clinic.

ADDITIONAL READINGS

Ariel, G.R.: Computerized dynamic resistive exercise. In Landry, F., and Orban, W.A.R., editors: Biomechanics of sports and kinanthropometry, Miami, 1978, Symposia Specialists.

Rasch, P.J., and Burke, R.K.: Kinesiology and applied anatomy, ed. 6, Philadelphia, 1978, Lea & Febiger.

Terauds, J., editor: Science in weightlifting, Del Mar, Calif., 1979, Academic Publishers.

PART FOUR

Moving beyond to future utilization and prediction

CHAPTER 24

Assessments and predictions

No one book can describe and analyze all the movements of which human beings, animals, fish, and birds are capable. Even if a book were able to do so for existing movements, the new movements or combinations of movements that are being discovered or created would soon cause such a book to be incomplete. Furthermore, since it may take decades for the existing movements of all species to be identified, much less recorded and analyzed, this task becomes monumental.

Therefore the preceding chapters in this book included descriptions of a limited, though broad, selection of movement patterns and included approaches to the analyses of these patterns. By nature these patterns represented examples from all three general categories of work, leisure, and activities of daily living. Further classifications were made with respect to movements on land, in the air, and in the water. Any new or unfamiliar skill will have some similarities to one or more of the movements described in these previous chapters.

Thus the theoretical model presented in Chapter 2 offers a means for dealing with unfamiliar and unusual movements, as well as with common and familiar ones. This scientific approach to the investigation of unknown movements can provide the link between the analyst and the performer. No preconceived ideas about the performance will interfere with an unbiased approach to the improvement of performance. Considerations depicted in the model—anatomic, mechanical, and environ-mental—provide an all-encompassing approach to the analysis of motion. Too often the analyst does not consider all aspects of the movement.

This chapter is designed to synthesize and extend the knowledge, concepts, and applications of the preceding chapters to enable the reader to advance beyond the scope of the book in analyzing new skills, making applications to new areas, and developing predictions of better ways of moving.

PROCEDURES FOR ASSESSMENT OF BASIC ANATOMY OF MOVEMENT

One starts with the identification of the anatomic or external axes of rotation for the movements being performed. The plane of each movement is then identified, as well as the type of joint about which the body part is rotating. Possible muscles that might be contracting to produce or to facilitate the movement, as in the stabilization of a joint or other body part, should be listed. These speculations are based on the plane of motion, as well as on attachments of muscles and their anatomic action, that is, flexion, extension, medial and lateral rotation, and abduction and adduction. The mechanical effectiveness of the muscle force, angle of pull, muscle length, and muscle cross section should be evaluated with respect to the force and velocity requirements of the movements. For example, the following elements contribute to mechanical effectiveness: (1) arm motion, (2) wrist, hand, and finger action, (3) adequate range of motion, and (4) proprioceptive feedback and reflexes.

Arm motion. The motion of the arm affects the velocity and accuracy of a movement. Medial rotation of the arm (extended elbow and shoulder reflexed) during shot putting, throwing, and striking furnishes much more power to the movement than does an outward rotation of this limb. Effective use of the latissimus dorsi (arm muscle with origin on the back) and the pectoralis major (arm muscle with origin on the chest) must be made by this rotation, especially in throwing actions and rope climbing. Chinning and lifting movements are more powerful when the palms of the hands are held upward in a forearm-supinated position.

The tendon of the long head of the biceps is inserted into the bicipital tuberosity of the radius. When the radius and ulna are uncrossed with the forearm in supination, the biceps pulls directly against the radius, and all of its power is directed toward flexion. The contraction of the biceps produces no rotational force against the forearm when the hand is in supination. This is the strongest position for elbow flexion. However, when the radius is rotated across the ulna with the palm of the hand in pronation, the tendon of the biceps is wrapped around the shaft of the radius. In this position, part of the power of the contraction of the biceps is applied toward supinating the forearm and the remainder toward flexing the elbow. The strongest action of the biceps in flexing the elbow is with the palm held in supination and with the elbow half flexed. This position should be employed in turning a screw when a screwdriver is used. The insertion of the brachialis is into the anterior surface of the ulna. The brachialis pulls directly in flexing the elbow. The brachioradialis is another flexor of the elbow. Because it is inserted into the lower end of the radius, its effort arm is long, and it has a better

mechanical advantage than does the biceps. The action of the brachioradialis is strongest when the forearm is in pronation because in this position the perpendicular distance from the axis of motion is greatest. These results have been found in laboratory situations.

Extension of the elbow is accomplished by the three heads of the triceps and the anconeus. The action of the flexors is approximately one and one-half times stronger than that of the extensors in most people. However, because of their great use of the extensors, gymnasts have been shown to have developed these muscles to equal the strength of the flexors. The action of these anterior flexors of the elbow is coordinated with that of the triceps and supinators, which cross the posterior portion of the elbow. All act together in movements that involve combinations of flexion and rotation of the forearm.

Pure supination of the forearm is a more powerful movement than is pronation (when the arm is in a flexed position). However, in many overarm movements, such as throwing a ball, the medial rotation of the humerus is accompanied by pronation of the forearm.

Wrist, hand, and finger action. The contribution of the action of the wrist, hand, and fingers to the performance of certain movements is self-evident. The action that can be made with the human hand and fingers, especially the thumb grasp, is one of the factors that have set the human being part from other mammals. The main muscles that help determine the strength of wrist and finger actions are attached above or below the elbow or both. Consequently the size of the hand is not correlated positively with the strength exhibited by it.

The many bones that compose the wrist (eight small carpal bones arranged in two rows and closely held together by ligaments), hand (five metacarpals), fingers (three phalanges to each finger), and thumb (two phalanges) have the potential for a great range of motion. These 26 bones, each in turn moving through its own range of motion, have an accumulated action like that of a whip crack. The great shooter in basketball, the top hitter in baseball, and the top passer in football are so relaxed that these bones appear to "rattle around" as action takes place. The key here is that these performers know how to relax the muscles that might restrict the joint action.

The wrist strength in flexion is nearly double that in extension, and the power of extension is lessened when the wrist is in the flexed position. The hand of the opponent in jujitsu can be rendered nearly helpless if the wrist is held in flexion.

During extreme flexion of the wrist it is almost impossible to curl the fingers strongly in full flexion. The reason is that the finger extensors, passing over the wrist joint, are too short to allow full finger flexion. A similar situation exists when the wrist is hyperextended. The range of hyperextension of the fingers is restricted because the length of the finger flexors passing over the wrist limits the movement. An involuntary adjustment to this relationship between finger and wrist action can be seen; when the fingers are voluntarily flexed, as in making a fist, the action is likely to be accompanied by wrist extension.

Range of motion. A person's or an animal's range of motion (ROM) is determined by its species, parental inheritance, nutrition, injury, functional and habitual use, and anthropometry. The ROM should be nearly identical for right and left sides of the body and should be limited, with respect to most joints, by the meeting of body parts that form these joints. Although several research studies have listed "normal" ROM values, one should refrain from using them as criteria for ideal ROM fitness levels, since most norms represent unacceptable values. The subjects have been sedentary adults, tense college students, or athletes with specific but narrow exercise programs. The best subjects to use for the setting of desirable ROM values would be physically active persons who

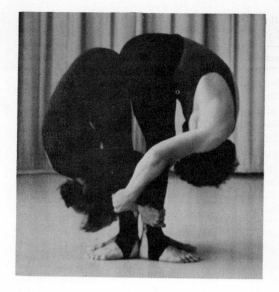

Fig. 24-1. Examples of adults who have maintained trunk and hip mobility.

have attempted to maintain extensive ROM levels in all their joints. These subjects are likely to be ballet and interpretive dancers (Fig. 24-1), yoga specialists, and "fitness exercisers." Table 24-1 provides ROM values that are realistic, yet of a high level, to be used as norms.

The ROM at a joint may be evaluated to determine whether or not limitations in motion exist. Basic anatomy provides the capability for movement solely because of structure. Success is dependent on the motion to be performed. The action of the foot and its relationship to the lower leg with respect to ROM will be used as an example of evaluation of adequate ROM.

The lower leg differs in structure a great deal from the forearm because of its weight-bearing function. The lower leg does not have the great rotatory motility of the forearm. The tibia is the major heavy weight-supporting bone of the lower leg. The tibia is enlarged at each end to form the articulation at the upper end with the femur and at the lower end with the talus (or astragalus) of the foot.

Table 24-1. Expected amplitudes of motion (in degrees) at each joint about each cardinal axis of physically active persons

Joint about which movement occurs	Flexion	Extension	Adduction	Abduction	Medial rotation	Lateral rotation
Shoulder (humeral-scapular)	180	60	45	180	← 180 →	
Elbow	150	10	N	N	N	N
Radial-ulnar	N	N	N	N	← 190 →	
Wrist	70	90	45	45	N	N
Metacarpal-phalangeal	90	30	30	20	N	N
Fingers (interphalangeal)	90	5	N	N	N	N
Hip	130	20	45	45	70	90
Knee	140	15	N	N	← 20 →	
Ankle	30	60	20	10	N	N
Metatarsal-phalangeal	30	90	N	15	N	N

N, negligible.

The hinge joint formed by the articulation of the tibia and fibula with the talus has practically no side-to-side motion because the projecting processes from the tibia and fibula reach down past the joint and embrace the talus tightly.

Although the axes through both the knee and ankle joint are horizontal in the normal upright standing position, these axes are not parallel to each other. With the knee joint in a frontal plane the axis of the ankle joint runs from posterolateral to anteromedial. Because of this arrangement it is natural for plantar flexion of the foot to be accompanied by lateral displacement and for dorsiflexion to be accompanied by medial movement of the foot. Thus coaches and teachers should expect that in running, walking, kicking, and jumping movements the toes will point slightly to the outside rather than straight ahead in the direction of the movement.

The long base of support offered by the foot makes possible a wide range of movements of the upper body without the balance of the body being seriously affected. The rear of the foot projects about 7.6 cm (3 in) behind the center of the line of support and about 17.78 cm (7 in) in front. It is therefore much more difficult to topple the body forward than to topple it backward.

The extra length added to the leg by the extension of the foot increases the effectiveness of the leg action in walking, running, jumping, and kicking. Even the simple act of reaching upward is increased by about 7.6 cm by rising on the toes. Not only is the extra length of the foot an advantage to leg movements, but the musculature of the foot is also an additional source of power in performance.

The kinesthetic sensations arising from the muscles and tendons of the foot aid in maintaining balance. When the feet are numbed by poor circulation or get too cold, these sensations are lost, and the ability to maintain balance is impaired.

The foot is an arch supported by two pillars, the ball and the heel of the foot. One pillar is anterior and the other posterior to the keystone of the arch, the talus, which bears the weight of the body. The arch serves as a half-elliptic spring that acts to absorb the shock when the body lands on the feet. The force of the shock is dissipated as the arch is flattened during walking. The force is also lessened by distributing it over a larger foot area through the arch. If the foot were flat, the force of landing would be transmitted directly to the small area immediately under the ankle: injury could result. The arch also places the toes in a good position for gripping the ground.

The ROM in the tarsometatarsal segment of the foot is approximately 10 to 20 degrees in dorsiflexion and 30 degrees in plantar flexion (dorsiextension). Swimmers and ballet dancers develop considerably more flexibility in this segment to be good performers. Tarsometatarsal mobility is also useful in walking, running, and jumping, since it adds to the total range of motion.

The first metatarsal bone of the foot supports nearly one third of the weight of the body in standing, and at times during running and jumping it bears more than half the weight load. The metatarsals are the long lever arms of the foot machine. The longer these levers, the greater is the linear range of movement and also the greater is the speed that can be developed if the power source is adequate for the load to be moved.

In walking, the forepart of the foot moves upward in dorsiflexion during the forward swing to clear the ground. The foot moves downward in plantar flexion after the heel strikes the ground to grip the ground and push off with the toes. Since the great toes carries at least one third of the load during the foreward propulsion phase of walking and running, it should be strongly activated to increase the effectiveness of the movement.

Morton mentions structural stability in relation to the present conformation of the foot. He states that "structural stability is manifested in the foot's arched contour, even in individuals under complete anesthesia. As the foot will resist any forcible effort to flatten it under such circumstances, this rigid arch is obviously not dependent upon the muscles."* However, he states that "foot balance is dependent upon the interrelated presence of both structural (bones and ligaments) and postural (muscle) stability, . . . and any appreciable defect in either element will be manifested by an unbalanced posture, irrespective of the integrity of the other element."*

During the act of walking, according to Morton,

_____

*Morton, D.J.: The human foot, Morningside Heights, N.Y., 1942, Columbia University Press.

the body weight is transferred from the heel along the axis of balance, which is near the center longitudinal line of the foot, and thence medially toward the great toe. The bottom of the foot contains large pads that serve to cushion the weight-bearing focal points. The plantar surface of the toes aids in gripping the ground during walking, running, and jumping.

Proprioceptive feedback and reflexes. Finally, the role of the proprioceptive feedback system and reflex systems should be assessed. Is there a reflex pattern that can be used to facilitate the motion, such as the myotatic stretch reflex? How complex is the neurologic patterning for the particular movement? Dance sequences usually require a high level of neuronal functioning during the learning phases. Likewise, strategy sports such as basketball require sequence of movements to be made at short time intervals and with continuity of motion. Remember, too, that reflexes might interfere with a movement, such as turning the head when performing a sidearm pattern.

INTERACTION OF MECHANICAL AND ANATOMIC CONSIDERATIONS

As movement occurs, the anatomy of the body with respect to spatial relationships, of one tissue to another, also changes. Since muscles, tendons, and ligaments hold bones together, the integrity and therefore vulnerability of the joint vary with the position of the joint.

A joint is most likely to be dislocated when bony contact is decreased. Bony contact is least at the midpoint of the range of the joint's movement. With a force greater than can be borne by a joint, the greatest damage will be done to one stabilized by bone and ligaments. Various areas of the body, their potential for action, and precautionary measures to avoid injury are discussed in the following discussions of the skull, the shoulder-arm complex, the hip joint, and the knee joint.

Skull. The skull is made up of 21 bones. The mandible (lower part of the face), which is a movable bone, is part of the head. Although the 21 other bones are held together tightly, they can be separated by a blow. A football player who uses the head to block an opponent or uses it in attempting to drive over a tackler must strike the opponent with the frontal bone of the skull (frontal eminence and top front part). In this position the head is a perpendicular continuation of the body. If the head is turned a few degrees off the perpendicular (to one side), the player tends to follow the head; thus it is much easier to be pushed aside, injury is more likely to occur, and forward momentum is lessened. Moving the neck gently from side to side prior to a physical performance tends to improve balance in action and helps relieve muscle tension. The awareness of body position is thus greatly increased. The mandible, the movable bone of the head, is connected to the skull in such a manner that it can be driven into the brain from a blow such as might be sustained in boxing. The boxer must protect himself by keeping the chin down against the chest in moving about exchanging blows with the opponent. If a blow is received with the chin down, there is less chance that the condyles will be driven up into the brain.

Shoulder-arm complex. Because at the shoulder the bones are held together only by surrounding muscles, this area must be protected from blows. A football player must be careful when blocking with the shoulder to have the protection of all the available muscles. This means not only that the arms should be across the body with the hands against the middle of the chest, so that the deltoideus muscles are used as protectors, but also that the chest and back muscles that attach to the humerus, such as the pectoralis muscles and latissimus dorsi, aid in protecting or holding the humerus in the best position to prevent injury. A dislocated shoulder (acromioclavicular separation) often results when the arm is in a poor position, that is, extended away from the body when a blow is received.

On the other hand, the anatomy of the shoulder is such that the humerus swings from a movable base. The base is formed by the scapula and clavicle, together with the muscles and ligaments that form the capsule within which the ball-shaped head of the humerus fits into the concavity of the glenoid fossa of the scapula. The radius of the glenoid fossa is smaller than that of the head of the humerus. Conversely, the humeral head is considerably larger than that of the glenoid surface, but the radius of curvature of the glenoid fossa is greater than that of the humeral head. A fibrocartilaginous ring enlarges the articular surface further, so that the head of the humerus is allowed great freedom of movement. Also the capsular ligament is firm at the distal portion and loose at the proximal part to permit freedom of movement. This great freedom of movement enables people to play many sports that involve a quick, wide range of arm movements. This great freedom of arm movement depends on strong musculature to keep the joint intact if strenuous demands are made on it.

The best position of the shoulder for withstanding a blow is with the humerus held downward and rotated medially because the head of the humerus is tied into the glenoid fossa by the capsular ligament, which is reinforced above by the coracohumeral and coracoacromial ligaments. These ligaments are not adequate to keep the shoulder joint in normal position when undue forces from the outside act on it. The protective support of the shoulder joint, then, is dependent mainly on the tonus of the surrounding muscles.

In addition to the deltoideus, the latissimus dorsi, the levator scapulae, the pectoralis muscles, and the teres major, the long head of the biceps brachii passes through the capsular sac, acting to strengthen the joint further. The long head of the triceps arises from a prominence immediately below the glenoid surface of the scapula.

The hand can be extended farthest from the shoulder when the arm, with extended forearm, is abducted 135 degrees because the humerus moves farther out of its socket at this point. A basketball player on defense often places one arm in this position to attempt to block an opponent's pass or shot better. A basketball player who wishes to have the highest reach in a jump leans to the opposite side to bring the abducted arm to the vertical position.

The range of motion of the shoulder-arm complex is large in forward and sideward movements and restricted in backward movements. With the elbow extended from 90 degrees of abduction the arm can be moved backward in the transverse plane 30 degrees beyond the body line. The arm can be carried sideward and upward only to the vertical with the humerus medially rotated. With outward rotation, which swings the scapula forward and opens the face of the glenoid fossa and also swings the greater tubercle forward and away from the costal surface of the scapula, the arm can be elevated past the vertical from 20 to 30 degrees. With the elbow flexed 90 degrees and the shoulder rotated medially, rarely can the arm be abducted beyond the horizontal; with the shoulder rotated laterally, abduction can be continued beyond the vertical.

Hip joint. The proper function of the hip is important in movement. The articulation between the head of the femur and the acetabulum of the hip bone is a ball-and-socket joint. This hip joint permits movements of flexion, extension, abduction, adduction, circumduction, and medial and lateral rotation of the thigh. It is generally believed that the limit to which dancers, high jumpers, and high hurdlers can flex and abduct the thighs is determined for the most part by the flexibility of the ligaments and muscles, not normally by the arrangement of the bones of the hip joint. For the most part the integrity of the joint is maintained by the pressure of the atmosphere against the partial vacuum in the hip joint. This is contrasted with the shoulder, in which the integrity of the joint is dependent on the musculature that surrounds it.

Since many of the large muscles that move the femur and have their origin on the pelvis have medial rotation as a secondary function to such actions as adduction and flexion, medial rotation of the thigh is a strong action. When great power is needed, such as when a fullback in football charges through the line, medial rotation of the thigh is used. Of course, the foot is turned slightly inward as a result of this movement. Also the knee is often flexed. However, when a performer such as a male sprinter tries too hard when running, he may find that the primary and secondary functions of the large muscles of the hip tend to neutralize one another, and he "ties up." The six lateral

rotators of the hip (which are situated between the posterior portion of the pelvis and the greater trochanter of the femur) are then activated and cause the hip to turn outward. The runner's stride is shortened when the hips and feet point outward. The legs move more slowly, and he performs far from his optimal level. These lateral rotators are the piriformis, obturator externus, obturator internus, gemellus superior, gemellus inferior, and quadratus femoris. This group of small muscles has lateral rotation as its special action. Medial rotation is a secondary function of some of the large muscles, as mentioned previously.

Runners and jumpers have special need of the gluteal muscles—the gluteus maximus, gluteus medius, and gluteus minimus. They function most strongly in extension. The powerful gluteus maximus does not function strongly either until the hip is flexed (with the trunk inclined forward to a 45-degree angle to be most effective), bringing the gravitational line in front of the hip, or until a strong resistance from the supporting surface is encountered, such as in running, jumping, climbing, and lifting. The gluteus maximus is also brought into strong action during the crouch start in sprinting. Persons who are climbing up a hill flex the trunk to activate the gluteus maximus. Elderly people incline the trunk forward while climbing stairs, as do bicyclists, for the same reason.

It is amazing how the body is designed so that the most effective use may be made of its parts. The several joints of the upper and lower limb enable a performer to transfer momentum from one joint to another. (The flea has five joints in the legs and is able to jump many times its own height.)

Knee joint. The knee joint and the actions that it may accomplish are unusual. It is free yet firm, stable yet versatile, and massive yet shapely. The absorption of stresses and strains, most of which are imposed on it from the upper body, is only a secondary function. The primary function of knee action is to impart motion to the lower leg in kicking and to the thigh in locomotion.

The knee joint, situated between the hip and ankle joint in the long, weight-bearing lower extremity, meets the rotatory stresses imparted by the femur by means of strong ligaments that bind the bones together. The knee joint is surrounded by fascia, tendons, and ligaments. The anterior portion of the knee joint is bound by the capsular and patellar ligaments. They allow an extreme range of motion to be accomplished in flexion of the knee. The posterior aspects of the knee are joined by the short popliteal ligament, which checks hyperextension of the joint. Sideward displacement is prevented medially by the tibial and laterally by the fibular collateral ligaments. In the middle of the knee joint lie the anterior and posterior cruciate ligaments, crossing each other like the lines of the letter X. The anterior cruciate ligament checks inward rotation. Outward rotation tends to uncross and relax the cruciate ligaments. These ligaments bind the femur and tibia together and prevent extreme motion of the tibia forward and backward and inward in rotation.

Participation in modern dance and football seems to put undue stress on the cruciate ligaments. Frequently the ligaments are not able to withstand the stress that occurs in these activities, and a knee injury results.

The relatively small surfaces of the head of the tibia are deepened for articulation with the large condyles of the femur by two semilunar fibrocartilages called *menisci*. These two crescent-shaped cartilages are thickest at the edges, attached to the outside of the joint, and free at the inside borders. The upper and lower surfaces of each semilunar meniscus are concave and are invested with a smooth synovial membrane, which serves to lubricate the knee joint. Motion in the knee is thus an articulation between the condyles of the femur and the upper surfaces of the semilunar menisci and the condyles of the tibia and the lower surfaces of the menisci. The knee is designed for two separate functions. When the leg is flexed less than 20 degrees, the joint is stable because of the restrictions of the surrounding ligaments. When the knee is flexed beyond 20 degrees, the posterior reinforcing ligaments are relaxed because the condyles are closed together in the rear. The knee joint then becomes loose and free for axial functions. How-

ever, the flexed knee is not adapted to heavy weight-bearing functions.

Each meniscus covers approximately the peripheral two thirds of the corresponding articular surface of the tibia. The semilunar menisci are commonly torn or loosened by a severe blow or twist that may occur in strenuous activity such as football, in a fall, or in a blow from some external object. If one meniscus is removed surgically, the other becomes the major weight-bearing surface, and its susceptibility to injury is increased. The removal of both semilunar menisci does not necessarily restrict the strength or range of movement of the knee joint. In giving way to the blow or twist, the menisci absorb some of the force. With the menisci removed this factor of safety is absent, and a severe blow or twist of the limb is more likely to damage the surrounding ligaments or to shatter the articulating surfaces of the bones.

The patella, one of the sesamoid bones in the body, lies within the tendon of the quadriceps femoris muscle. The patella is fastened to the tibia by the heavy patellar ligament. The angle of pull of the quadriceps is improved by the patella, and it is a protective shield defending the upper front of the knee joint. During flexion the patella occupies the deep groove between the two condyles of the femur. When the knee is extended by the action of the quadriceps, the patella is drawn strongly upward through the long recess (groove) in the front part of the femur. With the pulling up of the patella by the strong contraction of the quadriceps muscle in, for example, a kicking action, the pads that lie beneath the tendon lift up the synovial lining of the joint capsule. Thus the lining is pulled out of the way of the closing in of the bones (femur and tibia), and impingement between the condyles of the joint is prevented. Bursae above and below the patella act as protective cushions and elevate the patellar tendon, which improves its position mechanically to act.

PREDICTION AND PROFILING

Anatomic characteristics may be tabulated to produce a profile that can be compared to sports profiles, age profiles, or work profiles, and so on.

For decades the height and weight charts have been used to provide limited profiles of the growth and development of children. These charts did not provide enough information about the child to predict success or failure in movement. Unless there is a dysfunction of the movement systems, all movements of which a species is capable can be performed by all members of that species. There are, however, limitations of potential, just as a person's intelligence level limits cognitive functioning. Capitalizing on movement strengths and minimizing movement weaknesses are possible only after a thorough assessment of an individual's profile is made. This assessment would include the following:

1. Anthropometric characteristics: length, widths, girths, skinfolds, and ratios of these variables, such as the height-to-weight ratio, height-to-weight (cubed) ratio, and biacromial-to-biiliac ratio.
2. Physical performance: muscle strength, movement time (angular and linear movement of a limb or the body), reaction time, impulse production, range of motion, maximal work, maximal power, and tension control.

Since this assessment includes such a large number of factors, there may be many combinations that produce profiles which are "biomechanically ideal" for success in a particular type of movement, sport, or environment. The environment has been studied to some extent in the animal world. For example, distinct profiles exist for the large cats living in the jungles (tigers, leopards, and panthers) and those living in the open spaces (lions and cheetahs). Limited profiles have been done with human beings, but this assessment may have value in the future selection of persons best able to survive in outer space travel.

Many of the profiling factors can be changed. Exercise programs and other training or educational programs, such as for tension control, can be developed to enhance the profile of the individual for activities of daily living, work, a particular sport, dance, or single-movement pattern.

The construction of a profile allows a teacher, coach, or trainer, as well as the performer, to truly individualize the learning situation. An understanding of the particular characteristics of an individual, combined with an assessment of the performance of that individual, may facilitate the improvement of skill. For example, loss of body weight may be the only requirement to bring success to the performer (remembering that $F = ma$). An understanding of inadequate strength, excess body weight, or excess height (as for some industrial jobs) allows one to realize why persons modify their movement patterns from the norm in an attempt to bring success to the movement. These modifications may be partially successful, entirely successful, or unsuccessful. An understanding of anatomic, mechanical, and environmental considerations will help to create successful modifications.

The differences in performance patterns between skilled and unskilled performers account for the contraction of different muscle groups. Should the forces of the performance be greater than the body tissues can tolerate, the injuries to unskilled performers will occur in different muscles and body parts than in skilled performers. The injury rate to the unskilled, especially in skiing, exceeds the injury rate to the skilled. Thus the process of profiling can prevent needless injuries by predicting movement problems, modifications likely to be attempted, and modifications that should be made in the movement or the physical environment or both.

FORCES AND IMPLICATIONS FOR SAFETY

The six significant forces acting on the body have been identified as weight, normal reaction, friction, buoyancy, drag, and lift. The first three are more apt to produce injury to the body than are the latter three. For example, friction is the primary factor involved in abrasions and blisters occurring in falling, sliding, bicycle riding, longterm locomotion activities, and frequent turning movements so often prevalent in dance and basketball. Persons wearing prostheses also are plagued with problems of friction between the stump and prosthesis. New shoes, changes of terrain, and the use of hoes and other tools all present the possibility of "friction burns." Analysis and improvement of movement must consider the severity of friction.

The normal force produced during running, jumping, leaping, and other aerial activities may produce trauma to the bones and joints. Body weight usually is a consideration in the magnitude of normal force. Accelerations decrease or increase the normal force.

If the normal force is a result of a collision, as in football tackling, being hit by a hockey stick, or an accidental collision with another body, the bone may be fractured. For example, when blocking a soccer or football kick, the blocker collides with the leg of the kicker, which may cause the latter's tibia to break. In some cases the muscles tear or the tendons are avulsed because they continue to exert a force on a bone that is fixed by the force of the blocker.

Analyses of movements must include an estimation of forces so that adequate safety measures may be taken. Three examples of such biomechanical assessments and solutions to excessive force requirements are presented: changes in the volleyball spiking pattern, in the design of an archery bow, and in executing the headstand.

Volleyball spike assessment. The classic rotary volleyball spike has been replaced by an anteroposterior planar spike (Fig. 24-2). An analysis of the anteroposterior spike shows that the upper trunk and striking arm produce a moment of force about the hips and vertebral column, specifically the lumbosacral junction. This moment of force occurs as a result of positioning of the arm for the forward swing and the action-reaction by the legs, which serves to increase the posterior curvature of the lower back. The hyperextended position of the trunk causes an increase in the compression stress to the vertebral disks.

Although a forceful swing of the arm to strike

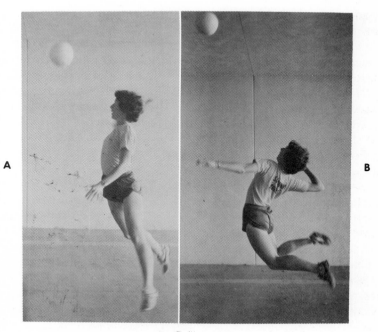

Fig. 24-2. Volleyball spiking patterns. **A,** Transverse rotation method. **B,** Hyperextension method.

the volleyball will create flexion at the hips as the legs rotate forward (facilitated by reactive force), a less forceful swing of the arm will require that the strong anterior muscles of the trunk and at the hip move the trunk from the hyperextended position to the pike, or erect, position.

Injuries to the back occurred as a result of the adoption of this anteroposterior spiking pattern without a concomitant adoption of a strength-conditioning program specific to this new style of performance. Subsequent program changes to include strength development of anterior trunk muscles, especially the rectus abdominis, reduced these injuries to the back.

Thus one of the prerequisites to the adoption of a new movement pattern should be a thorough analysis of the following:

1. Changes in spatial characteristics of the pattern
2. "New" muscles that will be utilized (not found in old pattern)
3. Nature and extent of forces acting on the body

Thus the question could be asked, "Will the body tolerate the repetition of the new skill without strength or ROM enhancement?" It is not enough to analyze the movement with respect to the increased force created by the body to act on external objects.

Archery assessment. The changes in archery bow design occurred because it was evident that the forces created by the body were not adequate for the goal. The average archer could not develop enough force to project the arrow at speeds necessary to meet the criteria of accuracy and distance set forth in competition and hunting. A pulley system type of bow was constructed (Fig. 24-3) to provide success to the average archer and reduce the stress to the upper back muscles. This type of bow possesses mechanical advantages that allow a person to draw a bow equivalent to a 222-N (50-lb) bow, with a force less than that used in drawing a 133-N (30-lb) bow. Thus the arrow can be projected horizontally rather than at an angle with the horizontal, since greater potential (kinetic) energy is created.

Headstand. There are three common methods of executing a headstand: the tripod, the kickup, and the draw-up, or leg pull-up. Most persons would agree that the leg pull-up method is the most difficult, but there may be a question concerning which is the easiest. By far the more important question is, Which is the safest? The major criterion for safety is the degree of danger to the spinal column, in either the lumbar region or the cervical region. By estimating the forces and moments of force on these parts of the spine produced in the three methods of performing the headstand, one can more scientifically decide on a teaching progression, spotting techniques, and mechanical principles to be comunicated to the learner.

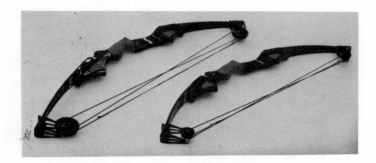

Fig. 24-3. Pulley type of archery bow that provides a mechanical advantage during draw.

Since accelerations produce forces and are proportional to the masses, a comparison of the accelerations should be made. Segmental alignment is the second important factor, and the amount of muscle effort is the final factor to consider. Table 24-2 shows such a comparison.

Thus the crucial problem in both the kickup and the pull-up is being able to achieve an extended trunk at the peak of the headstand. The kickup has the added advantage of providing practice in developing and recognizing optimal force production and kinesthetic awareness. If the feet are close to the hands at the start, the kickup is more vertical than rotatory, and the center of gravity of the body experiences a small displacement rather than a large one.

PROTECTIVE EQUIPMENT

Since sports situations produce high-frequency use of force, as well as high magnitudes of force, the necessity of protective equipment has arisen, especially in collision situations. Inherent in the analysis of a movement pattern is the identification of the external force during collisions. The following questions may be posed by the movement analyst:

1. Does the force of the collision approach or exceed human tolerances?
2. Does collision occur frequently?
3. Is there a high rate of injury for this collision?

If the answer is yes to any of these questions, protective equipment should be considered.

Selection of adequate protective equipment should be based on the following criteria:

1. Protective equipment must fit the anatomy of all performers. Quite often protective equipment is designed for the average person and is unsatisfactory for some persons.
2. Protective equipment must allow freedom of movement. For example, shoulder pads used in football sometimes restrict the movement of the players to the detriment of performance.

Table 24-2. Comparison of three methods of performing headstand

Tripod	Kickup	Leg pull-up
Center of gravity above base of support at start	Center of gravity outside base of support at start	Center of gravity well outside base of support
Minimal acceleration	Greatest acceleration of the methods	Minimal acceleration
Negligible moment arms exist	Moderate moment arms	Maximal moment arms
Minimal displacement of center of gravity of body in anteroposterior or frontal plane	Moderate displacement of center of gravity of body in anteroposterior plane; with unskilled might be moderate in frontal plane as well	Maximal displacement of center of gravity of body in anteroposterior plane; negligible in frontal plane
Moderate muscle effort, mainly of trunk muscles and extensors at hip	Minimal muscle effort, mainly leg muscles, except that abdominal muscles need to contract to counteract the kickup	Strong abdominal muscles needed, as well as trunk muscles
Some individuals have difficulty assuming tripod position (the obese in particular, and persons with weak arms)	Starting position easy to assume if feet are placed near the hands to minimize anteroposterior displacement and start the center of gravity high	Difficult to lift feet from floor

3. Protective equipment must attenuate the "excess" force. Analysis of the protective equipment after hours or seasons of use should be made to check attenuation characteristics.

Persons with physical impairments and those with muscular weaknesses may need some type of protective equipment for activities of daily living. The tolerances of their body tissues may be much lower than those of the athletic population. In particular, the frictional forces may cause injury to hands of persons with these impairments but may have no effect on hands of athletes. Anatomic considerations, again, are of vital concern to the movement analyst in identifying the forces and level of safety of movement patterns.

MODELING AND SIMULATION

One of the approaches to the analysis of movement is termed modeling. Physical models may be constructed to represent parts of, or the total, living body. The movement, in particular a collision, may be studied without submitting the living body to danger. Automobile and snowmobile collisions, football tackling and blocking, karate blows, and fluid dynamics of ski jumping, running, and swimming are among the applications of physical models. Although physical models provide a safe means of discovering new facts about the model's response to movements and impacts, there still exists the inability to exactly duplicate the live, "unpredictable" human body and thus to exactly predict the effect on a living body.

With advances in computer technology, mathematic models have become more prevalent than physical models. (See Miller for an excellent overview of modeling.) The magnitude and types of stresses causing deformation of body tissues, including bones, can be mathematically derived by incorporating morphometric data, as well as movement data, into the modeling program. Once again, however, the validity of the output is dependent on the validity of the input.

Two of the more promising applications of modeling to sport movement analysis is the use of the rigid-body mathematic model (1) to predict the highest goal achievement possible or the safest way of performing with respect to a particular movement pattern and (2) to create a better movement pattern through simulation techniques.

The following are three examples of such mathematic modeling and simulation:

1. Movies of speed skaters were analyzed by Marino to determine values of various kinematic variables characteristic of the ice skating start. The start was then simulated by means of mathematic modeling to predict maximal performance. The following changes in performance were determined to be within the performance limits of humans and would produce an increase of 0.5 m/sec: stride rate of 3.3 m/sec increased to 3.7, and take-off angle of 52.7 degrees decreased to 46 degrees. The limitation of this prediction, however, is the inability to measure interaction of the variables and individual differences among performers. For example, the impulse in the horizontal direction may be reduced as a result of these changes, and the net result will not show an increase in horizontal speed.

2. Chaffin has developed a safe lifting load (SLL) criterion based on his SLL model. The model simulates loads to be lifted at various distances from the body (base of support). The muscle moments of force and reaction forces are derived, and a SLL for each situation is predicted. The SLL is determined primarily by the magnitude of the forces acting at the weakest link in the human body, the junction of the fifth lumbar and sixth sacral vertebrae. Although the SLL model is primarily a biomechanical one, the estimations of human tolerances, which are the basis for the SLL model, are derived from epidemiologic, metabolic, cardiovascular, and biomechanical data.

3. The necessity of obtaining as much actual information from the living body for use in the interpretation of a mathematic model has been illustrated well by Putnam in her analysis of the "ideal" hiking position in a sailing dinghy. The mathematic model calculates muscle torques (moments of force) at the knee and hip and compares

three hiking positions. These are positions taken by the sailor, in which part of the body is outside the sailboat, acting as a counterbalance to the yawing of the boat because the wind is rotating it on its side. Actual reaction forces as measured by a force platform and maximal voluntary torques at the hip and knee joints in simulated hiking positions were used to compare modeling data with individual capabilities. It was noted that some individuals had greater strength in hip flexors than in knee extensors, whereas other individuals showed the reverse relationship. Thus, although one of the three hiking positions analyzed was less effective in creating adequate reactive forces than the other two, the preference for use of one of these two is dependent on the individual.

• • •

Although only three examples have been given, it is evident that mathematic modeling and simulation provide an avenue for greater insight into movement analysis. These techniques also have reaffirmed the importance of a total analysis, the need to consider individual differences, and the need to accept new information indicating new ways to move.

ANALYSIS OF INNOVATIVE MOVEMENT PATTERN OR PROPOSED CHANGE IN PERFORMANCE

When one proposes a change in one phase of a movement pattern, this change will influence other phases, to the detriment or enhancement of the performance. For example, instructions to increase the running speed before a long jump may result in an inadequate time in which the person can extend the leg during the jump phase. Thus one must inform the performer of the need to attempt to increase the extension speed of the jump.

If one applies the principle stating that the longer the distance through which one can accelerate an object, the greater will be the velocity imparted to that object, then the shot-putter should execute two or three revolutions and the hammer thrower should add one or more revolutions to the

movement pattern. Once again, however, another principle must be considered: rotatory movements may produce forces that are beyond the limit of the performer and may thus interfere with the final movement pattern. In the case of the shot-putter, the person has difficulty transferring the rotatory motion (horizontal plane) into a vertical plane. In the case of the hammer thrower, the person cannot counteract the centrifugal force of additional rotations.

Thus one might state that movements are a compromise in which the best combinations of applications of biomechanical principles are used. Consider the following examples.

1. A greater reach in swimming can create greater propulsion. The greater reach, however, creates a greater roll, which in turn creates greater drag and opposes propulsion. A compromise is achieved.

2. Jumping as high as possible during a basketball lay-up reduces susceptibility to being blocked and enables the performer to apply less force by the hand and arm muscles. Conversely, a vertical jump reduces the speed of the horizontal movement toward the basket and enables the opponent to be in a position to block the shot. In addition, greater muscle effort by the leg muscles is required to perform a vertical jump.

The theoretical model presented in Chapter 2 may be taken one step farther by drawing a debit and credit sheet. List the advantages (credits) of a proposed change or innovation, and then list the disadvantages (debits). For example, in golf, if a person swings beyond the horizontal plane on the backswing, the theoretical gain in distance because of increased distance of force application on the downswing may be 10% (credit). The actual outcome may be a loss in distance because the golfer tends to move out of the plane and adds another lever when the backswing goes beyond the horizontal. Thus the inconsistency in the point of impact may change the direction of the ball (debit). In a second example, if a jumper uses an extended leg to swing into a high jump, greater vertical acceleration results (credit), but this movement also creates a large backward component (debit). The flexed-leg upswing creates little backward force (credit) but less vertical force (debit). Different individuals use different amounts of flexion at the knee to create the most advantageous resultant force for themselves.

SPACE FLIGHT

Some mention of space flight research and its relevance to biomechanics is beneficial. At this time, life in outer space has been experienced for a period of over 3 consecutive months. The objectives of missions into outer space included the evaluation of human capabilities and of basic biologic processes during prolonged existence in space, which has zero gravity. The following changes noted in the astronauts involved in United States space missions and in simulated experiments have implications for kinesiologists:

1. Loss in body weight
2. Anatomic and anthropometric changes, such as flexion of upper trunk, flexion of legs, extension of thoracolumbar spine, appearance of a quadruped
3. Lower body negative pressure; that is, the fluid pressure and volume shifted cephalically, raising the center of gravity of the body and placing stresses on the body
4. Mineral loss in bones and consequent bone strength loss
5. Muscle strength decrements, especially in antigravity muscle groups and weight-bearing groups
6. Reduced work tolerances
7. Need to relearn simple tasks (indicated to be possible)
8. Disturbances in vestibular function

Physical exercise programs reduced these decrements in function. Devices were developed, such as a shoe cleat locking into a grid floor, to produce reaction forces so that movements could occur within the spacecraft chamber.

THE FUTURE

The kinesiology student and researcher of the future will have at their disposal significant technologic advances. What is done today by the graduate student in the laboratory will be done by the undergraduate student of tomorrow. The future undergraduate student will have (or must have) a working knowledge of mechanics, mathematics (including calculus), and computer science. These sciences will be prerequisites for entrance into a graduate program in biomechanics. The best graduate programs now have these requirements for admission.

Many beginning kinesiology students will soon be able to investigate problems once thought worthy of being studied only by the most sophisticated graduate students. The president of California Polytechnic State University in the early 1960s said that every 10 years the advancement of knowledge has been so rapid that the level of study has moved downward as much as 4 years in ranking.

Certain concepts and principles will be followed in making the future more attuned to reality. Some of these are as follows:

1. The beginning student, the practical user such as a coach, and the advanced researcher will work "hand in glove" in solving problems. In this way the young student will have an opportunity early to be familiar with many research situations.

2. The idea that an experienced and knowledgeable person who has played and coached a sport may become a researcher is both intriguing and sometimes necessary. This type of person brings to the laboratory insights not always available to the less experienced investigator. This researcher-coach may continue to be a practitioner. Thus the young student should gain much knowledge about a movement before investigating it.

3. The earlier a young student can determine his or her interest, the better equipped he or she will be to enter the chosen field of endeavor. Accumulated knowledge over a number of years adds to the expertise of an individual. This idea might be carried farther and transmitted into a concept that a sport or movement should be studied from an early age to better conduct research into its many facets. The demand for insightful people to help in the

understanding of a movement and to suggest ways to improve performance is increasing.

The young student must be aware of the increased technology that is available. Some of it will be used much sooner than is now imaginable. The following possibilities are listed:

1. Holography. It will be possible to produce three-dimensional photographs in the form of holograms, and analysis of a movement will be done in a more effective manner. This is possible now but is very expensive.

2. Mathematic models of movements. As previously mentioned, such models are being developed, and certain variables, such as length of stride, are being manipulated to determine the effect on the total performance. This is done without having the subject perform the variables. Young students of kinesiology should be aware of this possibility.

3. Scanning apparatus. In the medical field scanning apparatus is now available that could be used to determine the centers of gravity in live human beings. Most of the center of gravity data have been found with the use of cadavers, a method that is not without error.

The above examples are only a few of the many pieces of research apparatus that will entrance the young student in the future. The student should make ample preparation for the eventuality of this occurrence.

Future students of sports sociology, exercise physiology, sports psychology, biomechanics (kinesiology), and perhaps other sciences will join together to study human beings in sports environments. The excitement of such a happening is worthy of having a proper foundation. The promise of the future in this area is bright.

REFERENCES

Chaffin, D.B.: A computerized biomechanical model: development of and use in studying gross body actions, J. Biomech. **2**:429, 1969.

Marino, G.W.: Kinematics of ice skating at different velocities, Res. Q. **48**:93, 1977.

Miller, D.I.: Modelling in biomechanics: an overview, Med. Sci. Sports **2**:115, 1979.

Putnam, C.A.: A mathematical model of hiking position in a sailing dinghy, Med. Sci. Sports **2**, Autumn, 1979.

ADDITIONAL READINGS

Ariel, G.B.: Equipment safety and effectiveness. In Lowenthal, D.T., Bharadwaza, K., and Oaks, W.W., editors: Therapeutics through exercise, New York, 1979, Grune & Stratton, Inc.

Bajd, T., and Trnkoczy, A.: Attempts to optimize functional electrical stimulation of antagonistic muscles by mathematical modelling, J. Biomech. **12**:921, 1979.

Cooper, J.M.: Research in biomechanics, National College Physical Education Association for Men, Jan., 1976.

Cooper, J.M.: What we know about man and how he moves, National College Physical Education Association for Men, Jan., 1976.

Dillman, C.J., and Sears, R.G.: Proceedings kinesiology: a national conference on teaching, Champaign, 1977, University of Illinois Press.

McMahon, T.A., and Greene, P.R.: The influence of track compliance on running, J. Biomech. **12**:893, 1979.

Mersereau, M.R.: The use of normalized kinetic energy values in the analysis of developmental motor patterns. In Gedvials, L.L., and Kneer, M.E., editors: Proceedings of the National Association for Physical Education of College Women/National College Physical Education Association for Men, National Conference, Chicago Circle, 1978, University of Illinois Press.

Miller, D.I.: Body segment contributions to sport skill performance: two contrasting approaches, Res. Q. Exercise Sport **51**:219, 1980.

National Association for Sport and Physical Education, Kinesiology Academy: Guidelines and standards for undergraduate kinesiology, JOHPER **51**:19, 1980.

Nelson, R.C.: The new world of biomechanics of sport, National College Physical Education Association for Men, 1972.

Sapega, B.A., Minkoff, J., Nicholas, J.A., and Valsamis, M.: Sport-specific performance factor profiling, fencing as a prototype, Am. J. Sports Med. **6**:232, 1978.

Appendixes

APPENDIX A

International System of Units

The International System of Units (Système International, or SI) is now the universal system. It is sometimes referred to as the metric system, since distance (meters) is one of the most common items measured. The basic units of measurement for the movement analyst are those measuring time, distance, force, and mass. These form the basis for all the other kinematic and kinetic measures.

Table A-1 lists the SI standard unit and common multiples or fractions for each of the measures together with equivalents from the English system of measurement, the system previously used exclusively in the United States. Table A-2 lists some commonly used units that are derived from mathematical manipulation of the basic units or from a combination of time, force, distance, and mass units.

Table A-1. SI units

SI unit	English equivalent
Linear distance	
Meter (m)	3.28 feet (ft)
Millimeter (mm), 0.001 m	0.0394 inches (in)
Centimeter (cm), 0.01 m	0.3937 inches
Kilometers (km), 1000 m	0.621 miles
Angular distance	
Radian (rad)	57.296 degrees (°)
2π rad	360 degrees or 1 revolution
Time	
Minute (min)	Same
Second (sec), $1/60$ min	Same
Hour (hr), 60 min	Same
Force	
Newton (N)	0.225 pounds (lb)
Kilonewton (kn)	225 pounds
Mass	
Kilogram (kg)*	0.0685 slugs*
Gram (gm), 0.001 kg	0.0000685 slugs

*Note that 1 kg is equal to 1 Nsec²/m; 1 slug is equal to 1 lb-sec²/ft.

Table A-2. Derived units

SI unit	English equivalent
Velocity	
Meter per second (m/sec)	3.28 ft/sec or 0.447 mph
Acceleration	
Meter per second per second (m/sec²)	3.28 ft/sec² or 0.447 miles/hr²
Linear momentum (mV)	
Kilogram-meter per second (kgm/sec) (equal to newton-second)	0.225 lb/sec
Impulse (Ft)	
Newton-second (Nsec)	0.225 lb/sec
Moment of force (torque)	
Newton-meter (Nm)	0.738 ft-lb
Work (energy)	
Joules (J) (equal to newton-meter)	0.738 ft-lb
Power	
Watt (W) or newton-meter per second (Nm/sec)	0.738 ft-lb/sec
Moment of inertia (I)	
Kilogram-meter² (kgm²)	0.738 slug-ft²
Angular momentum (I)	
Kilogram-meter² · radian per second (kgm² rad/sec)	0.738 slug-ft² rad/sec
Pressure (Pa)	
Pasqual	
Kilopasqual	
Newton per centimeter²	0.689 lb/in²

APPENDIX B

Trigonometry, vectors, and problems

It is possible to solve many force and velocity problems by drawing vector diagrams. However, the degree of accuracy is dependent on the exactness of the drawing and measuring. In addition, this approach is time consuming when compared to the quicker, more accurate method using trigonometry. The word *trigonometry* literally means the *measurement of triangles*. Most problems in motion analysis involve the use of right triangles.

A right triangle is one containing an internal right angle (90 degrees). It should be recalled the *sum of the three internal angles of a triangle always equals 180 degrees*. Also, an *angle less than 90 degrees is called an acute angle* and one *greater than 90 degrees is an obtuse angle*. Two angles are said to be *complementary* if their sum equals 90 degrees. Thus in a right triangle it is apparent that the two acute angles are complementary. (If the sum of two angles equals 180 degrees, they are said to be supplementary.)

To understand the trigonometric functions, one must first be able to identify the parts of a right triangle. The following diagram of a right triangle will be used for the purpose of explanation.

The six component parts of the triangle consist of three angles and three sides. In the diagram

Prepared by Jim Richards, Indiana University, 1979.

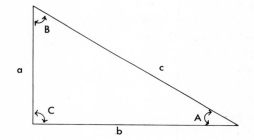

above, it should be noted that the longest of the three sides *(c)* is opposite the right angle *(C)*. This longest side is called the hypotenuse. Since the hopotenuse is always opposite the right angle, it is very easy to identify. The other two sides are called the *legs* of the right triangle. A side may also be referred to as the *side opposite* a particular angle. In the diagram, the side opposite angle *A* is side *a*. The side opposite angle *B* is side *b*. *Adjacent side* is a term used to identify the side that, along with the hypotenuse, forms a given angle. Thus the side adjacent to angle *A* is side *b*. Likewise, the side adjacent to angle *B* is side *a*. It is important to understand that the hypotenuse never changes; which side is opposite or adjacent depends on which angle is being considered.

Of the six trigonometric functions, four will be

described here. These functions are based on the relationships between the angles and sides of the triangle.

The *sine* of an angle (pronounced "sign" and abbreviated *sin*) is defined as the ratio of the side opposite to the hypotenuse. Thus the sine of angle *A* is the length of side *a* divided by the length of side *c*, the hypotenuse (sin $A = a/c$) and the sine of angle *B* is the length of side *b* divided by the length of side *c* (sin $B = b/c$).

The second trigonometric function is the *cosine (cos)*, defined as the ratio of the side adjacent to the hypotenuse. For angle *A* the cosine is *b/c;* for angle *B* it is *a/c*.

The *tangent (tan)* is defined as the ratio of the side opposite to the side adjacent. The tangent of angle *A* is *a/b,* and the tangent of angle *B* is *b/a*.

The *cotangent (cot)* is the ratio of the side adjacent to the side opposite. The cotangent of angle *A* is *b/a;* the cotangent of angle *B* is *a/b*.

These trigonometric functions have a specific, constant value for any given angle regardless of the size of the triangle. Since the values are constant, they can be compiled in tables such as Table B-1.

Since one angle in a right triangle is fixed, only five parts can vary (three sides and two angles). If either one angle and the length of one side or the lengths of two sides are known, the remaining parts can be calculated. The sides can be used to represent distance, magnitude of force, velocity, or other physical properties (vectors).

EXAMPLE: Assume that the hypotenuse is 6 cm in length and angle *A* is 40 degrees. Find (1) angle *B*, (2) side *a,* and (3) side *b*.

1. Angle *B* can be determined very readily since it is complementary to angle *A*, which is 40 degrees:

$$90 - A = B$$
$$90 - 40 = B$$

2. To find side *a*, we must select the trigonometric function that involves side *a* (which is unknown) and side *c*, the hypotenuse (which is known). The sine of angle *A* equals side *a* (opposite) over side *c*.

$$\sin A = \frac{a}{c}$$

Since *c* is known to be 6 cm and sin *A* can be obtained from Table B-1, the only unknown is side *a*.

$$\sin 40 = \frac{a}{6\ cm}$$
$$.6428 = \frac{a}{6\ cm}$$
$$6 \times .6428 = a$$
$$a = 3.86\ cm$$

3. The same procedure is used to find side *b*.

The following problems are included as practice exercises. It may be helpful to make a sketch of each triangle to better understand the problem.

1. GIVEN: Hypotenuse = 10 cm; one angle = 30 degrees
   FIND: Both legs (sides) of the triangle
2. GIVEN: One angle = 55 degrees; side opposite = 4 m
   FIND: Hypotenuse and adjacent side
3. GIVEN: Hypotenuse = 4 in; one side = 3 in
   FIND: Both acute angles
4. GIVEN: One leg = 3 m; other leg = 5 m
   FIND: Both acute angles and hypotenuse
5. GIVEN: A ball projected at an angle of 25 degrees with the horizontal; an initial resultant velocity of 10 m/sec (resultant equals hypotenuse)
   FIND: Vertical and horizontal components of the velocity
6. GIVEN: At take-off, long jumper with a forward velocity of 32 ft/sec and a vertical velocity of 12 ft/sec
   FIND: Angle of take-off and resultant velocity

Table B-1. Trigonometric functions*

Degrees	Sines	Cosines	Tangents	Cotangents	Degrees
0	.0000	1.0000	.0000		90
1	.0175	.9998	.0175	57.290	89
2	.0349	.9994	.0349	28.636	88
3	.0523	.9986	.0524	19.081	87
4	.0698	.9976	.0699	14.301	86
5	.0872	.9962	.0875	11.430	85
6	.1045	.9945	.1051	9.5144	84
7	.1219	.9925	.1228	8.1443	83
8	.1392	.9903	.1405	7.1154	82
9	.1564	.9877	.1584	6.3138	81
10	.1736	.9848	.1763	5.6713	80
11	.1908	.9816	.1944	5.1446	79
12	.2079	.9781	.2126	4.7046	78
13	.2250	.9744	.2309	4.3315	77
14	.2419	.9703	.2493	4.0108	76
15	.2588	.9659	.2679	3.7321	75
16	.2756	.9613	.2867	3.4874	74
17	.2924	.9563	.3057	3.2709	73
18	.3090	.9511	.3249	3.0777	72
19	.3256	.9455	.3443	2.9042	71
20	.3420	.9397	.3640	2.7475	70
21	.3584	.9336	.3839	2.6051	69
22	.3746	.9272	.4040	2.4751	68
23	.3907	.9205	.4245	2.3559	67
24	.4067	.9135	.4452	2.2460	66
25	.4226	.9063	.4663	2.1445	65
26	.4384	.8988	.4877	2.0503	64
27	.4540	.8910	.5095	1.9626	63
28	.4695	.8829	.5317	1.8807	62
29	.4848	.8746	.5543	1.8040	61
30	.5000	.8660	.5774	1.7321	60
31	.5150	.8572	.6009	1.6643	59
32	.5299	.8480	.6249	1.6003	58
33	.5446	.8387	.6494	1.5399	57
34	.5592	.8290	.6745	1.4826	56
35	.5736	.8192	.7002	1.4281	55
36	.5878	.8090	.7265	1.3764	54
37	.6018	.7986	.7536	1.3270	53
38	.6157	.7880	.7813	1.2799	52
39	.6293	.7771	.8098	1.2349	51
40	.6428	.7660	.8391	1.1918	50
41	.6561	.7547	.8693	1.1504	49
42	.6691	.7431	.9004	1.1106	48
43	.6820	.7314	.9325	1.0724	47
44	.6947	.7193	.9657	1.0355	46
45	.7071	.7071	1.0000	1.0000	45
Degrees	**Cosines**	**Sines**	**Cotangents**	**Tangents**	**Degrees**

*For angles larger than 45 degrees, be sure to use the headings that appear at the *bottom* of the columns.

PROBLEMS*

1. In the following triangle, label the sides (opposite, hypotenuse, and adjacent) with respect to angle *a*.

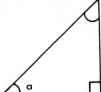

2. In the following triangle, complete the appropriate ratios.

sin *a* = _____
cos *a* = _____
tan *a* = _____

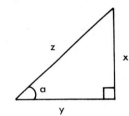

3. Using Table B-1, find the following.
   sin 30°   cos 30°   tan 40°
   sin 60°   cos 60°   tan 60°

4. In the following triangle, find the value of angle *a*.

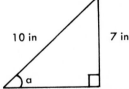

5. If angle *a* is 20 degrees and side *A* is 10 inches long, find sides *B*, and *C* and angle *b*.

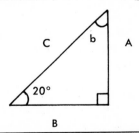

*Prepared by Jim Richards, Indiana University, 1979.

6. Find the two unknown sides and one unknown angle in the following triangle.

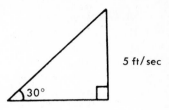

7. A woman walks 8 miles east, turns left, and walks 16 miles north. What is her resultant displacement?

8. The side of a mountain makes a 20-degree angle with the horizontal. If a man walks 1 mile up the mountain, how much has he increased his elevation?

9. A football is kicked with a resultant velocity of 12 m/sec at a 20-degree angle to the ground. What are the horizontal and vertical components of the velocity?

10. Without using trigonometric functions, determine the length of the hypotenuse (also called the resultant side) in the following triangle.

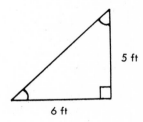

11. A man walks 36 km east and then 10.4 km north. What is his resultant displacement?

12. An automobile travels on a road 50 degrees north of east. If the car goes 17 miles, what are the north and east components of the displacement?

13. The side of a mountain makes a 30-degree angle with the horizontal surface of the earth. If a man walks 2 miles up the mountain side, what is his vertical elevation above the horizontal surface?

14. Find the resultants of the four following vectors:
    a. 100 cm at 0 degrees
    b. 80 cm at 40 degrees
    c. 110 cm at 130 degrees
    d. 160 cm at 210 degrees
15. A runner changes speed from 20 ft/sec to 28 ft/sec in 4 seconds. What is the acceleration? The average velocity? The total distance traveled?
16. A stone is dropped from the top of a vertical cliff. It strikes at the foot of the cliff 3 seconds after it was dropped. How high is the cliff? With what velocity did it strike?

17. If the wheels on an automobile have a diameter of 60 cm, how far does the car move when the wheels in contact with the road turn through 9 radians?
18. If a plank 12 ft long of uniform cross-section and density and weighing 120 lb is place so that 5 ft of it extends over the bank of a creek, how far out on the plank can a boy weighing 75 lb walk without tipping the plank? What is the minimum weight of stone that must be place on the end on shore to permit the boy to walk to the end over the creek without tipping?
19. A player jumps into the air with both arms

extended vertically overhead. Just before the maximum height is reached one arm is forcibly lowered so that the center of gravity is lowered 2 to 4 cm in the body. Do the fingertips of the other hand go higher or lower as a result? How much?

20. If a jumper jumps 2 ft high and takes off at an angle of 20 degrees with the horizontal, how fast is he going forward after the takeoff?

21. If the shot is put at an angle of 42 degrees with the horizontal and with a velocity of 10.8 m/sec in the direction of the put, what will be its upward velocity at the moment of release? What will be its forward velocity? What will be its time of flight from the point of release to the return to the same level at which it was released? How high will the shot go?

22. At the moment of take-off, a broad jumper has a forward velocity of 9 m/sec. Her vertical velocity is 3 m/sec. What is the angle of her takeoff? How high does her center of gravity rise?

23. If the shot were projected horizontally at a speed of 40 ft/sec from a height of 32 ft, how soon would it hit the ground? How far from the starting point would it hit in horizontal distance?

Muscle attachments and muscle actions

Table C-1. Attachments of muscles of upper limb

Muscle	Proximal attachment	Distal attachment
Levator scapulae	Transverse processes of atlas and axis; posterior tubercles of transverse processes of third and fourth cervical vertebrae	Vertebral border of scapula between medial angle and triangular smooth surface at root of spine
Pectoralis minor	Upper margins and outer surfaces of third, fourth, and fifth ribs near their cartilage; aponeuroses covering intercostales	Medial border and upper surface of coracoid process of scapula
Rhomboideus major	Spinous processes of second, third, fourth, and fifth thoracic vertebrae; supraspinal ligament	Lower part of triangular surface at root of spine of scapula; to inferior angle with arch connected to vertebral border by thin membrane
Rhomboideus minor	Lower part of ligamentum nuchae; spinous processes of seventh cervical and first thoracic vertebrae	Base of triangular smooth surface at root of spine of scapula
Serratus anterior	Outer surfaces and superior borders of upper eight or nine ribs; aponeuroses covering intervening intercostales	Ventral surface to vertebral border of scapula
Subclavius	First rib and its cartilage at their junction in front of costoclavicular ligament	Groove on undersurface of clavicle between costoclavicular and conoid ligaments
Trapezius	External occipital protuberance and medial third of superior nuchal line of occipital bone from ligamentum nuchae, spinous process of seventh cervical and spinous processes of all thoracic vertebrae, and corresponding portion of supraspinal ligament	Superior fibers—posterior border of lateral third of clavicle; middle fibers—medial margin of acromion and superior lip of posterior border of spine of scapula; inferior fibers—converge into aponeurosis inserted into tubercle at apex of smooth triangular surface on medial end of spine
Coracobrachialis	Apex of coracoid process in common with biceps brachii; intermuscular septum between two muscles	Into impression at middle of medial surface and border of body of humerus between origins of triceps brachii and brachialis

Table C-1. Attachments of muscles of upper limb—cont'd

Muscle	Proximal attachment	Distal attachment
Deltoideus	Anterior border and upper surface of lateral third of clavicle; lateral margin and upper surface of acromion and lower lip of posterior border of spine of scapula as far back as triangular surface at its medial end	Deltoid prominence on middle of lateral side of body of humerus
Infraspinatus	Medial two thirds of infraspinous fossa; ridges on its surface; infraspinous fascia, which covers it	Middle impression on greater tubercle of humerus
Latissimus dorsi	Spinous processes of lower six thoracic vertebrae; posterior layer of lumbodorsal fascia, by which it is attached to spines of lumbar and sacral vertebrae; supraspinal ligament; posterior part of crest of ilium; external lip of crest of ilium lateral to margin of sacrospinalis; three or four lower ribs	Bottom of intertubercular groove of humerus, extending higher on humerus than tendon of pectoralis major
Pectoralis major	Anterior surface of sternal half of clavicle; half breadth of anterior surface of sternum as low down as attachment of cartilage of sixth or seventh rib; cartilages of all true ribs; aponeurosis of obliquus externus abdominis	Crest of greater tubercle of humerus
Subscapularis	Medial two thirds of subscapular fossa; lower two thirds of groove on axillary border of bone; some fibers from tendinous laminae that intersect muscle and are attached to ridges on bone; others from aponeurosis that separates muscle from teres major and long head of triceps brachii	Lesser tubercle of humerus and front of capsule of shoulder joint
Supraspinatus	Medial two thirds of supraspinous fossa; strong supraspinous fascia	Highest of three impressions on greater tubercle of humerus
Teres major	Oval area on dorsal surface of interior angle of scapula; fibrous septa interposes between muscle and teres minor and infraspinatus	Crest of lesser tubercle of humerus
Teres minor	Dorsal surface of axillary border of scapula for upper two thirds of its extent and from two aponeurotic laminae, one of which separates it from infraspinatus, the other from teres major	Lowest of three impressions on greater tubercle of humerus; directly into humerus immediately below this impression
Anconeus	Back of lateral epicondyle of humerus	Side of olecranon and upper fourth of dorsal surface of body of ulna

Continued.

Table C-1. Attachments of muscles of upper limb—cont'd

Muscle	Proximal attachment	Distal attachment
Biceps brachii	Long head, from supraglenoid tuberosity at upper margin of glenoid cavity; short head from apex of coracoid process in common with coracobrachialis	Rough posterior portion of tuberosity of radius
Brachialis	Lower half of front of humerus extending below to within 2.5 cm of margin of articular surface; from intermuscular septa more extensively from medial than lateral	Tuberosity of ulna and rough depression on anterior surface of coronoid process
Brachioradialis	Upper two thirds of lateral supracondylar ridge of humerus and from lateral intermuscular septum, being limited above by groove for radial nerve	Lateral side of base of styloid process of radius
Triceps brachii	Long head, infraglenoid tuberosity of scapula; lateral head, posterior surface of body of humerus and lateral border of humerus and lateral intermuscular septum; medial head, posterior surface of body of humerus below groove for radial nerve, extending from insertion of teres major to within 2.5 cm of trochlea, medial border of humerus, and back of whole length of medial intermuscular septum	Posterior portion of upper surface of olecranon; band of fibers continues downward on lateral side over anconeus to blend with deep fascia of forearm
Pronator quadratus	Pronator ridge on lower part of volar surface of body of ulna; medial part of volar surface of lower fourth of ulna; strong aponeurosis that covers medial third of muscle	Lower forth of lateral border and volar surface of body of radius; deeper fibers into triangular area above ulnar notch of radius
Pronator teres	Humeral head immediately above medial epicondyle, tendon common to origin of other muscles, intermuscular septum between it and flexor carpi radialis, the antibrachial fascia; ulnar head, medial side of coronoid process of ulna	Rough impression at middle of lateral surface of body of radius
Supinator	Lateral epicondyle of humerus; radial collateral ligament of elbow joint and annular ligament; ridge on ulna that runs obliquely downward from dorsal end of radial notch; tendinous expansion that covers surface of muscle	Lateral edge of radial tuberosity and oblique line of radius as low down as insertion of pronator teres; back part of medial surface of neck of radius; dorsal and lateral surfaces of body of radius midway between oblique line and head of bone
Flexor carpi ulnaris	Humeral head, medial epicondyle of humerus; ulnar head, medial margin of olecranon and upper two thirds of dorsal border of ulna and intermuscular septum between it and flexor digitorum sublimis	Pisiform bone and prolonged from it to hamate and fifth metacarpal bones by pisohamate and pisometacarpal ligaments; transverse carpal ligament

Table C-1. Attachments of muscles of upper limb—cont'd

Muscle	Proximal attachment	Distal attachment
Flexor carpi	Medial epicondyle by common tendon; elbow joint fascia; intermuscular septa between it and pronator teres laterally, palmaris longus medially, and flexor digitorum sublimis beneath	Base of second metacarpal bone and slip to base of third metacarpal bone
Extensor carpi radialis brevis	Lateral epicondyle of humerus; radial collateral ligament of elbow joint; strong aponeurosis that covers it; intermuscular septa between it and adjacent muscles	Dorsal surface of base of third metacarpal bone on radial side
Extensor carpi radialis longus	Lower third of lateral supracondylar ridge of humerus; lateral intermuscular septum; common tendon of origin of extensor muscles of forearm	Dorsal surface of base of second metacarpal bone on radial side
Extensor carpi ulnaris	Lateral epicondyle of humerus by common tendon; dorsal border of ulna in common with flexor carpi ulnaris and flexor digitorum profundus; deep fascia of forearm	Prominent tubercle on ulnar side of base of fifth metacarpal bone
Palmaris longus	Medial epicondyle of humerus by common tendon; intermuscular septa between it and adjacent muscles; antibrachial fascia	Central part of transverse carpal ligament; palmar aponeurosis
Abductor digiti quinti	Pisiform bone; tendon of flexor carpi ulnaris	Ulnar side of base of first phalanx of little finger; ulnar border of aponeurosis of extensor digiti quinti proprius
Abductor pollicis brevis	Transverse carpal ligament; tuberosity of navicular; ridge of greater multangular	Radial side of base of first phalanx of thumb; capsule of metacarpophalangeal articulation
Abductor pollicis longus	Lateral part of dorsal surface of body of ulna; interosseus membrane; middle third of dorsal surface of body of radius	Radial side of base of first metacarpal bone
Adductor pollicis	From capitate bone; bases of second and third metacarpals; intercarpal ligaments; sheath of tendon of flexor carpi radialis	Ulnar side of base of first phalanx of thumb; lateral portion of flexor brevis and abductor pollicis brevis
Extensor digiti quinti proprius	From common extensor tendon; intermuscular septa between it and adjacent muscles	Joins expansion of extensor digitorum communis on dorsum of first phalanx of little finger
Extensor digitorum communis	Lateral epicondyle of humerus; intermuscular septa between it and adjacent muscles; antibrachial fascia	Second and third phalanges of fingers
Extensor indicis proprius	Dorsal surface of body of ulna below origin of extensor pollicis longus; interosseus membrane	Joins tendon of extensor digitorum communis, which belongs to index finger
Extensor pollicis brevis	Dorsal surface of body of radius below that muscle; interosseus membrane	Base of first phalanx of thumb
Extensor pollicis longus	Lateral part of middle third of dorsal surface of body of ulna below origin of abductor pollicis longus; interosseus membrane	Base of last phalanx of thumb

Continued.

Table C-1. Attachments of muscles of upper limb—cont'd

Muscle	Proximal attachment	Distal attachment
Flexor digiti quinti brevis manus	Convex surface of hamulus of hamate bone; volar surface of transverse carpal ligament	Ulnar side of base of first phalanx of little finger
Flexor digitorum profundus	Upper three fourths of volar and medial surfaces of ulna; depression on medial side of coronoid process; upper three fourths of dorsal border of ulna; ulnar half of interosseous membrane	Bases of last phalanges
Flexor digitorum sublimis	Humeral head, medial epicondyle of humerus, ulnar collateral ligament of elbow joint, intermuscular septa between it and adjacent muscles; ulnar head, medial side of coronoid process; radial head, oblique line of radius	Sides of second phalanx about its middle
Flexor pollicis brevis	Lateral portion, lower border of transverse carpal ligament and lower part of ridge on greater multangular bone; medial portion, ulnar side of first metacarpal bone	Lateral portion, radial side of base if first phalanx of thumb; medial portion, ulnar side of base of first phalanx
Flexor pollicis longus	Grooved volar surface of body of radius; adjacent part of interosseous membrane; medial border of coronoid process or medial epicondyle of humerus	Base of distal phalanx of thumb
Interossei dorsales	Each of four muscles arising by two heads from adjacent sides of metacarpal bone of finger into which muscle is inserted	Bases of first phalanges; aponeuroses of tendons of extensor digitorum communis
Interossei volares	Each of three muscles arises from entire length of metacarpal bone of one finger	Side of base of first phalanx; aponeurotic expansion of extensor communis tendon to same finger
Lumbricales manus	First and second from radial sides and volar surfaces of tendons of index and middle fingers respectively; third from contiguous sides of tendons of middle and ring fingers; fourth from contiguous sides of tendons of ring and little fingers	Into tendinous expansion of extensor digitorum communis, covering dorsal aspect of finger after passing to radial side of corresponding finger
Palmaris brevis	Transverse carpal ligament and palmar aponeurosis	Into skin on ulnar border of palm of hand
Opponens pollicis	Ridge on greater multangular; transverse carpal ligament	Whole length of metacarpal bone of thumb on radial side
Opponens digiti quinti manus	Convexity of hamulus of hamate bone; contiguous portion of transverse carpal ligament	Whole length of metacarpal bone of little finger along its ulnar margin

Table C-2. Attachments of muscles of lower limb

Muscle	Proximal attachment	Distal attachment
Adductor brevis	Outer surface of inferior ramus of pubis	Line leading from lesser trochanter to linea aspera and into upper part of linea aspera
Adductor longus	Front of pubis at angle of junction of crest with symphysis	Linea aspera between vastus medialis and adductor magnus, with both of which it usually blends
Adductor magnus	Small part of inferior ramus of pubis; inferior ramus of ischium; outer margin of inferior part of tuberosity of ischium	Linea aspera and upper part of its medial prolongation below; adductor tubercle on medial condyle of femur
Gemelli	Outer surface of spine of ischium; upper part of tuberosity of ischium	With obturator internus into medial surface of greater trochanter
Gluteus maximus	Posterior gluteal line of ilium, rough portion of bone, including crest immediately above and behind it; posterior surface of lower part of sacrum and side of coccyx; aponeurosis of sacrospinalis, sacrotuberous ligament, fascia of gluteus medius	Iliotibial band of the fascia lata; gluteal tuberosity between vastus lateralis and adductor magnus
Gluteus medius	Outer surface of ilium between iliac crest and posterior gluteal line above and anterior gluteal line below; gluteal aponeurosis covering its outer surface	Oblique ridge that runs downward and forward on lateral surface of trochanter
Gluteus minimus	Outer surface of ilium between anterior and inferior gluteal lines; behind from margin of greater sciatic notch	Anterior border of greater trochanter
Gracilis	Anterior margins of lower half of symphysis pubis and upper half of pubic arch	Upper part of medial surface of body of tibia below condyle
Iliacus	Upper two thirds of iliac fossa; inner lip of iliac crest; behind, from anterior sacroiliac and iliolumbar ligaments and base of sacrum; in front, reaching anterior superior and inferior iliac spines and notch between them	Lateral side of tendon of psoas major; some fibers being prolonged onto body of femur about 2.5 cm below and in front of lesser trochanter
Obturator externus	Rami of pubis, interior ramus of ischium; medial two thirds of outer surface of obturator membrane; tendinous arch that completes canal for passage of obturator vessels and nerves	Trochanteric fossa of femur
Obturator internus	Inner surface of anterolateral wall of pelvis; pelvic surface of obturator membrane except in posterior part; tendinous arch that completes canal for obturator vessels and nerve; to a slight extent from obturator fascia that covers muscle	Forepart of medial surface of greater trochanter above trochanteric fossa
Pectineus	Pectineal line and to slight extent from surface of bone in front of it; between iliopectineal eminence and tubercle of pubis; from fascia covering anterior surface of muscle	Rough line leading from lesser trochanter to linea aspera

Continued.

Table C-2. Attachments of muscles of lower limb—cont'd

Muscle	Proximal attachment	Distal attachment
Piriformis	Front of sacrum by three fleshy digitations attached to portions of bone between first, second, third, and fourth anterior sacral foramina; margin of greater sciatic foramen; anterior surface of sacrotuberous ligament	Upper border of greater trochanter behind, but often partly blended with, common tendon of obturator internus and gemelli
Psoas major	Anterior surfaces of bases and lower borders of transverse processes of all lumbar vertebrae; sides of bodies and intervertebral fibrocartilages of last thoracic and all lumbar vertebrae by five slips, each of which is attached to the adjacent upper and lower margins of two vertebrae and to intervertebral fibrocartilage; series of tendinous arches that extend across constricted parts of bodies of lumbar vertebrae between slips	Lesser trochanter of femur
Psoas minor	Sides of bodies of twelfth thoracic and first lumbar vertebrae; fibrocartilage between them	Pectineal line and iliopectineal eminence; iliac fascia
Quadratus femoris	Upper part of external border of tuberosity of ischium	Upper part of linea quadrata, that is, line extending vertically downward from intertrochanteric crest
Sartorius	Anterosuperior iliac spine and upper half of notch below it	Upper part of medial surface of tibia nearly as far forward as anterior crest; behind tendon of gracilis; capsule of knee joint; fascia on medial side of leg
Tensor fasciae latae	Anterior part of outer lip of iliac crest; outer surface of anterior superior iliac spine and part of outer border of notch below it between gluteus medius and sartorius; deep surface of fascia lata	Between two layers of iliotibial band of fascia lata about junction of middle and upper thirds of thigh
Biceps femoris	Long head, on back of tuberosity of ischium and lower part of sacrotuberous ligament; short head, lateral lip of linea aspera within 5 cm. of lateral condyle and lateral intermuscular septum	Lateral side of head of fibula and by small slip into lateral condyle of tibia
Semimembranosus	Upper and outer impression on tuberosity of ischium above and lateral to the biceps femoris and semitendinosus	Horizontal groove on posterior medial aspect of medial condyle of tibia; back part of lateral condyle of femur; fascia of popliteus muscle; tibial collateral ligament and fascia of leg
Semitendinosus	Lower and medial impression on tuberosity of ischium by tendon common to it and biceps femoris; from aponeurosis that connects two muscles 7.5 cm from their origin	Upper part of medial surface of body of tibia nearly as far forward as its anterior crest
Popliteus	Depression at anterior part of groove on lateral condyle of femur; to small extent from oblique popliteal ligament of knee joint	Medial two thirds of triangular surface above popliteal line on posterior surface of body of tibia

Table C-2. Attachments of muscles of lower limb—cont'd

Muscle	Proximal attachment	Distal attachment
Rectus femoris	Anterior inferior iliac spine; groove above brim of acetabulum	Base of patella
Vastus medialis	Lower half of intertrochanteric line, middle supracondylar line, tendons of adductors longus and magnus, and medial intermuscular septum	Medial border of patella and quadriceps femoris tendon, an expansion going to capsule of knee joint
Vastus intermedius	Front and lateral surfaces of body of femur in its upper two thirds and from lower part of lateral intermuscular septum	Deep part of quadriceps femoris tendon, which is inserted in base of patella
Vastus lateralis	Upper part of intertrochanteric line, anterior and inferior borders of greater trochanter, lateral lip of gluteal tuberosity, and to upper half of lateral lip of linea aspera	Lateral border of patella, blending with quadriceps femoris tendon
Articularis genu	Anterior surface of lower part of body of femur	Upper part of synovial membrane of knee joint
Gastrocnemius	Medial head, depression at upper and back part of medial condyle and from adjacent part of femur; lateral head, impression on side of lateral condyle and from posterior surface of femur immediately above lateral part of condyle; both heads, subjacent part of capsule of knee	Unites with tendon of soleus and forms with it tendo calcaneus, which is inserted into middle part of posterior surface of calcaneus
Peroneus brevis	Lower two thirds of lateral surface of fibula; medial to peroneus longus; intermuscular septa that separates it from adjacent muscles	Tuberosity at base of fifth metatarsal bone on lateral side
Peroneus longus	Head and upper two thirds of lateral surface of body of fibula; deep surface of fascia; intermuscular septa between it and muscles on front and back of leg	Lateral side of base of first metatarsal and lateral side of first cuneiform
Peroneus tertius	Lower third or more of anterior surface of fibula; lower part of interosseous membrane; intermuscular septum between it and peroneus brevis	Dorsal surface of base of metatarsal bone of little toe
Plantaris	Lower part of lateral prolongation of linea aspera; oblique popliteal ligament of knee joint	With tendo calcaneus into posterior part of calcaneus
Soleus	Back of head of fibula; upper third of posterior surface of body of bone; popliteal line; middle third of medial border of tibia; tendinous arch placed between tibial and fibular origins of muscle	Tendo calcaneus into middle part of posterior surface of calcaneus
Tibialis anterior	Lateral condyle and upper half or two thirds of lateral surface of body of tibia; adjoining part of interosseous membrane; deeper surface of fascia; intermuscular septum between it and extensor digitorum longus	Medial and under surfaces of first cuneiform bone; base of first metatarsal bone

Continued.

Table C-2. Attachments of muscles of lower limb—cont'd

Muscle	Proximal attachment	Distal attachment
Tibialis posterior	Posterior surface of interosseous membrane except for its lowest part; lateral portion of posterior surface of tibia between commencement of popliteal line above and junction of middle and lower thirds of body below; upper two thirds of medial surface of fibula; deep transverse fascia; intermuscular septa separating it from adjacent muscles	Tuberosity of navicular bone; sustentaculum tali of calcaneus; three cuneiforms; cuboid; and bases of second, third, and fourth metatarsal bones
Abductor digiti quinti	Lateral process of tuberosity of calcaneus; undersurface of calcaneus between two processes of tuberosity; forepart of medial process; plantar aponeurosis; intermuscular septum between it and flexor digitorum brevis	With flexor digiti quinti brevis into fibular side of base of first phalanx of fifth toe
Abductor hallucis	Medial process of tuberosity of calcaneus; laciniate ligament; plantar aponeurosis; intermuscular septum between it and flexor digitorum brevis	Tibial side of base of first phalanx of great toe
Adductor hallucis	Oblique head, bases of second, third, and fourth metatarsal bones and sheath of tendon of peroneus longus; transverse head, plantar metatarsophalangeal ligaments of third, fourth, and fifth toes and transverse ligament of metatarsus	Lateral side of base of first phalanx of great toe, fibers of two heads blending
Extensor digitorum brevis	Forepart of upper and lateral surfaces of calcaneus; lateral talocalcanean ligament; common limb of cruciate crural ligament	Dorsal surface of base of first phalanx of great toe; lateral sides of tendons of extensor digitorum longus of second, third, and fourth toes
Extensor digitorum longus	Lateral condyle of tibia; upper three fourths of anterior surface of body of fibula; upper part of interosseous membrane; deep surface of fascia; intermuscular septa between it and tibialis anterior on medial side and peronei on lateral side	Second and third phalanges of four lesser toes
Extensor hallucis longus	Anterior surface of fibula for about middle two fourths of its extent medial to origin of extensor digitorum longus; interosseous membrane to similar extent	Base of distal phalanx of great toe; base of proximal phalanx
Flexor digitorum longus	Posterior surface of body of tibia from immediately below popliteal line to within 7 or 8 cm of its lower extremity; fascia covering tibialis posterior	Bases of last phalanges of second, third, fourth, and fifth toes
Flexor digiti quinti brevis	Base of fifth metatarsal bone; sheath of peroneus longus	Lateral side of base of first phalanx of fifth toe
Flexor digitorum brevis	Medial process of tuberosity of calcaneus; central part of plantar aponeurosis; intermuscular septum between it and adjacent muscles	Sides of second phalanx of each of lesser toes

Table C-2. Attachments of muscles of lower limb—cont'd

Muscle	Proximal attachment	Distal attachment
Flexor hallucis brevis	Medial part of undersurface of cuboid bone; contiguous portion of third cuneiform; prolongation of tendon of tibialis posterior	Medial and lateral sides of base of first phalanx of great toe
Flexor hallucis longus	Inferior two thirds of posterior surface of fibula with the exception of 2.5 cm at its lowest part; lower part of interosseous membrane; intermuscular septum between it and peronei laterally and from fascia covering tibialis posterior medially	Base of last phalanx of great toe
Interossei dorsales pedis	Surfaces of adjacent metatarsal bones	Bases of first phalanges; aponeurosis of tendons of extensor digitorum longus
Interossei plantares	Bases and medial sides of bodies of third, fourth, and fifth metatarsal bones	Medial sides of bases of first phalanges of same toes; aponeuroses of tendons of extensor digitorum longus
Lumbricales pedis	From tendons of flexor digitorum longus as far back as their angles of division; each of four muscles springing from two tendons except first	Expansions of tendons of extensor digitorum longus on dorsal surfaces of first phalanges
Quadratus plantae	Lateral head, lateral border of inferior surface of calcaneus in front of lateral process of its tuberosity, long plantar ligament; medial head, medial concave surface of calcaneus	Two heads joining to be inserted into lateral margin and upper surface and undersurface of tendon of flexor digitorum longus; slips usually sent to tendons going to second, third, and fourth toes

Table C-3. Muscle actions of the upper limb*

Muscle	Shoulder girdle						Upper arm						Lower arm			
	El.	Dep.	Pro.	Ret.	Rot. up	Rot. down	Fl.	Ext.	Abd.	Add.	Med. rot.	Lat. rot.	Fl.	Ext.	Sup.	Pro.
Levator scapulae	X															
Pectoralis minor		X	X			X										
Rhomboideus major		X		X		X										
Rhomboideus minor		X		X		X										
Serratus anterior			X		X											
Subclavius		X														
Trapezius	Superior	Inferior		X		Middle and inferior										
Coracobrachialis							X			X						
Deltoideus							Anterior	Posterior	X							
Infraspinatus												X				
Latissimus dorsi								X		X	X					
Pectoralis major							X			X	X					
Subscapularis											X					
Supraspinatus									X							
Teres major								X		X	X					
Teres minor								X				X				
Anconeus														X		
Biceps									Long	Short			X		X	
Brachialis													X			
Brachioradialis													X	X		
Triceps								Long		Long				X		
Pronator quadratus																X
Pronator teres													X			X
Supinator															X	

Muscle	Lower arm				Hand				Thumb				Fingers			
	Fl.	Ext.	Sup.	Pro.	Fl.	Ext.	Abd.	Add.	Fl.	Ext.	Abd.	Add.	Fl.	Ext.	Abd.	Add.
Flexor carpi ulnaris	X				X			X								
Flexor carpi radialis	X			X	X		X									
Extensor carpi radialis brevis						X	X									
Extensor carpi radialis longus	X					X	X									
Extensor carpi ulnaris		X				X		X								
Palmaris longus	X				X											
Abductor digiti quinti manus													Proximal finger phalanges		Little finger	
Abductor pollicis brevis									Draws thumb to plane at right angles to palm							
Abductor pollicis longus							X				Carries thumb laterally from palm					
Adductor pollicis												Approximates thumb to palm				
Extensor digiti quinti proprius						X								Little finger		
Extensor digitorum communis		X				X								X	In ext.	
Extensor indicis proprius						X								Index finger		
Extensor pollicis brevis						X				X						
Extensor pollicis longus						X				X						
Flexor digiti quinti brevis manus													Little finger			

*Information based on Goss, C.M., editor: Gray's anatomy of the human body, ed. 29, Philadelphia, 1973, Lea & Febiger.

Key: *Abd.*, Abducts; *Add.*, adducts; *Dep.*, depresses; *El.*, elevates; *Ext.*, extends or extension; *Fl.*, flexes; *Lat.*, lateral; *Med.*, medial; *Pro.*, pronates or protracts; *Ret.*, retracts; *Rot.*, rotates or rotation; *Sup.*, supinates.

Continued.

Table C-3. Muscle actions of the upper limb—cont'd

Muscle	Lower arm				Hand				Thumb				Fingers			
	Fl.	Ext.	Sup.	Pro.	Fl.	Ext.	Abd.	Add.	Fl.	Ext.	Abd.	Add.	Fl.	Ext.	Abd.	Add.
Flexor digitorum profundus	X												Middle and proximal phalanges			
Flexor digitorum sublimis					X											
Flexor pollicis brevis												Proximal phalanx				
Flexor pollicis longus					X				Proximal X							
Interossei dorsales manus										X			First finger	Second and third phalanges	X	
Interossei volares										X			First finger	Second and third phalanges		X
Lumbricales manus									X	X			First finger	Second and third phalanges		
Palmaris brevis													Corrugates skin on ulnar side of hand			
Opponens pollicis												X				
Opponens digiti quinti manus												X	Deepens hollow of palm			

Table C-4. Muscle actions of the lower limb*

Muscle	Thigh						Lower leg			
	Fl.	Ext.	Abd.	Add.	Rot. med.	Rot. lat.	Fl.	Ext.	Rot. med.	Rot. lat.
Adductor brevis	X			X		X				
Adductor longus	X			X		X				
Adductor magnus	Upper part	Lower part		X	Lower part	Upper part				
Gemelli			In flexion			X				
Gluteus maximus		X		Lower part		Lower part				
Gluteus medius			In extension		Anterior fibers					
Gluteus minimus			In extension		Anterior fibers					
Gracilis	X			X	X				X	
Iliacus	X				Slight					
Obturator externus			In flexion			X				
Obturator internus			In flexion			X				
Pectineus	X			X		X				
Piriformis			X			X				
Psoas major	X				Slight					
Psoas minor			Tensor of iliac fascia							
Quadratus femoris				X		X		X		
Sartorius	X			X		X	X			
Tensor fasciae latae			X		X					
Biceps femoris		X					X			In flexion
Semimembranosus		X					X		Slight	
Semitendinosus		X					X		X	
Popliteus							X		In flexion	
Rectus femoris	X							X		
Vastus medialis								X		
Vastus internus								X		
Vastus lateralis								X		
Articularis genu	Occasionally blended with vastus intermedius									

*Information based on Goss, C.M., editor: Gray's anatomy of the human body, ed. 29, Philadelphia, 1973, Lea & Febiger.
Key: *Abd.*, Abducts; *Add.*, adducts; *Ever.*, everts; *Ext.*, extends; *Fl.*, flexes; *Inv.*, inverts; *Lat.*, laterally; *Med.*, medially; *Pro.*, pronates; *Rot.*, rotates; *Sup.*, supinates.

Continued.

Table C-4. Muscle actions of the lower limb—cont'd

Muscle	Lower leg				Foot				Toes			
	Fl.	Ext.	Rot. med.	Rot. lat.	Plantar fl.	Dorsi-fl.	Inv.	Ever.	Fl.	Ext.	Abd.	Add.
Gastrocnemius	X				X							
Peroneus brevis					X			X				
Peroneus longus					X			X				
Peroneus tertius						X		X				
Plantaris	X				X							
Soleus					X							
Tibialis anterior						X	X					
Tibialis posterior					X		X					
Abductor digiti quinti									X		X	
Abductor hallucis									X		X	
Adductor hallucis									X			X
Extensor digitorum brevis										X	X	

Table C-4. Muscle actions of the lower limb—cont'd

Muscle	Foot				Toes			
	Plantar fl.	Dorsi-fl.	Inv.	Ever.	Fl.	Ext.	Abd.	Add.
Extensor digitorum longus		X				X		
Extensor hallucis longus		X				X		
Flexor digitorum longus	X				X			
Flexor digitorum brevis					X		X	
					Little toe		Little toe	
Flexor digitorum quinti					X			X
Flexor hallucis brevis					X			
Flexor hallucis longus	X				X			
Interossei dorsales pedis					X	X	X	
Interossei plantares					X	X		X
Lumbricales pedis					X	X		
Quadratus plantae					X			

APPENDIX D

Projectiles

Projection of an object or of oneself is the outcome—the product—of many motor skills. Since the velocity and the angle of projection imparted to the projectile by the performer determine the degree of skill, the instructor who can measure them has a device that can profitably be added to instructional procedures. For example, if greater velocity is desired, changes in joint action can be suggested. If velocity is measured before and after the changes have been made, the instructor can evaluate suggestions and the learner has had the opportunity to experience the effect of some lever action, thereby adding to understanding of body mechanics.

Since air resistance is negligible when the body projects itself and when it projects many objects, the path of flight of these projectiles is determined by two forces: the force imparted by body levers and the force of gravity. If the time of flight is known, the effect of gravity can be determined. The following discussion applies only to those projections for which air resistance is neglible; it does not apply to projectiles such as a javelin, discus, badminton shuttlecock, or ball that is spinning rapidly.

EFFECT OF GRAVITY

The effect of gravity* on unsupported objects is the same regardless of the weight of the object.

---

*Metric system would mean a distance of $\frac{16.1}{3.28} = 4.9$ m

The constant acceleration of gravitational force pulls the object downward a distance that equals in feet 16.1 t^2, in which t represents the time in seconds during which gravity has been acting on the object. In 1 second an object would be pulled downward 16.1 ft (16.1 × 1²); in 0.5 second the distance would be 4.025 ft (16.1 × 0.5²). If the velocity and direction imparted by body levers are known, the path of flight can be determined. In Fig. D-1 the horizontal line represents the projection of an object by means of force imparted by the body, a velocity of 80 ft/sec in a horizontal direction. Each dot represents an additional 8 ft in flight and also an additional 0.1 second of time. The effect of gravity at each time interval is represented by the vertical lines. The lower ends of the vertical lines mark the path of flight resulting from the two forces. The path of flight can be determined in like manner whenever the velocity and direction imparted by body force to an object are known.

DETERMINATION OF VELOCITY AND ANGLE

When the body projects itself or an object, neither the velocity nor the angle of projection is known. However, information can be obtained in such situations, and with this information velocity and angle can be determined. The needed items of information are (1) the starting point of flight, (2) the end point in its relation to the start—that is, the horizontal distance from the starting point and the vertical distance between the two points—and (3) the time of flight.

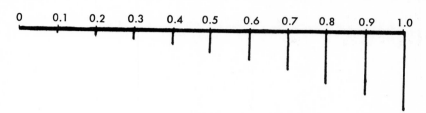

Fig. D-1. Gravitational effect at each 0.1 second on object projected horizontally at 80 ft/sec. Each 0.4 in represents 8 ft.

Velocity. If a ball resting on the ground (starting point) were kicked and landed 80 ft from the starting point (horizontal distance 80 ft, vertical distance 0 ft) in 2.1 seconds (time), the effect of gravity during this time would be 71.001 ft (16.1×2.1^2). Had gravity not pulled the ball downward, it would then have been 71 ft above the landing point. The horizontal distance, 80 ft, and the vertical line, 71 ft, form two sides of a right-angled triangle. The path that the ball would travel had gravity not pulled it down is that connecting the starting point and the upper end of the 71-ft vertical, the hypotenuse of the triangle. Its length is the square root of the sum of the squares of the sides ($80^2 + 71^2$), or 107 ft, the distance that the ball would have been projected by the force imparted by the body. This is 50.9 ft/sec ($107 \div 2.1$).

Had the ball landed on a downslope 20 ft below the starting point and had the horizontal distance and the time been the same, the calculations would differ. The vertical line of gravitational force would be the same length, but the lines of the triangle would be 80 ft horizontally and 51 ft vertically ($71 - 20$). The length of the hypotenuse in this case would be the square root of the $51^2 + 80^2$, 94.87 ft, and the velocity 45.18 ft. Had the ball hit a wall at a height 20 ft above the starting point and 80 ft away from it in the same time, the

vertical line completing the triangle would be 91 ft in length ($71 + 20$), the hypotenuse 121.16 ft, and the velocity 57.69 ft/sec. These examples show that the measure of the horizontal distance of a throw or a jump is not a valid measure of the force exerted by the body levers.

Other mathematic calculations can be used to determine the length of the hypotenuse, and they are presented in the next paragraph.

Angle. Once the horizontal and the vertical distance of the triangle have been determined, the angle of projection can be found by calculation and reference to the values of natural trigonometric functions. The vertical length of the triangle divided by the horizontal length is the value for the tangent. In the first illustration $71 \div 80 = 0.8875$, the tangent of an angle of 41° 35′; the downslope tangent value is 0.6375, and the angle is 32° 31′; in the third situation the tangent value is 1.1375, and the angle is 48° 41′.

• • •

With trigonometric relationships the measures of angles and velocities can be obtained in many ways; those which require the least calculation can be used. As one example the angles of projection might have been determined before the velocities. When the angle is known, another trigonometric value might be used to determine the length of the

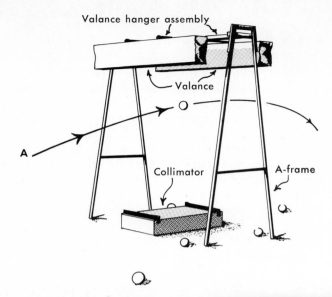

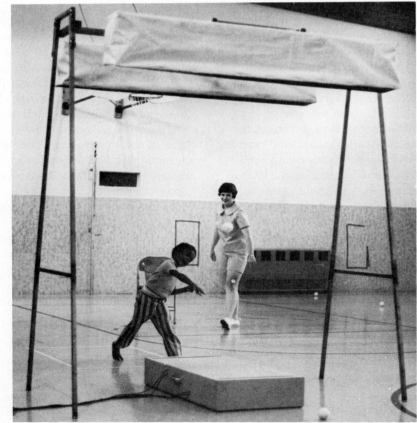

Fig. D-2. A, Velocimeter, a device used to measure precise horizontal velocity of projectiles. **B,** Velocimeter used indoors to measure the velocity of ball thrown by child. (Courtesy Kinesiology Research Laboratories, University of Wisconsin.)

hypotenuse, which is equal to the length of the vertical side divided by the sine of the angle. In the first of the situations the sine of an angle of 41° 35' is 0.6637: 71 ÷ 0.6637 = 107. In the downslope the angle was 32° 31'; the sine value is 0.5375, and 51 ÷ 0.5375 = 94.8. In the last situation the sine value is 0.751, and 91 ÷ 0.751 = 121.

In teaching situations in which velocities of projections are measured frequently, instructors have prepared tables that give the velocity and angle for specific distance and time measures. These measurements are usually based on a given vertical height, and although not accurate to a fine degree they are sufficiently so to measure individual progress and to determine group averages.

Although velocity can be measured satisfactorily for most class situations, investigators often want a method of measurement that will be accurate to a finer degree. Research needs frequently promote the development of new devices. The need for a precise measure of the velocity of projectiles led to the development of the velocimeter shown in Fig. D-2, which records the time during which a projectile travels 1 m horizontally. This instrument is easily portable and can be set up in less than 5 minutes without tools. As shown in Fig. D-2, *B*, it can be used indoors; it is equally efficient out of doors in full daylight. The large area between the stands supporting the valance enables it to be used to measure a variety of throwing and kicking skills and the velocity of batted balls, such as those used in tennis, golf, and baseball.

LOCATION OF HIGH POINT OF FLIGHT

If an object is projected horizontally or downward, the highest point of its flight will be the starting point. If it is projected upward, gravity will immediately decrease vertical velocity, and the high point will be reached when the downward velocity imparted by gravity is equal to that of the upward velocity imparted by the body. The velocity caused by gravitational force is always 32.2 t (the time value in seconds). Thus the high point is reached when vertical velocity − 32.2 t = 0. The time to the high point is vertical velocity ÷ 32.2.

In the first situation in kicking, the velocity was 50.9 ft/sec, and the angle was 41° 35'. It is now convenient to consider this velocity as the hypotenuse of a triangle. It has a vertical and a horizontal component. The vertical component is the hypotenuse times the sine of the angle—in this case 50.9 × 0.6637 = 33.78. The high point will be reached when t = 33.78 ÷ 32.2, or 1.049+. The time for total flight was 2.1 seconds, and the high point is reached midway in flight. This will always be the case when the vertical distance between the beginning and end of flight is zero.

When the vertical distance between the beginning and end of flight is not zero, the time to the high point will not be half the flight time. In the downslope situation, the vertical component of the velocity imparted by the body is 0.5375 × 45.2 = 24.29 ft/sec. The time to the high point is 24.9 ÷ 32.2 = 0.754 second. In this situation the drop after the high point continues after the level of the starting point is reached. In the third situation the vertical component of velocity is 0.751 × 57.69 = 43.32 ft/sec. The time to the high point is 43.32 ÷ 32.2 = 1.345 seconds. Here the drop does not reach the level of the starting point.

The horizontal distance to the high point can be calculated with the cosine value of the velocity imparted by the ball. The distance from the starting point will be the horizontal component of the velocity multiplied by the time to the high point. When the projection velocity in each of the three kicking situations is multiplied by the cosines of the angles, the horizontal components are as follows:

    1. (Cosine 0.7479) × 50.9 = 38.068 ft/sec
    2. (Cosine 0.8432) × 45.2 = 38.112 ft/sec
    3. (Cosine 0.6602) × 57.69 = 38.086 ft/sec

The horizontal distance to the high point in each case is as follows:

    1. 38.068 × 1.05 (time to high point) = 39.97 ft
    2. 38.112 × 0.754 (time to high point) = 28.74 ft
    3. 38.086 × 1.345 (time to high point) = 51.23 ft

If the exact height of the high point is desired, it is obtained by multiplying the vertical velocity by the time to the high point and subtracting from the product, the 16.1 t² value for this time.

The processes described can be used to determine the position of the projectile at any time in its flight. When the projection has a downward component, the 16.1 t² value is added, instead of subtracted, in determining the height, and the resulting sum would be subtracted from the starting height.

Knowledge of velocity, angle, and position at any time in flight can be applied to many situations and will enable the instructor to set specific goals for development of skill in a given situation. One illustration is that of developing skill in a tennis serve. Most beginners are likely to direct the ball upward; yet a velocity of 80 to 90 ft/sec can be achieved by the average adult. Suppose that the height at which the ball is impacted is 8 ft and the ball has a velocity of 80 ft/sec. The net is approximately 40 ft from the impact, and the ball would reach it in 0.5 second. The 16.1 t² value for this time is 4.025 ft, so that, as the ball reaches the net, it would be 3.975 ft above the ground, thus clearing the net by 0.975 ft. The ball would reach the ground when the 16.1 t² value was 8 ft; $8 = 16.1 \, t^2$; $t^2 = \dfrac{8}{16.1} = 0.4969$; t = 0.704 second. The horizontal distance would be $80 \times 0.704 = 56.32$ ft, which is well within the service court.

Angle, velocity, and ball position have been applied by Mortimer in determining the projection most likely to make a basket from the free throw line when the starting point is 5 ft above the floor. She recommends a velocity of 24 ft/sec and an angle of 58 degrees.

OPTIMAL PROJECTION ANGLE
FOR GREATEST DISTANCE

A projection angle of 45 degrees is often recommended as the optimum when the greatest possible distance is desired. This is true only when the vertical distance between the starting point and the end of the flight is zero. Bunn has shown this in discussing the projection of the shot put.

When the vertical distance between the start and the end of flight and the velocity of projection are known, the angle that results in the greatest distance is one in which the following applies:

$$\text{Sine}^2 = \frac{\text{Velocity}^2}{2 \, (\text{velocity}^2 - gh)}$$

In this formula, g is 32.2, and h is the vertical distance between the start and end of flight. If the start is higher than the end, h will be a minus quantity.

Bunn gives a table of the distances that the shot put would reach if projected at angles from 37 through 44 degrees when released at a height of 7 ft at velocities from 20 to 50 ft/sec. If the shot were given a velocity of 30 ft/sec, the determination of the optimal angle would be as follows:

$$\text{Sine}^2 = \frac{30^2}{2 \, [30^2 - (32.2 \times -7)]}$$

In this case the end of the flight is below the starting point, and h has a minus value.

$$\text{Sine}^2 = \frac{900}{2 \, (900 + 225.4)}$$

$$\text{Sine}^2 = \frac{900}{2250.8} = 0.39985$$

In this case the sine = 0.6323, which is the value for an angle of 39° 13'. For a 39-degree angle and for a 40-degree angle Bunn's table gives a distance of 34.42 ft, the longest for the angles included in his table.

In jumping for distance the center of gravity is higher at the beginning of flight than it is at landing. At the beginning of flight the body is extended, the arms are raised, and in an adult 6 ft tall, the height of the center of gravity can be estimated as 3 plus ft. If the landing is made with the thighs horizontal and some inclination of the legs, it will be assumed for this illustration that the center of gravity is 1.5 ft lower than it was at the beginning of flight. If the velocity of projection is 16 ft/sec, the optimal angle for greatest distance will be one in which the following applies:

$$\text{Sine}^2 = \frac{16^2}{2 \, [16^2 - (32.2 \times -1.5)]}$$

$$\text{Sine}^2 = 0.4206$$

In this case the sine = 0.6485. This is the value for an angle of 40° 26'.

If the velocity is 12 ft/sec and the other measures remain the same, the optimal angle is 37° 43'. If the positions of the center of gravity are determined at the beginning and end of flight, as they can be from film, the value of h can be more accurately determined. The velocity of the center of gravity can also be determined from these film measures (Chapter 13). In calculating the angle of projection in better-than-average performers we have found that this angle is less than 45 degrees; this is another example of the body's making necessary adjustments without the person's being aware that it is doing so.

SUMMARY OF CALCULATIONS

For ready reference the calculations discussed here and others that are related and useful are summarized here.

Range is the horizontal distance between the starting and landing point; time means the time in flight.

1. Horizontal velocity = Range ÷ Time.
2. In determining vertical velocity (V. vel.) consideration must be given to the vertical distance (VD) between the starting and the landing point.
   When VD is 0:
   $$V. \text{ vel.} = 16.1 \ t^2 \div \text{Time}$$
3. When the starting point is higher than the landing point:
   $$V. \text{ vel.} = (16.1 \ t^2 - VD) \div \text{Time}$$
   Note that, if $16.1 \ t^2$ is less than VD, the minus quantity indicates that the projection is below the horizontal.
4. When the starting point is lower than the landing point:
   $$V. \text{ vel.} = (16.1 \ t^2 + VD) \div \text{Time}$$
5. For the projection velocity (Proj. vel.):
   a. When the horizontal velocity (Horiz. vel.) and vertical velocity components are known:
   $$(\text{Proj. vel.})^2 = (\text{Horiz. vel.})^2 + (V. \text{ vel})^2$$

b. When the angle of projection is known:
   Proj. vel. = V. vel. ÷ Sine, or
   Proj. vel. = Horiz. vel. ÷ Cosine.
6. The angle of projection can be determined by use of trigonometric relationships. For the angle of projection:
   a. Tangent of the angle = V. vel. ÷ Horiz. vel.
   b. Sine of the angle = V. vel. ÷ Proj. vel.
   c. Cosine of the angle = Horiz. vel. ÷ Proj. vel.
7. The high point (h.p.) of the projection can be located by finding first the time to the high point.
   Time to high point = V. vel. ÷ 32.2
8. The distance of the high point above the starting point = (V. vel. × Time to h.p.) − 16.1 (time to h.p.)^2
9. The horizontal distance from the starting to the high point = Horiz. vel. × time h.p.

The relationships used in finding the high point can be used to locate the projectile at any time and at any point in flight. For example, a tennis ball was projected from a height of 7 ft and 40 ft from the net at a velocity of 50 ft/sec and at an angle of 10 degrees above the horizontal. Where was the ball when it reached the net? The horizontal and vertical velocity components must be known. They can be found by rearranging the equations in 5b:

$$V. \text{ vel.} = \text{Proj. vel.} \times \text{Sine}$$
$$\text{Horiz. vel.} = \text{Proj. vel.} \times \text{Cosine}$$

For an angle of 10 degrees the sine is 0.173; the cosine is 0.984. In the described tennis situation the numerical values are as follows:

$$V. \text{ vel.} = 50 \times 0.173, \text{ or } 8.65 \text{ ft/sec}$$
$$\text{Horiz. vel.} = 50 \times 0.984, \text{ or } 49.2 \text{ ft/sec}$$

Following is the time to the net:

$$40 \div 49.2, \text{ or } 0.81 \text{ second}$$

During this time the vertical velocity has moved the ball upward; gravitational force has moved it downward. The combined effect will be as follows:

$$(8.65 \times 0.81) - 16.1 \ (0.81)^2$$
$$7.00 - 10.573, \text{ or } 3,573 \text{ ft}$$

Table D-1. Gravity distance*

Time	0.00	0.01	0.02	0.03	0.04	0.05	0.06	0.07	0.08	0.09
0.0	0.000	0.001	0.006	0.014	0.025	0.040	0.057	0.078	0.013	0.13
0.1	0.161	0.194	0.231	0.272	0.315	0.362	0.412	0.465	0.521	0.58
0.2	0.644	0.710	0.779	0.851	0.927	1.006	1.088	1.173	1.262	1.35
0.3	1.449	1.547	1.648	1.745	1.861	1.972	2.086	2.204	2.324	2.44
0.4	2.576	2.706	2.840	2.976	3.116	3.260	3.387	3.556	3.709	3.86
0.5	4.025	4.187	4.353	4.524	4.694	4.870	5.048	5.230	5.416	5.60
0.6	5.796	5.980	6.188	6.290	6.584	6.802	7.014	7.227	7.444	7.66
0.7	7.889	8.116	8.346	8.579	8.816	9.056	9.299	9.545	9.795	10.04
0.8	10.304	10.573	10.825	11.091	11.360	11.632	11.970	12.186	12.468	12.75
0.9	13.041	13.332	13.627	13.925	14.226	14.530	14.838	15.148	15.462	15.77
1.0	16.100	16.432	16.750	17.080	17.414	17.750	18.090	18.433	18.779	19.12
1.1	19.481	19.837	20.196	20.558	20.923	21.292	21.664	22.039	22.417	22.79
1.2	23.184	23.602	23.963	24.357	24.755	25.156	25.560	25.967	26.378	26.79
1.3	27.209	27.629	28.052	28.469	28.899	29.342	29.778	30.208	30.660	31.10
1.4	31.556	32.008	32.464	32.922	33.384	33.850	34.318	34.790	35.265	35.74
1.5	36.225	36.709	37.197	37.688	38.172	38.680	39.180	39.684	40.192	40.70
1.6	41.216	41.732	42.252	42.776	43.307	43.832	44.365	44.901	45.440	45.98
1.7	46.529	47.078	47.630	48.187	48.745	49.306	49.861	50.439	51.011	51.58
1.8	52.164	52.745	53.329	53.917	54.508	55.102	55.660	56.310	56.903	57.51
1.9	58.121	58.734	59.361	59.907	60.593	61.220	61.849	62.482	63.118	63.75
2.0	64.400	65.046	65.644	66.346	67.002	67.960	68.322	68.987	69.206	70.326
2.1	71.001	71.679	72.360	73.044	73.732	74.422	75.116	75.813	76.514	77.217
2.2	77.924	78.634	79.347	80.064	80.783	81.566	82.232	82.962	83.694	84.430
2.3	85.169	85.911	86.657	87.405	88.157	88.912	89.671	90.432	91.197	91.965
2.4	92.736	93.510	94.288	95.069	95.854	96.640	97.431	98.224	99.021	99.823
2.5	100.625	101.432	102.341	103.054	103.871	104.690	105.503	106.339	107.168	108.000
2.6	108.836	109.675	110.517	111.362	112.211	113.262	113.917	114.780	115.637	116.502
2.7	117.369	118.240	119.114	119.992	120.872	121.756	122.643	123.534	124.437	125.024
2.8	126.224	127.127	128.034	128.943	129.856	130.772	131.692	132.614	133.540	134.469
2.9	135.401	136.336	137.275	138.217	139.162	140.110	141.062	142.016	142.974	143.936
3.0	144.900	145.868	146.828	147.802	148.790	149.770	150.754	151.781	152.731	153.724
3.1	154.721	155.721	156.724	157.730	158.740	159.752	160.768	161.787	162.810	163.835
3.2	164.864	165.896	166.931	167.970	169.021	170.056	171.104	172.157	173.210	174.268
3.3	175.168	176.393	177.480	178.531	179.605	180.682	181.763	182.846	183.933	185.023
3.4	186.116	187.212	188.312	189.415	190.521	191.630	192.742	193.858	194.977	196.100
3.5	197.125	198.354	199.585	200.620	201.759	202.901	204.045	205.193	206.344	207.498
3.6	208.656	209.817	210.981	212.148	213.319	214.492	215.669	216.849	218.033	219.219
3.7	220.409	221.602	222.798	223.998	225.200	226.406	227.615	228.828	230.043	231.262
3.8	232.484	233.709	234.938	236.169	237.404	238.642	239.884	241.128	242.376	243.627
3.9	244.881	246.138	247.399	248.663	249.930	251.200	252.474	253.750	255.030	256.314
4.0	257.600									

*Distance in feet through which freely falling objects move in a given time, calculated as distance $= \frac{1}{2}gt^2$ ($g = 32.2$). Conversion to metric system: value in table, divided by 3.28.

At the time that the ball reaches the net it will be 3.573 lower than the starting point, or 3.427 ft above the ground and 0.427 ft above the net, which is 3 ft in height.

The question might also arise as to where the ball would be at a given time, such as 0.5 second after the flight began. From the starting point it would travel horizontally as follows:

$$49.2 \times 0.5, \text{ or } 24.6 \text{ ft}$$

Vertically it would travel as follows:

$$(8.65 \times 0.5) - 16.1 \ (0.5)^2$$
$$4.325 - 4.025, \text{ or } 0.3 \text{ ft}$$

In 0.5 second the ball would be 0.3 ft higher than, and 24.6 ft from, the starting point.

SPIN AND BOUNCE OF BALLS

The ball is the most frequently used implement in sports. These balls vary in size, shape, mass, and construction. Diameters range from a 1.25-cm marble to a 3-m push ball. Practically all balls used in sports are spheres with exception of the football and the lawn bowling ball. Balls vary in mass from the light pingpong ball to the heavy shot or hammer. Balls are constructed from many types of material such as rubber, leather, wood, celluloid, brass, lead, ivory, glass, agate, clay, and plastic. They may be hollow or solid and may contain substances that vary the weight and reaction of the ball. The cover may be smooth, fuzzy, dimpled, ribbed, or ridged. The ball may be ringed with metal or have holes for gripping. Each separate characteristic affects the manner in which the ball is delivered, the way it passes through space or along a surface, and how it reacts to the objects that it strikes. In addition, the handling of the ball further affects its behavior in space or on the surface and the way that it reacts to the objects with which it comes in contact.

The ball to be used for each game is prescribed by the rules, and because the characteristics of the ball are fixed, the player need not consider the relative merits of balls of different sizes, shapes, and types of construction. The player is concerned only with the action of the ball that has been prescribed for the game that is being played. The action of the ball is affected first by the force and second by the spin applied.

Effects of the direction of applied force

The force that a performer applies to a ball usually puts the ball in motion. If the force is applied through the center of gravity of the ball, the resulting motion will be linear. The direction of the linear motion may be horizontal or vertical, or it may have vertical and horizontal components. In situations in which the ball is moving through the air, the force of gravity changes the vertical velocity, and the direction of motion becomes curvilinear rather than linear. The effect of gravity on a projectile is discussed previously in this appendix.

Effect of spin on a ball in flight

The manner in which any ball passes through space and reacts to objects depends on the effect of the amount of spin of the ball. A ball thrown with a great deal of spin will move more slowly than another thrown at the same force but with only a slight spin. The reduction in speed because of the great amount of spin results in a lessening of the force of the ball in flight. The reason that the spin reduces speed is that a spinning ball offers more resistance to the air through which it travels.

A spinning ball seeks the line of least resistance in its flight through the air. A rapidly spinning ball creates a greater friction on one side of the ball than on the other. As a result the flight of the ball is curved. This phenomenon is illustrated in Fig. D-3. The extent of the curve when various balls are delivered with a common speed and rate of spin depends on the shape and mass of the ball. Light balls, such as ping-pong and tennis balls, curve widely. In heavy ones, such as medicine balls, the curve is too slight to be noticeable. Verwiebe has measured the curve of the baseball by having the pitched ball pass through five screens of fine thread placed at equal intervals between the pitcher's rubber and home plate. By measuring the different points on the screens where the ball passed

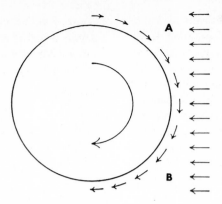

Fig. D-3. Rapidly spinning ball encounters more resistance at *A* than at *B* and in flight will curve toward *B*.

through, he was able to follow the path of the ball. He found that a baseball could be thrown in a curved path. A slow pitch broke into a curve sooner and wider than a faster pitch. A curve as wide as 15 cm (6 in) was measured.

The direction and amount of the curve of a thrown ball depends on the direction and amount of spin and the speed of the ball. One thrown with a spin from right to left will curve to the left as it follows the line of least resistance. In golf this is known as a *hook* and is caused when a right-handed golfer strikes the ball with the outside of the clubhead ahead of the inside of the clubhead. In a baseball pitch this is an *outcurve* when pitching to a right-handed batter. The right-handed pitcher delivering an outcurve throws the ball so that the fingers against the right side of the ball twist the ball from right to left.

The ball spinning from left to right will curve toward the right as it follows the line of least resistance. In golf the *slice* is caused by striking the ball with the heel of the clubhead ahead of the outside of the clubhead, imparting a spin to the right. In baseball this is the *incurve* and results from the push of the pitcher's index finger against the left side of the ball.

Top·spin causes the ball to fall rapidly. In this case since the line of resistance is in the same direction as the force of gravity, the effect of the spin on the curve is pronounced. A golf ball hit with a top spin drops quickly to the fairway and rolls a considerable distance.

A *backspin,* or undercut, will diminish the rate of falling of the ball. If the speed and rate of backspin result in an upward component greater than the force of gravity, the ball will continue to rise upward until the speed of the spin is diminished. A fastball in baseball may be thrown with a slight backspin by holding two fingers on top of the ball and allowing the fingers to slide downward as the ball is pushed forward. The fastball appears to maintain a horizontal flight during the 60-foot flight from the pitcher to the catcher.

Effect of spin on rolling balls

A rolling ball with a top spin, at the point of contact, pushes back against the surface on which it is rolling, and therefore the resulting forward push of the surface increases the forward velocity of the ball. Consequently, a ball with a top spin rolls farther than it would if it had no spin. Conversely, a ball spinning from bottom to top exerts a forward push against the surface, and the backward push from the surface will decrease the forward velocity of the roll. Thus a ball with a backspin does not roll as far as it would if it had no spin.

Effect of spin on bouncing balls

A ball that has no spin will rebound from a smooth surface at the same angle that it had when it hit the surface. If the approach is at an angle of 90 degrees, the rebound will be at the same angle; if the approach angle is 45 degrees, the rebound will be at an angle of 45 degrees with the surface. This is because all contacting parts of the ball push against the resisting surface with equal force. If the ball has rotatory motion, the contacting parts can push against the surface with different amounts of force.

A ball with a top spin rebounds at a lower angle than it would if it had no spin; a ball with a backspin rebounds at a higher angle. A ball spinning to the right or left rebounds in the direction of spin.

REFERENCES

Bunn, J.W.: Scientific principles of coaching, Englewood Cliffs, N.J., 1955, Prentice-Hall, Inc.

Mortimer, E.: Basketball shooting, Res. Q. **22**:234, 1951.

Verwiebe, F.L.: Does a ball curve? Am. J. Physics **10**:119, 1942.

APPENDIX E

Computer program for center-of-gravity data

Name: Joe Scheuchenzuber
Program: Body C/G Program
Language: FORTRAN

Purpose

The purpose of this program is to compute present body center-of-gravity data, given the available segmental end points. The program also includes the options of a plot of the movement of the segments and calculations of the velocity and acceleration for the center of gravity from frame to frame. The latter option should be used only for gross estimations because of the limitations of using film analysis for computing kinetic data.

Program input for each set of frames

Card 1
  Col. 1-2   Number of sets of data to be processed (any number)

Card 2
  Col. 1-3   Number of frames in set (up to 50)
  Col. 6-11 Multiplier for this set
              Form XX.XXXX or free form with decimal punched

Col. 16-25 Data type to be used in computation for this set of data
           Form (one of the following)
           DEMPSTER = Dempster
           B AND F = Braune and Fischer
           CLAUSER = Clauser
           H.RLESS= Harless
           BSTEIN (F) = Bernstein (female data)
           BSTEIN (M) = Bernstein (male data)
Col. 30-34 Weight of the subject for this set
           Form XXXX.X or free form with decimal punched
Col. 39-43 Weight of object for this set (if any) (none needed)
           Form XXX.XX or free form with decimal punched
Col. 48-53 Frame rate for the set
           Form XXXXX.X or free form with decimal punched
Col. 60   Punch 1 if printed segmental c.g. data is wanted.
Col. 61   Punch 1 if punched deck of segmental c.g. data is wanted.
Col. 62   Punch 1 if a printer plot of body c.g. data is wanted.
Col. 63   Punch 1 if a printer plot of right-side segmental c.g. data is wanted.
Col. 64   Punch 1 if a printer plot of left-side segmental c.g. data is wanted.

Additional information regarding this type of computer program can be obtained from the Biomechanics Laboratory of the School of Health, Physical Education and Recreation, Indiana University, Bloomington, Ind. 47401.

Col. 65   Punch 1 if velocity and acceleration data for body c.g. is wanted.

Program input for each frame (see figure)

Card 1

Col. 1   Punch 0 if top of head was taken on this frame.
Punch 1 if c.g. for head was taken on this frame.
Punch 2 if estimated body c.g. was taken on this frame.

Col. 4-10   Coordinate of X zero point
Form XXXX.XXX or free form with decimal punched

Col. 11-17   Coordinate of Y zero point
Form XXXX.XXX or free form with decimal punched

Col. 18-22   Number of frame analyzed (as counted from first frame) (actual frame number)

Seg.	Col.	Card 2 (X for segments below) Card 3 (Y for segments below)
1	1-4	Top of head or head c.g. or estimated body c.g.
2	5-8	Sternal notch or blank if not available
3	9-12	Crotch or blank if not available
4	13-16	Right shoulder
5	17-20	Right elbow
6	21-24	Right wrist
7	25-28	Right finger (Leave blank if not available.)
8	29-32	Left shoulder
9	33-36	Left elbow
10	37-40	Left wrist
11	41-44	Left finger (Leave blank if not available.)
12	45-48	Right hip
13	49-52	Right knee
14	53-56	Right ankle
15	57-60	Right toe (Leave blank if not available.)
16	61-64	Left hip
17	65-68	Left knee
18	69-72	Left ankle
19	73-76	Left toe (Leave blank if not available.)
20	77-80	Object—estimated c.g. of object (if any) or blank

Form: Each coordinate's form is XX.XX or free form with decimal punched
For each additional frame return to top of page.
For next set of frames return to Card 2 under Program input for each set of frames.
When punching data, note that Form XXX.XX means that the decimal is implied between the third and fourth digit and must not be punched unless necessary for change in magnitude of data.

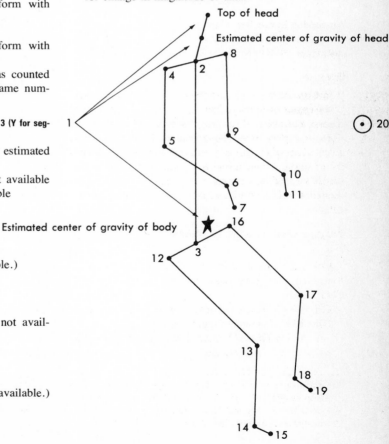

APPENDIX F

Glossary

acceleration Time rate of change of velocity. It may be positive or negative and may increase or decrease. When the velocity is constant, the acceleration is zero.

attenuation Reduction or absorption of force, energy, or some other factor.

axis Real or imaginary line about which a body, or segment of a body, rotates.

biomechanics The study of forces produced by and acting upon living bodies and the study of the subsequent motion or lack of motion.

braking force (retarding force) Force that acts to decelerate the body or body segment, such as placing the foot in such a manner that the forward propulsion of the body is slowed or stopped, or using muscle force to reduce the speed of the segment.

center of gravity That point at which the body will balance; the intersection of the three cardinal planes; the point about which an airborne body will rotate; also termed the center of mass. A moving body will have a changing center of gravity in direct relationship to the moving parts.

conservation of angular momentum The concept that angular momentum will remain the same as long as no external force is added or subtracted from the system. Thus the shortening of the radius of rotation (decreasing the moment of inertia) will increase the angular velocity to maintain angular momentum. It is the product of moment of inertia and angular velocity.

compression Stress that shortens a body, tends to push the particles together, or crush the body.

displacement Movement of a body from its place of origin; displacement is described vectorally.

energy Capacity for performing work. Potential energy is stored energy, and kinetic energy is energy of motion; both may be expressed as $\frac{1}{2}mV^2$ or Ft.

force That which produces motion or acceleration or has the capacity to do so.

frontal plane The vertical plane that divides the body anteroposteriorly.

general motion Motion that is both translatory and rotatory; it may be planar or multiplanar.

horsepower Unit for measuring power, usually of motors and engines; it is equivalent to 550 ft-lb/sec, or 702 watts.

impact Collision between two or more bodies; impact may be measured according to impulse or energy units.

impulse Product of force and the duration of the application of this force; the units are newton-seconds; impulse is synonymous with momentum.

inertia The property of a body to remain at rest or in a state of constant motion; the resistance of a body to any alteration in its state.

kinematics That portion of mechanics related to temporal and spatial characteristics of motion, without regard to the forces.

kinesiology The science of motion; therefore kinesiology is synonymous with biomechanics.

kinesthesis The proprioceptive sense of body and limb position in space, speed of movement, and force of movement; muscle, tendon, and joint receptors are the same organs.

kinetics That portion of mechanics related to the forces producing or modifying motion.

lever A rigid bar that rotates about an axis.

mass Measurement of the difficulty in setting a body in motion; it is expressed as the ratio of force of gravity to the acceleration of gravity and is measured in kilograms.

mechanics That branch of physics concerned with motion and forces causing motion or deformation of bodies.

moment of inertia A body's resistance to rotatory motion; the product of mass and radius squared (the radius is the distance from the axis to the center of gravity of the body).

momentum The force with which a body moves; the product of a body's mass and its velocity. Momentum synonymous with impulse.

myotatic reflex An involuntary response to fast and/or extreme range of motion causing the motion to be inhibited; for example, when adductors are lengthening rapidly, the reflex will cause them to shorten. This is considered to be a built-in safety mechanism, based on muscle spindle control. It is also termed the stretch reflex.

Newton's three laws of motion The basic rules governing motion as set forth by Sir Isaac Newton.

planar Occurring within one plane.

plane A surface in which if any two points are connected with a straight line, the line will lie wholly in that surface; there are three basic (cardinal) planes of movement.

power Work per unit of time.

radian A measure of angles or arcs, equivalent to approximately 57 degrees (that is, $1/2\pi$ of a circle). It is considered unitless.

reaction force Equal and opposite force to a force acting on a body; ground reaction and joint reaction forces are examples of external and internal reaction forces.

reflex An involuntary act or movement usually due to a nervous impulse transmitted by means of one synapse inward from a receptor to a nerve center and outward to a muscle.

rhythm Measurement of motion and the flow of cadences of motion. Each motion has its own unique sequencing in time.

rotatory Motion in which a body rotates about a point (fulcrum) or axis. The more distal body part will move the farthest, and the more proximal body part will move the shortest distance.

sagittal plane The vertical plane that divides the body mediolaterally.

scalar Quantities that have magnitude only and can be specified by a number and unit; examples include length, speed, energy, and mass.

shear stress that causes two contiguous parts of a body to slide relative to each other in a direction parallel to their plane of contact.

speed A scalar quantity denoting distance per unit of time, such as meters per second.

strain The amount of deformation per unit length caused by stress.

stress The molecular resistance of a body to a force, expressed as force per unit area.

tension Stress that elongates a body, tends to pull the particles apart.

translatory Pertaining to motion in which every particle of a body moves an equal distance; usually identified as linear or curvilinear motion.

transverse plane The horizontal plane that divides the body cephalocaudally.

vectors Quantities that have both magnitude and direction; examples include force, velocity, and acceleration.

velocity A vector quantity denoting speed in a given direction.

weight Gravitational force exerted on a body by the earth (in this gravitational field); the magnitude of weight is expressed in newtons and the direction is always downward.

work The product of force and the distance the point of application of work is moved in the direction of the force (Fd). The units are newton-meters or joules.

Index

A

Acceleration
  calculation of, 76, 177
  definition of, 11
  in throwing, 238-239
Activities of daily living, description of movements in, 6, 10, 368-379
Adaptation, neural, 159
Adductor muscle, action of, 127-128
Adenosine triphosphate, 107
ADL; *see* Activities of daily living
Aging, patterns of locomotion and, 318-319
Agonist muscle, 111-112
Air resistance, bicycling and, 303-304
Airborne activity
  basic principles of, 336-337
  description of movements in, 336-352
All-or-none law, 106-107
American Society for Testing Materials, 365
Anatomy, structure and forces in, 92-114
Angle of inclination, definition of, 189
Angular momentum, in gymnastics, 346
Animal Locomotion, 20
Antagonist muscle, 112
Anthropometry, movement and, 13
Aquatic activities, description of movements in, 324-334
Archery, assessment of forces in, 400
Archimedes' principle, 18, 324
Aristotle, 18, 200
Arm
  assessment of motion of, 391
  avoidance of injury to, 395-396
Arthrodia, 92
ATP; *see* Adenosine triphosphate
Axes of rotation in throwing, 239-241
Axon, function of, 145-146

B

Badminton, description of strokes in, 276-279
Balance
  dynamic, 47
  effects of, in skiing, 307-308

Balance—cont'd
  on hands, 45
Balance beam, activities on, 351
Balance point in human body, 36
Ball-and-socket joint, 92-93
Baseball, batting in, 273-276
Basketball, description of movements in, 265-268
Batting, baseball, description of movements in, 273-276
Bernoulli's principle, 74, 75, 329, 331
Biceps brachii muscle, action of, 124-125
Bicycle, design of, 304
Bicycling, description of movements in, 303-304
Biomechanics; *see* Kinesiology
Blood pressure, rise in, due to erect posture, 40
Body
  human
    anatomic differences in, 142-143
    evolution of, 37-38
    segments of, 141-142
    speed of parts of, 139-140
  significant forces on, 398-399
  types of rotation of, 340-343
Body dimension, movement and, 13
Body weight, effect of, in skiing, 306-307
Bone(s)
  in body lever systems, 116-143
  description of, 98-102
  effects of activity on, 101-102
  elasticity of, 99
  fractured, treatment of, 101
  modeling theories of, 99-102
  normal growth of, 100-101
  racial influences on, 102
  strength limits of, 102
  use of, in throwing, 240
Bone cells, types of, 100
Borelli, 48
Bowleg, causes of, 101
Bowling, description of movements in, 11-12, 252-254
Brachiation, 37
Brachioradialis muscle, action of, 125-126
Brain, physiology of, 144-145